IMMUNOLOGY AND IMMUNOPATHOLOGY OF DOMESTIC ANIMALS

IMMUNOLOGY and IMMUNOPATHOLOGY of DOMESTIC ANIMALS

Laurel J. Gershwin, D.V.M., Ph.D., Dip. A.C.V.M.
Professor of Immunology
Department of Pathology, Microbiology, and Immunology
School of Veterinary Medicine
University of California
Davis, California

Steven Krakowka, D.V.M., Ph.D.
Professor
Department of Veterinary Pathobiology
College of Veterinary Medicine
The Ohio State University
Columbus, Ohio

Richard G. Olsen, Ph.D.
Professor Emeritus
College of Veterinary Medicine
The Ohio State University
Columbus, Ohio

SECOND EDITION

with 87 illustrations

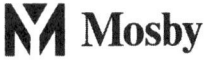

St. Louis Baltimore Boston Chicago London Madrid Philadelphia Sydney Toronto

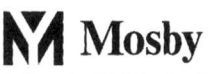
Dedicated to Publishing Excellence

Publisher: Alison Miller
Editor: Linda L. Duncan
Developmental Editor: Jo Salway
Project Manager: Gayle May Morris
Production Editor: Lisa Marcus
Design Manager: Susan Lane
Cover Design: GW Graphics

Illustrations: Felecia Paras, Biomedical Visuals, Columbus, Ohio; for first edition Cynthia Olsen.

SECOND EDITION

Copyright © 1995 by Mosby-Year Book, Inc.

Previous edition published in 1979 by Charles C. Thomas, Publisher.

All rights reserved. No part of this publication may be reproduced, stored in a retrieval system, or transmitted, in any form or by any means, electronic, mechanical, photocopying, recording, or otherwise, without prior written permission from the publisher.

Permission to photocopy or reproduce solely for internal or personal use is permitted for libraries or other users registered with the Copyright Clearance Center, provided that the base fee of $4.00 per chapter plus $.10 per page is paid directly to the Copyright Clearance Center, 27 Congress Street, Salem, MA 01970. This consent does not extend to other kinds of copying such as copying for general distribution, for advertising or promotional purposes, for creating new collected works, or for resale.

Printed in the United States of America
Composition by V&M Graphics, Inc.
Printing/binding by

Mosby-Year Book, Inc.
11830 Westline Industrial Drive
St. Louis, Missouri 63146

International Standard Book Number 0-8016-6398-9

95 96 97 98 / 10 9 8 7 6 5 4 3 2 1

Contributor

James S. Cullor, *D.V.M., Ph.D.*
Associate Professor
Department of Pathology, Microbiology, and Immunology
School of Veterinary Medicine
University of California
Davis, California

To my mother
Elizabeth Fitzgerald Bray
*(1915-1993)
whose love and encouragement
helped me to achieve my goals in veterinary medicine*

and to **Wicki**
*(1965-1994)
a very special horse*

L.J.G.

To my son
Ben

S.K.

To my wife
Melinda

R.G.O.

Preface

This book, the second edition, is intended to provide updated information on topics covered in the first edition. The book is intended to serve as a textbook for students of veterinary medicine, a reference for graduate students, and a source book for practitioners to update their immunological knowledge. Immunology is one of the most (if not the most) rapidly changing and expanding fields in applied biological sciences. The present trend in veterinary education to reduce time spent in didactic lecture courses and facilitate problem-based learning does not allow for expansion of the number of lecture hours in immunology. Thus we are faced with an increase in the information base and less time in which to teach it. Students and graduate veterinarians will be required to spend time reading texts to fully appreciate the immune system and its relationship to disease. This book will provide both basic and more advanced information that should serve both the student just acquiring a knowledge of veterinary immunology and the post-DVM who desires to understand the developments in understanding of the immune system that have occurred since he/she last studied immunology; for the DVM out of school ten years or more these developments are considerable!

Much of the information presented in the first edition by Drs. Krakowka and Olsen remains in the second edition. I have updated and added to the text as necessary to create a text that is as current as one can hope to achieve in a field that changes on a daily basis, as results of ongoing research are published.

The authors are deeply indebted to Ms. Felecia Paras, whose artistic talent is evident in many of the figures. Finally, the editorial expertise of Ms. Jo Salway is greatly appreciated; her dedication to the completion of the second edition made it happen.

Laurel J. Gershwin

Contents

PART ONE

Principles of Immunology

1 Innate Immunity   3

2 Antigens and Immunogens   6

3 The Lymphoid System and Cells of the Lymphoid System   13

4 Immunoglobulins   30
   Products of Activated B Lymphocytes

5 Cytokines   40
   Soluble factors of the immune response
   James S. Cullor

6 Complement System   47

7 Histocompatibility Antigens and Blood Group Antigens   55

8 Immune Response   62

PART TWO

Methods to Evaluate Immune Function

9 Assays for Innate Immune Defenses   71
   Neutrophils and Complement

10 Assays for Humoral Immunity, Including Serology   76

11 Assays for T Lymphocyte Function   99
    In vitro and in vivo assessment of lymphocyte functions and
    identification of lymphocytes and subpopulations of lymphocytes

PART THREE
Immunopathology

12 Inherited Immunodeficiencies, Myelomas, and Lymphomas 113

13 Immunologic Mechanisms in Immune-Mediated Diseases 129

14 Immune Complex Diseases 139

15 Autoimmunity 150

PART FOUR
Principles of Immunoprophylaxis

16 Immune Response and Infectious Disease 159

17 Vaccines, Vaccination, and Immunomodulators 169

PART ONE

Principles of Immunology

1 Innate Immunity

The immune system has evolved as a mechanism to protect the host from invasion by pathogenic organisms. Recognition of self and the ability to distinguish self from nonself is therefore basic to the normal function of the immune system. The foundation for immunology was laid by Edward Jenner in 1798 when he first observed that smallpox could be prevented by exposing susceptible persons to cowpox material, thereby immunizing them. The immune response generated as a result of infection or vaccination is an acquired one based on specific recognition and response.

Much knowledge about the immune system and its function, components, and regulation has been acquired since the days of Jenner's cowpox vaccine. Although the importance of specific immune responses is recognized and many new vaccines have been developed, some diseases are still not adequately prevented by vaccination. In some instances certain individuals or breeds fail to respond to vaccines as the rest of the population does. We recognize diseases in which the immune response is exuberant (allergy and autoimmunity), and we are still attempting to fully define the cause and/or methods of prevention for these ailments. There are many parallels between human immunology, mouse (experimental) immunology, and veterinary immunology, but there are also many differences. With the advent of monoclonal antibody technology and molecular cloning techniques, the development of immunologic reagents that allow veterinarians to evaluate immune function at the same level of sophistication as in human medicine has greatly increased during the past decade. This book contains much information unavailable when the first edition was published in 1979—an indication of the rapid expansion of the field of veterinary immunology. We look forward to an even greater expansion of this knowledge during the next decade.

Innate immunity

Before the development of an acquired immune response to a pathogen, there are innate immune mechanisms available to assist the host in curing itself. These innate immune mechanisms are nonspecific, that is, they are effective against a variety of pathogens and do not require prior exposure for their induction. An example of innate immunity is the phagocytic neutrophil. When bacteria gain entrance to a break in the skin and begin to multiply, neutrophils are attracted and engulf and kill the bacteria, forming pus in the process. Innate immunity consists of the protective cells and substances that are present for host defense without previous exposure of the host to an infective agent. This is in contrast to acquired immunity, which the host develops after contact with the infectious agent. Although innate immunity provides some degree of protection from disease, infectious organisms are often able to evade these defenses. These innate mechanisms of defense include mechanical barriers, secreted products, inflammatory cells, and physiologic functions (Figure 1-1). Other factors such as genetics and body temperature are important to the body's resistance to selective disease agents. The extent to which these mechanisms are protective is often modulated by factors such as age, hormonal status and nutritional condition.

System related innate defenses

Skin

The skin serves as a barrier to the external environment. The importance of this barrier is best illustrated in situations in which it is impaired. For example, during muddy and wet weather horses are more prone to develop thrush, a fungal infection of the hoof. During dry conditions the protective outer layers of cornified skin that form the sole of the hoof are impermeable and uninviting to fungal organisms. However, softened and weakened sole tissue is an inviting environment for growth of these organisms. Hence, thrush occurs in horses during wet months when the hoof is allowed to remain wet and muddy. The skin also has chemical defense mechanisms such as a low pH and fatty acids; these mechanisms, in addition to the desiccation that is naturally present on skin, discourage the growth of pathogenic microorganisms.

Another important component of the skin's resistance is the presence of a normal flora. These

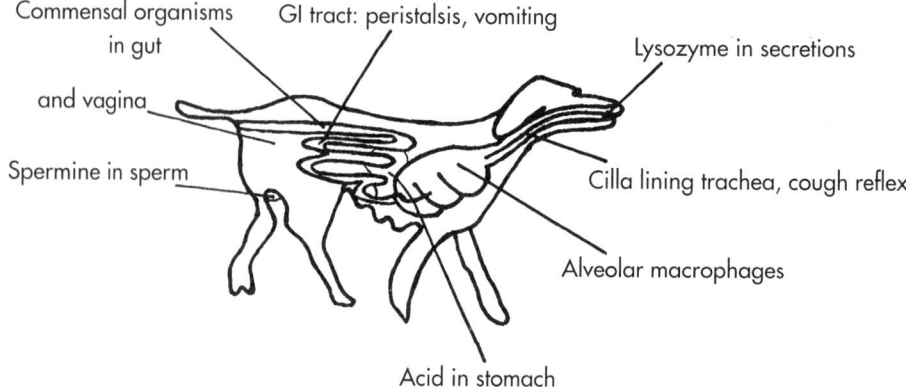

Figure 1-1 Biochemical and physical innate defenses.

nonpathogenic bacteria are normal residents of skin. They occupy a niche and thereby prevent other more harmful organisms from inhabiting that niche. Prolonged antibiotic therapy sometimes creates mucosal infections with fungal organisms, which are able to occupy the niche vacated by the antibiotic-susceptible normal flora.

Gastrointestinal tract

As with the skin, there is a barrier function in the gut mucosa. In addition, a mucous coat assists in making this barrier impenetrable to foreign organisms.

Certain physiologic functions of the gastrointestinal tract aid in eliminating toxins and pathogens; these are the vomiting and peristaltic reflexes. Diarrhea, often a response to the ingestion of an irritant, toxin or pathogenic organism, removes the source of its stimulation in an effective manner.

Chemical defenses in the gastrointestinal tract include a low pH in the stomach, proteolytic enzymes, and lysozyme, a substance that splits the bond in the cell wall of bacteria, thereby weakening its structure.

Indigenous flora are even more important in the gut than they are on the skin. The existence of commensal bacteria that occupy a niche is essential for prevention of the adhesion of pathogenic bacteria to the epithelial cells lining the gut. Pathogenic bacteria such as strains of *Escherichia coli* have pili, which bind tightly to receptors on these cells. These pathogenic strains must adhere to the receptors in order for them to cause disease. When sufficient numbers of nonpathogenic bacteria prevent this adherence, disease does not result.

Respiratory tract. Physiologic functions are extremely important defense mechanisms in the lung. The cough reflex removes foreign material quite efficiently and works with the mucociliary blanket, which moves the mucus from the lower respiratory tract up to the oropharynx for expulsion.

Deeper in the lung the alveolar macrophage engulfs and destroys particulates that are of 1 μm or less in size and that have advanced in the alveolar spaces.

Urogenital tract

In the vagina there are lactobacilli that create an acid environment, which is not conducive to the growth of many pathogens. In the urinary tract a low pH and the flushing action associated with periodic bladder emptying are important. Clinical treatment of cystitis uses both urine acidification and increasing urine flow as adjuncts to antibiotic therapy. The mammary gland also uses a flushing action to prevent milk stasis and growth of microorganisms. Additional innate defenses active in the mammary gland include the antibacterial chemical substances lactoferrin and lactoperoxidase.

Cells involved in innate immunity

Neutrophils

The primary line of cellular defense consists of the polymorphonuclear leukocyte (neutrophil). These cells are short lived, spending only about 12 hours in the blood-vascular system before exiting to the extravascular compartment. While in the tissues they live for 2 to 3 days, responding to chemotactic stimuli and traveling to the site of inflammation. Neutrophils phagocytose and kill invading microorganisms, forming a purulent exudate in the process. The importance of neutrophils as an innate defense mechanism is apparent when their function is compromised or they are absent (see Chapter 12). Assays to evaluate the function of neutrophils are described in Chapter 9.

Macrophages

The macrophage is an important cell because it bridges both innate and acquired immune systems. As a component of innate immunity, the macrophage engulfs and kills invading microorganisms. Unlike the neutrophil, the macrophage can repeatedly engulf and kill. The macrophage also serves as an antigen-presenting cell (see Chapter 8). After engulfing and digesting antigen, the macrophage takes a peptide from the antigen and displays it on the cell membrane in the groove of its own major histocompatibility antigen (MHC) Class II protein. It is within this context that helper thymus-derived (T)-lymphocytes are able to recognize and respond to the antigen, thereby stimulating an immune response. Thus the macrophage is important to innate immunity and provides a bridge to the acquired response.

Macrophages exist free and fixed within the body. The reticuloendothelial system is composed of fixed macrophages, which line sinuses and serve to sieve particulates from the blood percolating through these sinuses. In the liver, fixed macrophages are called Kupffer's cells. Macrophages exist in the intraglomerular mesangium of the kidney, exist as microglia in the brain, are associated with serosal surfaces, and appear as monocytes circulating freely in the blood. As mentioned above, macrophages serve an important function in the lung as alveolar macrophages, removing inhaled debris.

Complement as an innate defense mechanism

The complement system, which is described in detail in Chapter 6, can be associated with innate and acquired immune defenses. When a host is naive with respect to a particular pathogen and therefore has no specific antibody, the alternate complement pathway is evoked and damage can be done to the bacterial cell with complement components. In addition, by-products of the complement fixation reaction are chemotactic for neutrophils and assist in attracting them to the area.

Molecules that mediate innate immunity

Interferons

Interferons are molecules that are produced by many different cell types after a viral infection. Interferons are of two types, I and II. Type I interferon, alpha and beta interferon, is induced by viral infection and has antiviral effects. Interferons produced after viral infection bind to neighboring cells and induce production of antiviral proteins. These proteins are enzymes with kinase activity, and their role is to inactivate enzymes needed for viral protein and RNA synthesis, thus obstructing viral reproduction in the affected cell. Alpha interferon is produced by monocytes; beta interferon is produced by fibroblasts. Other effects of type I interferons include an inhibition of cell proliferation, enhancement of natural killer (NK) cell lysis, and modulation of MHC expression by increasing Class I expression and decreasing Class II expression. Type II interferon, gamma interferon, is produced by helper T lymphocytes after stimulation by antigen (not necessarily viral antigen). Gamma interferon is a cytokine with diverse effects, including macrophage activation (see Chapter 5).

Tumor necrosis factor

Tumor necrosis factor (TNF) is produced by macrophages after they are stimulated by bacterial lipopolysaccharide. Other sources include activated T cells, NK cells and mast cells. TNF binds to cell surface receptors to exert the following effects: neutrophil activation, macrophage stimulation, increased leukocyte adhesion, and increased MHC Class I expression. This cytokine can also cause induction of fever, synthesis of acute phase proteins, and activation of the coagulation system. It is an important molecule in the defense against gram-negative sepsis.

Interactions of innate and acquired immunity

Although innate mechanisms of immunity provide the first line of defense for the body, some of the reactions that occur without previous exposure to a pathogen are enhanced once an acquired immune response develops. An example is the effect of opsonization with antibody on the efficiency of phagocytosis by macrophages and neutrophils. Without specific antibody, phagocytosis occurs, but when there is specific antibody present to bridge the phagocyte and organism through Fc receptor binding, the uptake and killing are greatly improved. For some organisms opsonization is critical; these are bacteria with polysaccharide capsules that make phagocytosis very difficult without antibody. Other organisms are not readily killed by phagocytes; these are the facultative intracellular organisms, such as Brucella and Listeria. T-cell activation and the production of gamma interferon are required before macrophages are able to kill these organisms.

2 Antigens and Immunogens

Prevention of infectious disease by vaccination has been practiced for centuries. Jenner's classical studies on immunization against smallpox used material from cowpox lesions. These studies demonstrated that exposure of the immune system to a disease agent in a form that does not elicit disease creates an immunologic memory such that re-exposure to the agent in a virulent form fails to cause disease. However, exposure to an unrelated disease agent results in disease. Thus the immunologic memory created by vaccination is responsible for creating a specific protective response in the vaccinated individual that resembles the resistance acquired by contracting and recovering from the disease.

Antigens, or immunogens, are substances that provoke an immune response. The term *immunogenicity* is defined as having the ability to evoke an immune response, such as antibody production. Some antigens are strongly immunogenic; others are weakly immunogenic. The physical characteristics that determine immunogenicity include size, stability/rigidity, complexity, degradability, charge and foreignness.

CHARACTERISTICS OF AN EFFECTIVE IMMUNOGEN

Size is an important attribute of an antigen. Generally, molecules greater than 10,000 daltons (D) are good immunogens. Some smaller molecules such as insulin at 2500 D, can be weakly immunogenic. Very small molecules must be bound to a larger protein called a *carrier* in order to elicit an immune response. Such a molecule is referred to as a hapten.

A molecule must have a *stable* or *rigid structure* to be immunogenic, because the immune system responds to the stereochemical shape of macromolecules. For example, gelatin is a large molecule, but it lacks rigidity and is a poor immunogen.

Complexity, physical and chemical, is an important attribute of an antigen. Experiments have been performed using antigen proteins in a variety of forms, and the results have shown that complexity is important. For example, monomeric proteins do not produce a good immune response and aggregated proteins do. Synthetic polymers of the same amino acid (e.g., poly-l-lysine) as immunogen fail to elicit an immune response; whereas molecules made with increased complexity produced by alternating poly-l-lysine with poly-l-tyrosine are immunogenic.

It is important that a potential antigen be *degradable* in order for it to be immunogenic. An antigen that is a good immunogen is capable of being phagocytosed and degraded within the host. Large organic molecules that are not degraded are not immunogenic. The presence of D-amino acids within a protein structure decreases immunogenicity, because the enzymes in the macrophage are specific for L-amino acids and the macrophage must be able to process the antigen for presentation to thymus-derived T cells for elicitation of an immune response.

Charge is another attribute of a molecule that can affect immunogenicity. Excessive charge decreases immunogenocity, presumably because it can create repulsing interactive forces with antibodies and cellular receptors.

The most important attribute of an antigen is that it is *foreign* to the host. As stated in Chapter 1, the immune system is able to function because it can distinguish self from nonself. During early development of the immune system, clones of cells that have the potential for recognizing self-determinants are purged (clonal deletion). Thereafter the bursal-derived (B)-cell repertoire contains cells that can react with a diverse array epitopes, all of which are foreign to the host. However, the concept of foreignness is relative. For example, if we immunize a dog with bovine serum albumin, the dog's immune system will recognize the bovine proteins as foreign and will develop an immune response to them. If we immunize a cow with the same proteins, the cow's immune system will not recognize the proteins as foreign and will not make an immune response to them, even though the size, complexity and other factors are consistent with good immunogenicity. Occasionally there is a breakdown in self-tolerance and certain self-antigens are recognized as foreign to the host, resulting in autoimmune disease.

ANTIGENIC DETERMINANTS (EPITOPES)

The *antigenic determinant* is part of an antigen that is recognized by the receptor molecules of the immune system. Antigenic determinants are also called *epitopes* and are usually located on an exposed part of the molecule. The size of an antigenic determinant is usually 4 to 6 amino acids. Classic studies performed by Landsteiner showed that antibodies are so specific in their recognition of antigenic determinants that they can distinguish cis from trans configurations of chemical groups composing an antigenic determinant. Similarly, antibodies, whose production was stimulated by a molecule with the paraconfiguration of a chemical group, do not react as well with meta and ortho configurations.

The number of antigenic determinants present on a complete antigen is related to the molecular weight or size of the molecule. Complex antigens have a number of different antigenic determinants. Immunization of an animal with one of these compounds elicits the production of antibodies specific to each of the determinants. The antiserum obtained from the blood of the immunized animal contains a heterogeneous population of antibodies, some specific for each determinant.

The *accessibility* of an epitope is an important factor that determines the outcome of the immune response to that epitope. With synthetic polypeptides it has been shown that amino acid residues at the free ends of side chains elicit an immune response, while the same residues near the backbone of the molecule are "hidden" from immune recognition.

Although proteins are the most common antigens, other compounds, such as glycoproteins, lipoproteins, carbohydrates, and nucleic acids can also function as antigens. In the autoimmune disease systemic lupus erythematosus (SLE), antibodies are produced that react with DNA.

HAPTENS OR INCOMPLETE ANTIGENS

A *hapten* is an *incomplete antigen*; it cannot elicit an antibody response without being attached to a larger carrier molecule. Once the antibody response has been elicited, the hapten can bind to the antibody without the carrier. A hapten is generally a small chemical group and the carrier is a protein. Such a carrier is immunogenic by itself, and the antibody response elicited includes antibodies that are reactive with the carrier as well as those reactive with the hapten. The carrier is called a *complete antigen*; it need not be bound to another molecule to be immunogenic.

Haptens can be useful as diagnostic reagents. Skin testing for infection with *Mycobacterium bovis* is commonly performed in cattle by injecting a small amount of purified protein derivative (PPD) intradermally. The PPD reacts with sensitized lymphocytes in the infected animal, yet if the animal is uninfected, it will not elicit an immune response. This procedure takes advantage of the ability of the hapten to combine with immune reactants (antibodies and sensitized T lymphocytes), if they have already been produced, but hapten alone is unable to elicit responses.

The binding of a small molecule to protein in the host's skin or blood sometimes elicits an immune response that can lead to an allergic response. An example of such a hapten is a small drug moiety (such as the penicillin metabolite penicillinoyl) that can bind to serum proteins as a carrier to elicit the production of antibodies. These antibodies can then trigger an allergic response (see Chapter 13). Other examples of haptens binding to host proteins and becoming immunogenic include metals, plastics, and dyes. The contact hypersensitivity that dogs sometimes develop to carpet or to plastic in a food dish is the result of a hapten-carrier eliciting an immune response.

PROTEIN EPITOPES

Proteins are made up of amino acid chains that are folded into a three-dimensional configuration. There are two types of antigenic determinants: those for which the primary amino acid sequence is most important in determining binding and those whose three-dimensional configuration is most important. Configurational determinants are formed by the three-dimensional folding of the amino acid chain, which brings residues that may be far apart on the amino acid chain together at the surface of the folded protein. Such residues make contact with complementary residues on the antibody-combining site of the antibody molecule. Experimental data suggest that the maximum length of an amino acid chain that can fit into the combining site is 6 to 8 residues. The other type of antigenic determinant is that which is recognizable on the unfolded amino acid chain.

Protein epitopes have been divided into two types, sequential (continuous) and conformational (discontinuous) (Figure 2-1). Because of the globular nature of proteins, the majority of epitopes have some involvement of three-dimensional structure, the result of folding the peptide chain. Two amino acid residues located side by side within an antigenic determinant are more likely to be there as a result of the folding of the peptide chain than the native amino acid sequence. When three-dimensional protein structure is reduced by chemical treatment for sodium-dodecylsulfate (SDS)-polyacrylamide gel electrophoresis, anti-

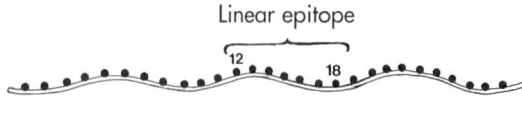

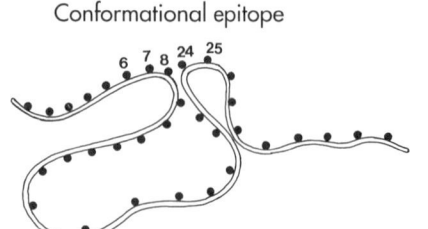

Figure 2-1 A linear epitope is composed of sequential amino acids, as in those numbered 12 through 18. A conformational epitope is composed of epitopes that are brought close together by folding of the protein, as illustrated by amino acids 6 to 8 and 24 and 25.

genic determinants based solely on secondary structure are lost. Studies that illustrate these principles have been done on the protein myoglobin, which contains both sequential and conformational epitopes. For example, a sequential determinant is formed by residues 15 to 22. Residues 4, 79, and 12 are part of a conformtional epitope.

The antibody response to protein epitopes, as demonstrated in the myoglobin system, is specific to both sequential and conformational epitopes. In one series of experiments, 60% to 70% of antibodies elicited by immunization with myoglobin recognized peptide fragments of myoglobin; the remaining 30% to 40% recognized the native structure. The specificity of antibodies for the protein configuration that elicited immunization is greater than that for altered forms of the protein.

CROSS-REACTIVITY: SHARED EPITOPES

The specificity of the antibody response refers to the ability of an antibody to distinguish between the antigen that elicits its production and other antigens. Generally, a single antibody is specific for a given antigenic determinant or epitope. When an antigen is complex and contains many epitopes, there will be a population of antibodies elicited that is specific for each of these. In nature there often exist closely related antigens, such that they share some epitopes and have others that are unique. The phenomenon of *cross-reactivity* occurs when an antibody raised by immunization with one antigen is able to bind with an epitope on another antigen (Figure 2-2). An antibody reacts most strongly with the antigen that elicits its production (the homologous antigen). However, often an antibody reacts less strongly with a related antigen. The phenomenon of cross-reactivity occurs when two antigens bear a similar antigenic determinant such that antibodies elicited by one antigen bind to the similar determinant on the other.

Cross-reactivity has important implications for in vitro testing and can be important in the pathogenesis of certain autoimmune diseases. Such cross-reactivity can be a helpful or an undesireable occurrence for the immunologist. For example, the human respiratory syncytial virus is closely related to and cross-reacts with the bovine respiratory syncytial virus. Commercially available antisera for detection of the human respiratory syncytial virus can thereby be used to detect the bovine strain. Another example of cross-reacting viral epitopes is the feline infectious peritonitis virus (FIP) and the transmissable gastroenteritis virus (TGE) that affects swine. These coronaviruses share antigenetic determinants such that TGE virus antigen can be used as antigen source for FIP testing. Cross-reactivity between coronaviruses can also prove to be a problem in diagnostic testing for the presence of FIP antibodies. Many cats are exposed to enteric coronaviruses that will cross-react with whole FIP virus on any in vitro assay that uses whole virus as antigen. This is a potential source of false-positive reactions. The cross-reactivity between the human myocardium and group B streptococci can cause autoimmune disease. Antibodies elicited during a streptococcal infection can bind to the myocardium and initiate an autoimmune reaction against heart tissue resulting in valve scarring and rheumatic heart disease in humans. A similiar phenomenon has been suggested in equine strangles.

ANTIGENS IN THE ENVIRONMENT

Antigens that are encountered by the animal within the usual environment consist of infectious agents (virus, bacteria, parasite, fungi), inhalants (pollens), food components, and sometimes allogenic and tumor cells. Most of these are complex antigens with many antigenetic determinants.

Although proteins are the most common chemical group to serve as antigens, carbohydrates are important as glycoproteins and glycolipids. Polysaccharides in the form of lipopolysaccharides, are important constituents of the bacterial cell wall.

Bacterial antigens

Bacteria are single-celled organisms that are comprised of a cell wall, cell membrane, and nucleic

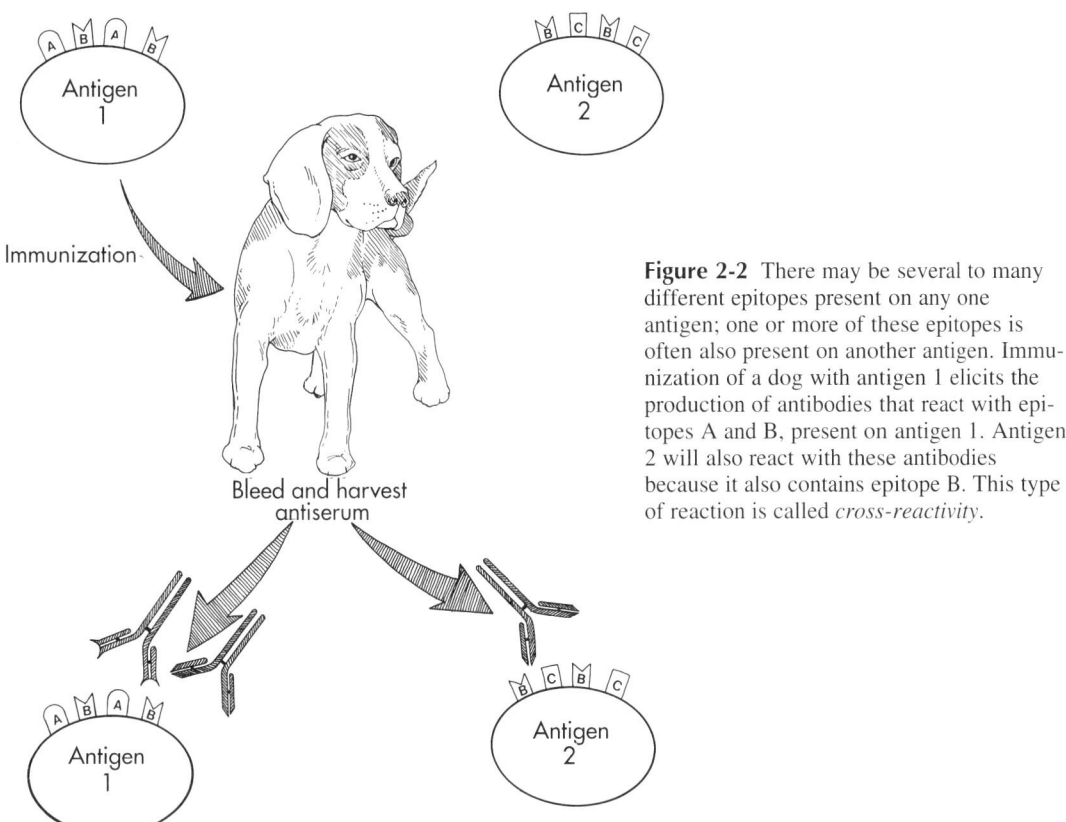

Figure 2-2 There may be several to many different epitopes present on any one antigen; one or more of these epitopes is often also present on another antigen. Immunization of a dog with antigen 1 elicits the production of antibodies that react with epitopes A and B, present on antigen 1. Antigen 2 will also react with these antibodies because it also contains epitope B. This type of reaction is called *cross-reactivity*.

acids; they can display a variety of appendages, such as fimbria, or pili, (protein), or capsule (polysaccharide). Some bacteria produce potent exotoxins (protein) that are immunogenic. Any or all of these bacterial components can act as antigens. Polysaccharide antigens on the gram-positive streptococcal cell wall are important in defining different serotypes of streptococcus, based on antisera raised against these differing determinants.

The gram-negative cell wall contains a backbone of protein and lipid A, which includes endotoxin, causing fever, leukopenia, and shock-like symptoms. The side chains forming the O antigen are made up of carbohydrates. Salmonella bacteria have a well characterized O antigen, which consists of oligosaccharide units that form a polysaccharide that surrounds the outer surface of the bacterial cell. Some antigenic determinants of the O antigen in Salmonella demonstrate cross-reactivity between the species of Salmonella. Yet other determinants are species specific. Another important antigen of Salmonella, called the H antigen, is made from the protein flagellin. The flagellar antigens elicit a strong antibody response. Development of antisera specific to the different antigenic determinants was used to establish the classification system of Kauffman-White. The Salmonella isolates are assigned to serogroups based on their reactivity with antisera, designating specific cell wall (O) antigens and flagellar (F) antigens.

Bacteria that produce polysaccharide capsules are better able to evade phagocytosis than non-encapsulated bacteria. Polysaccharide capsules contain repeating epitopes that are highly immunogenic. Once an antibody response has been elicited, opsonization occurs and phagocytosis is facilitated.

Immune responses can be elicited not only to antigens on an infecting organism but also to products produced by that organism. Often these antibodies are important for the protection of the host from subsequent infection. *Pasteurella haemolytica*, the gram-negative bacteria involved in bovine shipping fever pneumonia, produces a leukotoxin in log phase growth. Antibodies produced against surface determinants of the bacteria do not seem to assist in prevention of disease. A current approach to vaccination attempts to elicit antibodies against the leukotoxin. A well-accepted means of preventing the development of tetanus is the production of antibodies specific to the toxin of *Clostridium tetani*.

Viral antigens

Viruses are composed of a nucleocapsid that contains antigenic protein determinants. The nucleic acid, either DNA or RNA, is enclosed within the nucleocapsid. Some viruses have envelopes that may contain spikes or knoblike structures that can elicit an immune response, such as the hemagglutinin of the Influenza virus. Capsid proteins are generally good immunogens. Although most viral proteins are immunogenic, those on the surface of the virion are most important in protective immunity. Viruses reproduce within host cells, and some viruses bud from the cell membrane as a means of leaving the host cell. These viruses generally introduce virus-specific proteins into the cell membrane before budding. This enables cytotoxic T cells of the immune system to recognize and eliminate these infected cells.

A mechanism to evade the immune response occurs with Influenza virus. Antigenic determinants on the envelope glycoproteins, hemagglutinin, and neuraminidase, undergo frequent change such that antibodies that were protective against one viral strain fail to protect against infection with a new strain. This process is referred to as *antigenic shift*, and it leads to disease outbreaks in previously immune populations.

Parasite antigens

Parasites, such as the nematode *Dirofilaria immitis*, display an array of antigens, some of which are stage specific. Antigens on the third and fourth stage larvae elicit immune responses, as do microfilaria and adult forms. Currently there is interest in the potential use of antigens obtained during the molting process for immunization, with the idea that such antibodies might arrest parasite development.

Antigenic variation is a mechanism whereby an organism, such as a parasite, changes the antigenic determinants on its outer surface in an effort to evade the immune response. For example, the protozoan parasite *Trypanosoma cruzi* changes its antigens with each new wave of parasite production, thus enabling this hemoparasite to survive within an environment containing antibodies without being adversely affected. The new antigenic determinants elicit a new population of antibodies that are effective until the antigens are varied again.

Some parasite antigens are particularly able to elicit production of immunoglobulin E (IgE) antibodies. IgE antibodies degranulate mast cells and cause the release of vasoactive mediators, which assist in the elimination of the parasite.

Other antigens

A variety of antigens in the environment are potent inducers of IgE antibodies in certain individuals, including: pollens, molds, dust, ectoparasites, and some food components (nuts, shrimp, milk proteins, wheat, etc.). Other individuals fail to develop an immune response to these inhaled or ingested substances. Immunogenicity, therefore, depends on the genotype of the host to which it is presented. Other factors, such as the dose of antigen presented and its route of presentation, are important in determining the ultimate immune response to an antigen.

ANTIGENS PRESENT ON MAMMALIAN CELLS

Grafting of tissue from one individual to another invokes the problem of recognition by the recipient of foreign antigens on the donor tissue. When the tissue grafted is from one species to another, as in the case of a baboon heart into a human infant or the recent graft of a baboon liver into an adult human, the graft is called *xenograft*. Species-specific antigens present on the graft are recognized as foreign, and a rejection reaction is instigated unless the recipient is immunosuppressed. The existence of species-specific antigens on cells and proteins is useful for the identification of the origin of meat and blood samples. Immunologic tests with species-specific antisera are used in forensic investigations to differentiate human blood stains from those attributed to other species.

A graft between individuals within the same species, as in human-human or dog-dog transplants is called an *allograft*. These grafts can be successful if the major histocompatibility antigens (MHC) are matched (see Chapter 10). MHC antigens are highly polymorphic proteins on the surface of nucleated cells. The MHC class I antigens are composed of two noncovalently-associated subunits, an alpha chain that is anchored into the cell membrane (45 kilodalton [kD]) and a smaller (12 kD) molecule, known as beta-2 microglobulin. The class II proteins consist of two protein chains, both of which are anchored in the cell membrane. Matching these polymorphic proteins is essential for survival of a tissue graft (Figure 2-3C).

Other antigens found on mammalian cells include the tumor-specific and oncofetal antigens that are present on tumor cells. These antigens are not normally found on body cells or they are present in negligible amounts; and they can become targets for antitumor antibodies and cytotoxic T lymphocytes. Some tumor-associated antigens (TAA) are specific to a tumor type; others are present on a variety of tumor types. For example, chemically-induced tumors bear new antigens spe-

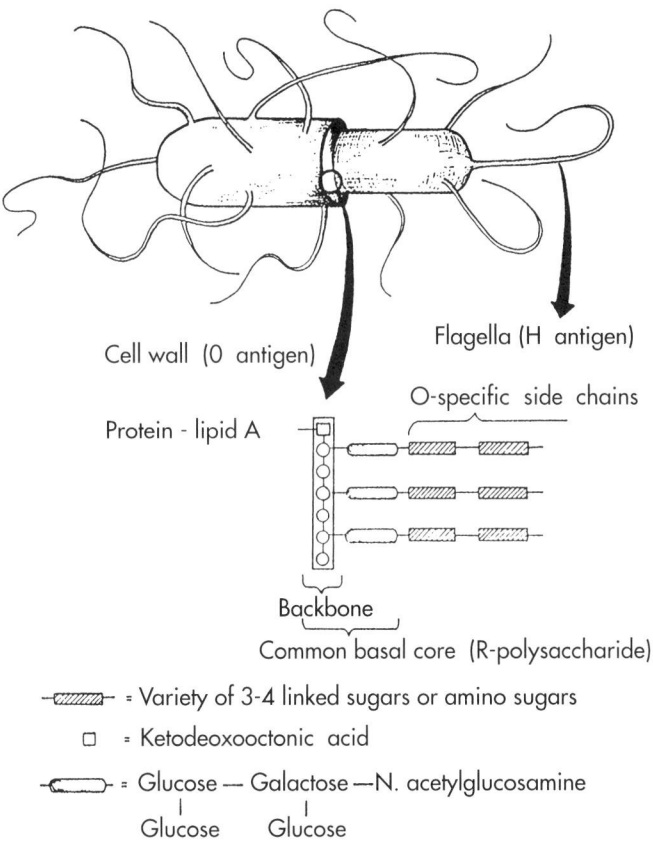

Figure 2-3 Antigens present on a gram-negative bacteria include the O (somatic) antigen of the cell wall and the H flagellar antigen (in motile species). Within the cell wall is the protein-lipid-carbohydrate complex that forms the endotoxin.

cific to a tumor. These antigens arise by a mutation of a cellular gene. Cytotoxic T-cell responses to such antigens are specific to the particular tumor type.

Oncofetal antigens are present on cells at various times during development. Some of these antigens are produced by certain tumors. Alpha-fetoprotein, a 70-kD polypeptide chain that resembles serum albumin, is produced by the fetal liver, yolk sac, and gastrointestinal tract. Serum levels are high in the fetus but virtually nonexistent in the adult. These antigens are found on some hepatomas and gastrointestinal tumors. Another oncofetal antigen is carcinoembryonic antigen (CEA), a 180-kD glycoprotein antigen. This antigen is associated with tumors of the gastrointestinal tract and shows some low-level cross-reactivity to polysaccharide blood group antigens.

Other cell surface antigens include the erythrocyte antigens, which vary from species to species (see Chapter 10). These antigens, can be immunogenic in those individuals that lack a particular determinant. Cross-matching blood before transfusion precludes the development of immune responses. Also present on erythrocytes of some species is an antigen called *Forssman antigen*. Species that are positive for Forssman antigen include the horse, sheep, dog, cat, mouse, and bird species. Negative species include the rabbit, rat, monkey, duck, guinea pig, and human species. No correlation has been made between the presence of this antigen and any particular function. However, if a rabbit is immunized with sheep erythrocytes, it will make antibodies to Forssman antigen as well as to other determinants.

Integral membrane proteins of leukocytes have been recognized and associated with particular functions. The recognition of these cell-surface markers has been achieved by use of monoclonal antibody reagents (see Chapter 4), which are capable of interacting with a single epitope on a cell surface. These markers have been designated *clusters of differentiation antigens*, or CD antigens.

Each CD antigen has a number; for example, CD4 designates the helper subset of T lymphocytes. Although it is not antigenic in the species of origin, the CD molecule is antigenic in the heterologous species, such as the mouse, used to produce the diagnostic monoclonal antibodies. These cell-surface molecules vary in size from less than 20 kD to greater than 150 kD; some are single chains, others are heterodimers.

SUPERANTIGENS

Certain bacterial products, including Staphylococcal enterotoxins, appear to have the ability to polyclonally activate T lymphocytes. This is not an antigen-specific reaction; it occurs as a result of the crosslinking between the T-cell antigen receptor and the MHC class II molecule on antigen-presenting cells, regardless of the nature of the T-cell antigen specificity. This stimulates a variety of different T cells to proliferate and thereby generates a polyclonal response. Superantigens are a current topic of immunologic research.

EPITOPES AND IMMUNOGENICITY IN SYNTHESIZING VACCINES

Most antigens must be presented to a helper T cell before they can elicit the production of antibodies. They are therefore called T-dependent antigens. A few antigens, such as the polysaccharide of the pneumococcus capsule, can directly stimulate B cells. These antigens usually elicit only an immunoglobulin M (IgM) response.

The epitopes recognized by the helper T cells are different than those recognized by B cells. T cells are able to distinguish single amino acid differences, and substitutions can make the difference between recognition and nonrecognition. Recognition of a B cell epitope is a property of immunoglobulin surface receptor present on that cell. The size of the B-cell epitope is therefore determined by the antigen-binding site on that surface Ig molecule. A B-cell epitope can be either linear or nonlinear and are often conformational, usually quite accessible on the surface of a globular protein or cell. B-cell epitopes are often hydrophilic.

A T-cell epitope is different from a B-cell epitope in several ways. The T-cell epitope is a linear peptide, which is presented to the T cell while bound to a MHC molecule. It must bind to the T-cell receptor and to the MHC molecule. The term *epitope* is used to refer to the part of the peptide that binds the T-cell receptor; the term *agretope* is used to describe the part that binds to the MHC molecule. The peptides binding to T cells are amphipathic, having a hydrophobic portion that is the agretope and a hydrophilic portion that is the epitope. The size of the peptide may vary from as few as 7 to as many as 20 amino acids. It is generally larger than the B-cell epitope.

Recent technological advances in protein sequencing and peptide synthesis have made it possible to construct antigenic peptides that include the epitopes needed for stimulating a good immune response without undesirable components of the organism for which the vaccine is constructed. A requirement for immunogenicity of a synthetic vaccine is the presence of both a B-cell epitope and a T-cell epitope. Induction of a humoral immune response requires the cognate interaction between hapten-specific B cells and carrier-specific T cells that recognize different nonoverlapping areas on the antigen. Studies using polyvalent synthetic vaccines have shown that induction of an immune response requires only one strong T-cell epitope. The T-cell epitope must be able to interact with class II molecules on the host cells. The technique of epitope mapping has increased our knowledge about T-cell and B-cell epitopes. In epitope mapping, a protein is digested into a set of overlapping peptides; these are then reacted with antisera specific to the particular protein. This technique has shown that T-cell epitopes are usually composed of a linear array of sequential amino acids, whereas B-cell epitopes may be composed of sequential or nonsequential amino acids. The requirement for T-cell epitopes to interact with both the T-cell receptor and with an MHC molecule means that it has two distinct interaction sites: the epitope, which interacts with the T-cell receptor, and the agretope, which interacts with either MHC class I or class II molecules. Synthetic T-cell epitopes may prove to be effective immunogens to elicit a protective cell-mediated immune (CMI) response.

SUGGESTED READINGS

Berzofsky JA, Cease K, Cornette J, et al: Protein antigenic structures recognized by T cells: potential applications to vaccine design, *Immunol Rev* 98:9-52, 1987.

Jolivet M, Lise L, Gras-Masse H, Tartar A, et al: Polyvalent synthetic vaccines: relationship between T epitopes and imunogenicity, *Vaccine* 8:35-40, 1990.

Rothbard JB, Gefter MI: Interactions between immunogenic peptides and MHC proteins, *Ann Rev Immunol* 9:527-565, 1991.

3 The Lymphoid System and Cells of the Lymphoid System

The cells involved in the immune response belong to the lymphoreticular system, which is comprised of two cellular populations, lymphocytes and macrophages. These cell populations perform different functions in the immune response. Lymphocytes and their progeny manifest specific reactions to various stimuli, such as the production of humoral antibodies against specific agents or the ability to differentiate and respond specifically to various foreign tissue antigens. Macrophages are nonspecific in that their products or functional behavior can be initiated by many different stimuli. The response observed is stereotypic for macrophages and not for specific antigen or stimulus.

Within these two cell groups, subpopulations of cells have been identified. For example, antibody production results from the stimulation and differentiation of a population of lymphocytes called bone marrow or bursial-derived (B) cells. The other major subset of lymphocytes, known as thymus derived (T) cells, have the ability to recognize and reject skin grafts as well as respond to certain antigens, such as tuberculin.

The functional attributes of macrophage subsets are not as well characterized. As a general concept, macrophages can be viewed as the chief means of degradation and inactivation of foreign substances. Current studies indicate that the material that escapes this physiological digestion process is highly immunogenic and that macrophage processing of antigens is a necessary step in the induction of the immune response in vivo.

In addition to antigen processing, macrophages actively participate immunological processes in vivo. For example, in a positive tuberculin test, the immunological specificity is provided by the T cells. Macrophages are attracted to the reaction site by humoral chemotactic factors as well as by products secreted by T cells following contact with antigen. These effector macrophages digest and inactivate antigen as well as products of tissue-breakdown, thus serving as agents of wound débridement.

Functional attributes of the various cellular populations are associated with specific anatomic regions in lymphoid tissues. Lyphoid tissues are classified as either central or peripheral organs. Central lymphoid organs, such as the bone marrow, thymus or bursa of Fabricius in avians, are identified as areas that produce major changes in lymphocyte development and differentiation. Peripheral lymphoid organs, such as spleen, lymph nodes, and Peyer's patches of the intestine, are populated by lymphoid cells that have achieved immune capability. Peripheral organs are designed to bring immunocompetent lymphocytes into contact with antigen and thus serve as the sites of development of the specific features of immunity (Figure 3-1).

DEVELOPMENT OF THE LYMPHOID SYSTEM

In the developing embryo, primitive lymphocytes are first identified in the yolk sac, along with other hematopoietic elements. Later in development, the liver achieves primacy as the major site of lymphocytic development. Eventually, the bone marrow becomes the primary source of lymphocytes. All of the blood cells originate from a common stem cell. The stem cell then becomes committed (in the case of lymphocytes) to differentiate along the lymphoid lineage. B and T lymphocytes are derived from this committed lineage.

Central lymphoid organs

Bone marrow

The source of hematopoietic elements, including lymphocytes, is found chiefly in the central cavities of developing long bones. A supporting network of primitive reticulin-producing cells, fibroblasts, collagen, adipose tissue fills these cavities. Enmeshed within this network are nests of *erythrocytes, granulocytes, monocytes* and *lymphocytes*, and their stem-cell (*myeloid*) precursors. The tissue is richly supplied with lymphatics and capillaries. Lymphocytes in the bone marrow are derived mainly from mitotic divisions of lym-

14 Principles of Immunology

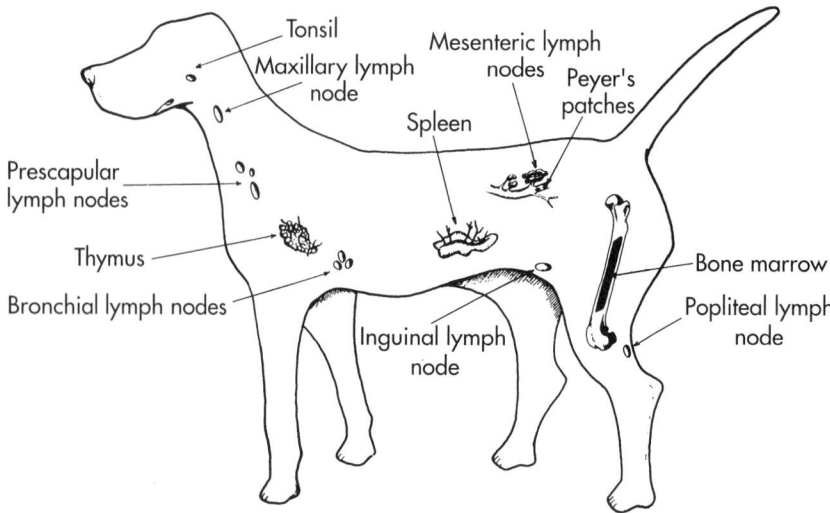

Figure 3-1 Peripheral and central lymphoid tissues of the dog.

phoblasts or prolymphocytes. After an undetermined number of replications in the marrow, lymphocytes leave this site chiefly by *efferent* lymphatics. Control mechanisms exist that regulate both the number of developing cells and the number leaving the marrow. However, these mechanisms remain to be delineated. Lymphocytes leaving the bone marrow are programmed for further development in one of two locations. Lymphocytes that are ultimately involved in antibody production migrate to the spleen and lymph nodes. Lymphocytes involved with cellular immunity must first pass through the thymus and then to the peripheral lymph nodes. Because the great bulk of this cellular migration occurs before birth in domestic animal species, lymphoid tissues of the neonate are well developed.

Thymus

The thymus, a multilobed lymphoid structure located in the thoracic mediastinum, extends from the base of the heart to the thoracic inlet (Figure 3-2). It reaches its maximum size in the young animal and undergoes progressive involution with age. The epithelial component of the thymus is derived from an outpouching of gut endoderm at the level of the third and fourth pharyngeal pouches. The supporting reticulin network is mesenchymal in origin and the lymphocytic portion (thymocytes) is derived from bone marrow. Appropriate homing of bone-marrow origin lymphocytes to the thymic region is dependent on the preexisting epithelial component. The histological unit of the thymus is the thymic lobule, which is further divided into an outer cortex and an inner medulla (Figure 3-3). The cortex is composed of dense aggregates of small lymphocytes, but the medulla is relatively acellular. The epithelial cells are most prominent in the lobule region and are arranged in whirls (Hassall's corpuscles) that often form keratohyalin. Primative myoephithelial cells also are present in this region and can be recognized by the presence of myofibrils.

The thymus is populated with marrow-derived lymphocytes during early in utero development. Thymocytes are detected at 60 to 80 days of gestation in horses, 40 days for calves and piglets, 35 days for sheep, 28 days for dogs, and 5 days for chickens. Only *efferent* lymphatics are present in the thymus, indicating that lymphocytes enter the thymus by the blood-vascular system. Afferent arterioles enter the lobule and divide the capillaries at the corticomedullary junction to supply both the cortex and the medulla. Capillaries are comprised of a complete layer of endothelial cells, a prominent basement membrane, and a complete outer layer of epithelial cells.

Under normal conditions, a physiological antigen barrier in the thymus prevents antigens from localizing and inciting an immune response in the thymus. In certain disease states, such as canine distemper, viral antigen gains access to thymic tissue and, in the recovery phase of infection, may stimulate the formation of a germinal center in the medulla.

Thymic lymphocytes, or thymocytes are highly active metabolically. Mitotic indexes of thymocytes in the cortex are four to ten times greater than mitosis in nonthymic lymphoid tissue. Many thymocytes produced by these mitotic divisions die without ever leaving the thymus. After an unknown number of divisions that culminate in

The Lymphoid System and Cells of the Lymphoid System 15

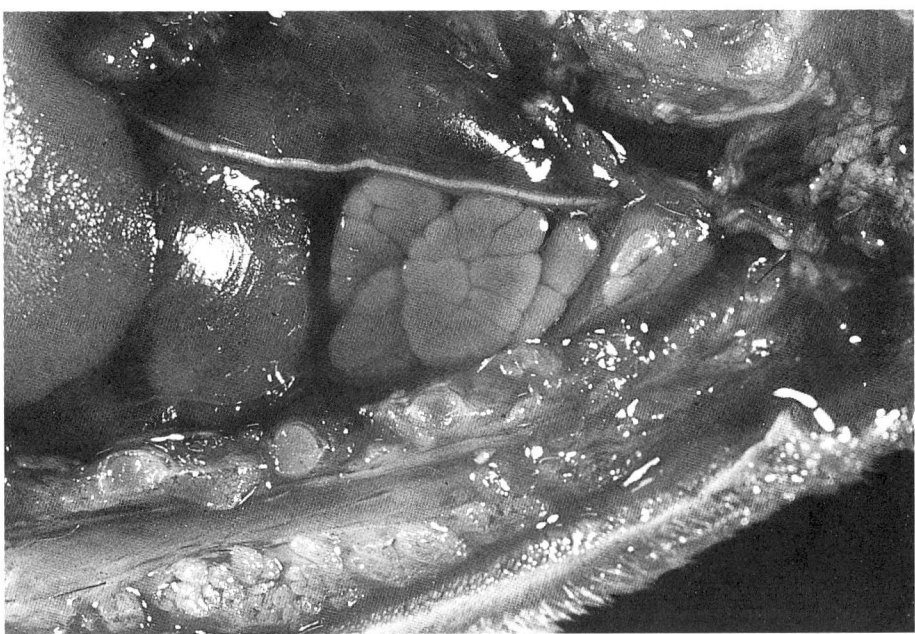

Figure 3-2 Location of the mammalian thymus. The thymus is located within the mediastinum and extends from the thoracic to the pericardial sac. Courtesy of Krakowka S, Hoover EA: *Modern veterinary practice*, 1977, Santa Barbara, Calif., American Veterinary Publications

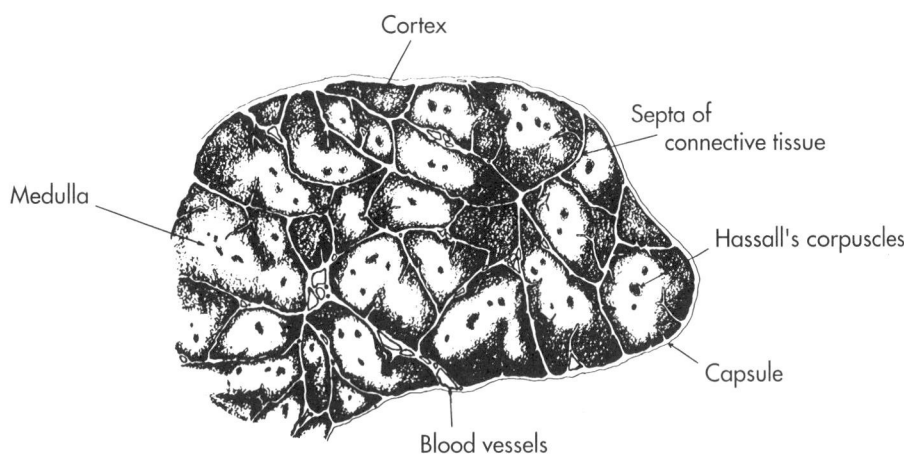

Figure 3-3 Histologic anatomy of the thymus; various features are labeled.

maturation, the differentiated cortical thymocytes leave the thymus by passing through the medullar lymphatics. The most immature thymocytes are present in the cortex, and the most mature thymocytes are found in the medulla.

While thymocytes are in the thymus, several important events occur. These events are proliferation, differentiation, and selection. While in the thymus, thymocytes begin to express the T-cell receptor for antigen. A wide variety of specificities are represented. In addition to the T cell-antigen receptor, the expression of CD4 and CD8 cell-surface molecules is also first seen in the thymic cortex. Although thymocytes proliferate quickly in the thymic cortex, a large number of them die before entering the medulla because of selection. The process of positive selection ensures that the mature thymocyte will be self-MHC restricted. This is an essential part of antigen recognition (see Chapter 7). Equally important to antigen recognition is negative selection, which removes autoreactive clones and renders the mature thymocytes tolerant of self-antigens. After positive and negative selection have occurred, the remaining T cells express T-cell receptors that react with foreign antigen in a self-MHC restricted manner.

During the process of differentiation in the thymus, the thymocytes come into contact with a variety of nonlymphoid cells. Among these are superficial cortical epithelial cells called *nurse cells*. The nurse cells surround thymocytes with membrane invaginations. In this environment the thymocytes come into contact with the self-MHC Class II molecules expressed on the epithelial surface, as well as the thymic hormones produced by these cells. Thymic hormones include a variety of well-characterized molecules including thymosin, thymulin, and thymopoietin. Much interest has centered on the potential use of these molecules for the restoration of T-cell function to persons with immunodeficient states, such as DiGeorge syndrome in humans. Thymosin is a thymic hormone with an estimated molecular weight of approximately 10,000 daltons (D). Secreted by the thymic epithelial cells, thymosin induces stem-cell differentiation to T-lymphocytes when cultured with bone marrow cells in vitro. Purified hormone induces T-lymphocyte maturation. Thymosin acts only on stem cells destined to become T-lymphocytes. Thymosin has no effect on lymphocytes from animals depleted of T cells by irradiation and/or neonatal thymectomy. Thymosin does not alter the activity of B cells directly.

Bursa of Fabricius

Unlike mammals, avian species have, in addition to a thymus, a well-defined central lymphoid structure that is intimately concerned with B-lymphocyte differentiation. This structure, called the bursa of Fabricius, is a dorsal diverticulum of the cloaca. Structurally it resembles the thymus, in that the bursa has intimate associations with gut epithelium and developing lymphocytes. During embryonic growth, the bursa develops after the thymus. The epithelial thymus develops on day nine and is populated by thymocytes by day twelve. The epithilial component of the bursa first appears on day fourteen, and lymphocytes are found by day seventeen.

Proof that the bursa is a central lymphoid organ was obtained by surgical or testosterone-induced bursectomies of developing chicks before day seventeen. Bursectomized chicks lost the ability to make immunoglobin in postnatal life, yet had intact lymphocytic function in the thymus. A lymphocyte-differentiating hormone, bursopoietin, has been identified. This polypeptide induces B-cell differentiation in a manner similar to the action of thymosin on T lymphocytes.

Many investigators have attempted to give mammalian gut-associated lymphoid tissue (GALT) an analagous role as an area of B-lymphocyte development equivalent to the bursa. The sheep has an extensive GALT system, which is currently considered quite similiar to the bursa in function. In other mammalian species, no such function has been attributed to the GALT, and it is thought that the bone marrow serves as the bursal equivalent.

Peripheral lymphoid organs

Lymph nodes

Lymph nodes are organized collections of lymphoreticular tissue located along lymphatic channels. The prime function is filtration and removal of bacteria and other material. A schematic cross-section of a lymph node is shown in Figure 3-4. The node is divided into cortex and medulla. Lymph enters the node at the capsular surface and exits at the hilus, the region in which arterioles enter and venules leave the node.

The medulla contains the large blood vessels that divide and, along with associated lymphatics and supporting network form lymph cords. Between the cords is a loose network of lymphatic sinuses that contains macrophages, lymphocytes, and plasma cells.

The cortex is distinguished from the medulla by a dense cellular mass of lymphocytes. In most species, nodes contain lymphocytes at birth. Within the cortex are large nodules, or germinal centers. The central portions of the centers are composed of larger, light-staining cells, often with mitotic activity. Germinal centers are sites of B-lymphocyte differentiation into antibody-producing plasma cells. B cells originate from the bone marrow. Following antigenic stimulation, these cells begin proliferating and differentiating toward plasma cells. As these B cells mature, they move to the peripheral area, or mantle, of the germinal center and then to the sinus areas in the medulla.

Between the outer cortex and inner medulla is the paracortical, or T-cell–dependent area, a zone of lymphocytes not involved in antibody production. T lymphocytes, either in the initial homing phase or in continuous recirculation between blood and lymph, enter this area through specialized vascular connections at the level of the postcapillary venules. They then percolate through the cortex and medulla to lymphatic sinuses in the medulla and leave the node through efferent lymphatics. T-cell–dependent areas are depleted by procedures that interfere with thymocyte development, such as neonatal thymectomy in rodents, or by techniques for destroying T cells, such as long term thoracic duct drainage or administration of antithymocyte serum.

Antigen-stimulated nodes rapidly increase in size and cellularity. Initial increases in cellularity

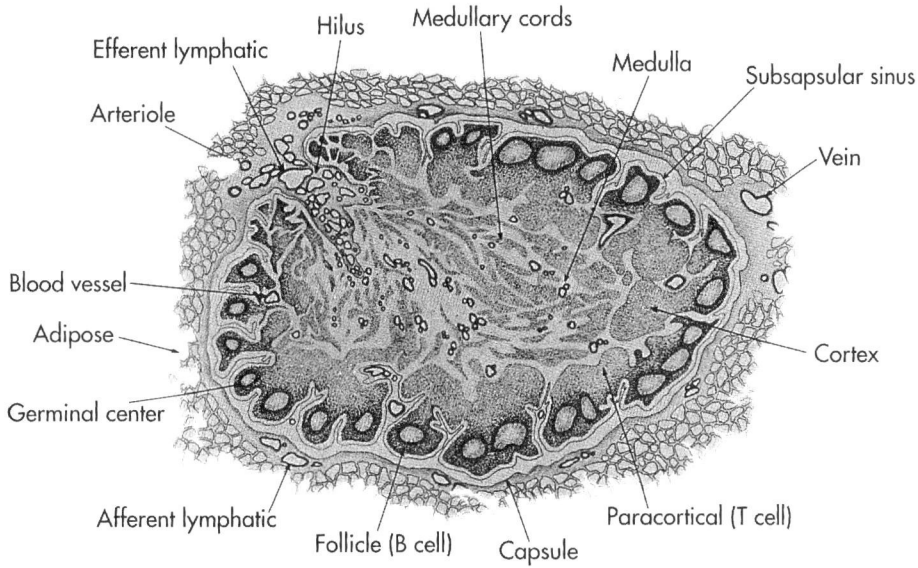

Figure 3-4 Cross section of a mammalian lymph node. B-cell (follicles) and T-cell (paracortical)–dependent areas are labeled.

are the result of enhanced "trapping" of circulating lymphocytes, particularly those from bone marrow. Further, there is a transient shutdown in the exit rate of lymphocytes from antigen-stimulated nodes. Later, antigen-mediated proliferation of clones of antigen-stimulated cells constitute the bulk of cells in the node. Thus lymph nodes, as well as other peripheral lymphoid organs, are dynamic and ever-changing in terms of their cellular components.

Filtration of lymph is a major function of lymph nodes. Macrophages, cells of the reticuloendothelial system derived from bone-marrow precursor cells, are the chief means of clearing foreign material from the lymph.

Spleen

The spleen is a large vascular organ located in the gastrosplenic ligament along the greater curvature of the stomach. Unlike lymph nodes, the spleen has no afferent lymphatics, so the sinusoidal network of the spleen is derived from capillaries and filled with blood. A dense collagenous capsule surrounds the organ, and trabeculae continuous with the capsule divide the substance of the spleen into lobules (Figure 3-5). Blood vessels enter and leave at the hilar region and follow the trabecular framework into the tissue, first as central arterioles, then as smaller straight arterioles, then as capillaries.

Because a major function of the spleen is vascular filtration of particulates and removal of damaged or aged erythrocytes, the capillary network of the red pulp is abundantly supplied with macrophages to perform this function. In addition, other blood elements (e.g., granulocytes and megakaryocytes) are found in this region.

Two distinct collections of lymphocytes are observed; together they comprise the erythrocyte-poor white pulp. Large lymphoid follicles, either as solid sheets of cells or as germinal centers being formed, are present at or near the divisions of central arterioles. These malpighian bodies are similar in all respects to B-cell–dependent areas of lymph nodes and are the sites of B-lymphocyte differentiation and secretion of immunoglobulin. The second portion of white pulp distinct from those lymphoid follicles is found surrounding the central arterioles, as in the form of periarteriolar lymphoid sheaths. These areas are populated by T lymphocytes. Procedures that interfere with development of thymocytes result in the depletion of these areas.

Lymphocytes follow a circulation pattern that alternates between the vascular and lymphatic compartments, which intimately involve both the spleen and the lymph nodes. T lymphocytes are a highly mobile population of cells, whereas B cells are relatively sessile and migrate only slowly within lymphatic tissues. The secretory products, however, have easy access to peripheral circulation as immunoglobulin. T lymphocytes, the majority of lymphocytes identifiable in peripheral blood, leave the vascular system and enter efferent lymphatics through postcapillary venules and secondary lymphoid organs. Eventually they pass

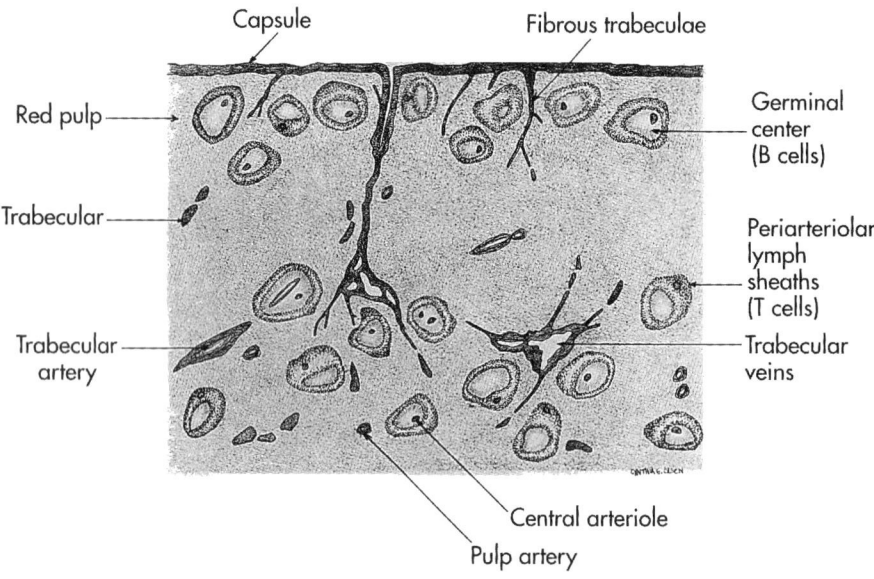

Figure 3-5 Cross section of a mammalian spleen. B-cell follicles and germinal centers and T-cell (periarteriolar lymphoid sheaths)-dependent areas are labeled.

from the thoracic duct to the anterior vena cava and back to the blood. Cannulation or resection of the thoracic duct interrupts this migration pattern and results in the depletion of thymus-dependent areas in lymphoid tissues. The net effect of this cellular migration pattern, coupled with the perfusion of almost all tissues with antibodies contained in the circulation or in mucosal secretions, is to provide a systematic and efficient method for the dissemination and recognition of immunologic material.

Other secondary lymphoid structures

Organized aggregates of lymphoid nodules exist in many locations in the body. These lymphoid areas are distinguished from lymph nodes by the lack of afferent lymphatics and a definite capsule. In the respiratory system there are various levels of organization of this lymphatic tissue. In the pharynx, tonsils and pharyngeal nodules are formed. These tissues are in intimate contact with pharyngeal epithelium. Both T lymphocytes and lymphoid follicles characteristic of B lymphocytes are present. Lymphoid nodules extend down the bronchial tree to the bronchiolar level, where lymphoid aggregates are found. The bronchus-associated lymphoid tissue (BALT) is more prominent in some species than in others. Mice have abundant BALT that consists of lymphoid aggregates, particularly at areas where bronchioles bifurcate. These are readily seen on histological section. The human, horse, and cow species have less distinct BALT.

Peyer's patches, analogous to tonsil, constitute the chief organized lymphoid structure in the gut. In addition, there are numerous solitary lymphoid nodules scattered throughout the lamina of the gut. Although a major function of lymphoid tissues located along mucosal surfaces is the production of a specific class of immunoglobulin called immunoglobulin A (IgA), other immunoglobulins are produced as well as T lymphocytes. The epithelial cells covering areas of Peyer's-patches consists of specialized cells ("M" cells) with micropinocytic properties that allow these cells to sample antigen. Under this area of specialized epithelium there are aggregates of T cells, B cells, and plasma cells. In sheep the Peyer's patches reach their maximum in two-month-old lambs; they then get smaller and are macroscopically involuted by fifteen months of age. It is currently thought that these lymphoid aggregates are a bursal equivalent for the sheep species. In areas of chronic inflammation, lymphoid nodules may develop in a variety of sites (Figure 3-6).

Species variation in the structure of lymphoid tissues

Chicken

The chicken and other avian species lack organized lymph nodes as described earlier for the mammalian species. Instead, lymphoid aggregates and nodules located along lymphatics and blood vessels serve as lymph node analogues.

Hemal Nodes in Ruminants

Ruminants, in addition to possessing the usual complement of lymph nodes, have organized lymphoid structures called *hemal lymph nodes,* which are scattered along small blood vessels. These structures do not contain lymphatics, although they superficially resemble lymph nodes. The capillary network within this tissue is similiar to that of the spleen, and it is reasonable to attribute similar blood-filtering and granulopoietic functions to them. The pig also possesses similar structures with the addition of lymphatics, which are intermediate between true hemal nodes and lymph nodes proper.

Lymph Node Structure of the Pig

The pig's lymph nodes, unlike other domestic animal species, are arranged such that the dense B-lymphocyte tissue is located deep in the node, whereas the loosely-arranged lymphatic tissue and sinuses corresponding to the medulla are located under the capsule. Coincident with this arrangement is the course of lymphatics. Afferent lymphatics enter the hilus, but efferent lymphatics leave the capsular surfaces.

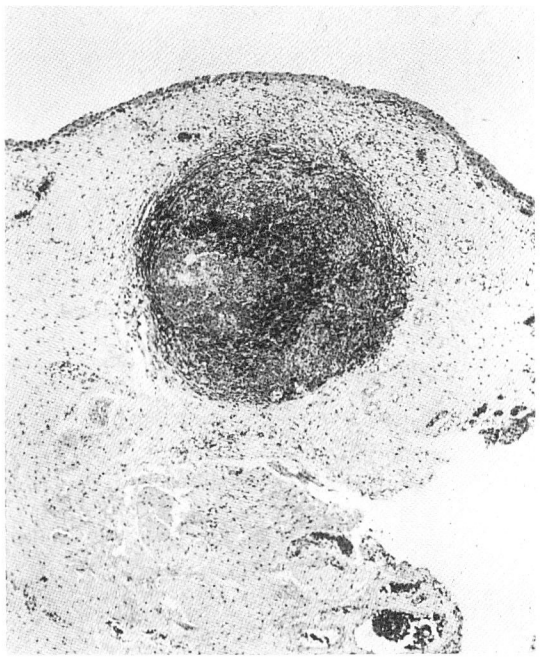

Figure 3-6 An organized lymphoid follicle underlying the transitional epithelium of the bladder in a dog with chronic cystitis (×16).

CELLS OF THE IMMUNE SYSTEM
(Table 3-1)

The cells of the immune system develop from stem cells in the bone marrow. From hematopoietic stem cell there is a common myeloid progenitor cell and a common lymphoid progenitor cell. The lymphoid lineage gives rise to the T and B lymphocytes that are important in the acquired immune response to antigen. The myeloid precursor gives rise to megakaryocytes (platelet precursors), the granulocytic cell series (neutrophilic, eosinophilic, and basophilic polymorphonuclear leukocytes), mast cells, and monocytes, which give rise to the macrophage. The erythroid lineage produces red blood cells. The events of hematopoiesis are regulated by cytokines.

The two types of cells that are considered phagocytes are the neutrophil and the macrophage. These cells have an important role in the innate immune response.

Phagocytic Cells

Phagocytic cells are important in both innate immune responses and acquired immunity. The two major types of phagocytic cells are the neutrophil and the monocyte/macrophage. While the macrophage plays an important role in both innate and acquired immunity, the neutrophil is an innate, or first line, defense mechanism.

Polymorphonuclear Leukocyte (Neutrophil)

The neutrophil is derived from bone marrow precursors and is closely related to the eosinophil and basophil, which are described later in this chapter. Neutrophils are released from the bone marrow into the blood-vascular system where they circulate for 12 to 18 hours, leaving the blood and traveling in tissue spaces for their remaining 2 or 3 days of life. Neutrophils respond to chemotactic stimuli by adhering to endothelial cells through adhesin molecules, diapedesing through the vessel wall, and then following the chemotactic gradient to an area of inflammation. The neutrophil is capable of phagocytosis and killing ingested organisms, and once it has performed these functions, the cell dies and becomes a component of the purulent exudate associated with bacterial infections. The remarkable importance of this defense mechanism is underscored by diseases in which neutrophils are either defective or in low number (such diseases are discussed in Chapter 12).

The neutrophil has a multilobulated nucleus and neutral staining granules, attributes from which its name is derived. Neutrophils are generally 10 to 12 μm in diameter.

Table 3-1 Selected cell membrane markers and receptors expressed on cells of the immune system

Cell membrane marker	Function/ synonym	mac	T	B	NK	Mast cell/baso	Eos	PMN
TCR: alpha, beta	Ag receptor	−	+	−	−	−	−	−
Ig	Ag receptor	−	−	+	−	−	−	−
CD3	Signal transduction	−	+	−	−	−	−	−
CD4	Adhesin: class II	−	+	−	−	−	−	−
CD8	Adhesin: class I	−	+	−	−	−	−	−
CD16	IgG Fc receptor	+	−	−	+	−/+	+	+
CD2	Adhesin: sheep rbc receptor	−	+	−	+	−	−	−
CD25*	TAC, IL-2 receptor	+	+	+	−	−	−	−
CD23*	IgE Fc$_{II}$ receptor	+	−	+	−	−	+	−
CD11b	MAC 1 (CR3)	+	−	−	+	−	+	+
CD18	Adhesin, beta$_2$ integrin	+	+	+	+	−/+	+	+

Ag, antigen; CD, cluster of differentiation antigen; Ig, immunoglobulin.
*on activated cells.

Mononuclear Cells/Macrophages

Monocytes/macrophages arise from stem cells of the bone marrow and enter the blood-vascular system to form freely circulating cells called promonocytes and monocytes. Monocytes/ macrophages join the resident phagocytic cells (macrophages) in the sinusoidal systems of the reticuloendothelial system or in the sinusoidal systems of the vascular sinuses of the spleen, liver, bone marrow, and lymphatic sinuses of lymph nodes. Freely circulating monocytes leave the blood-vascular system and become normal tissue residents in the lungs (alveolar), skin (Langhan's cells), and loose connective tissue (histiocytes).

Monocytes are large mononuclear cells that possess prominent kidney-shaped or pleomorphic nuclei. The cytoplasm is abundant, slightly basophilic, and contains indistinct cytoplasmic lysosomal granules. In histologic sections, cytoplasmic borders are indistinct. Activated collections of cells may fuse to form multinucleated giant cells or may exist as sheets of cells with abundant eosinophilic, vacuolated cytoplasm. In histologic sections, monocytes stain positively for cytoplasmic lysozyme and are diffusely positive for the enzyme serine esterase. Macrophages play a dual role in immune responses. The most widely known property of macrophages is that of phagocytosis and digestion of offending pathogens and tissue debris (Figure 3-7). Macrophages also function as the chief antigen-presenting cell (APC), which is crucial for the induction of an immune response.

Two general types of macrophages have been identified in lymph nodes. The sinusoidal or medullary macrophages line the lymphatic and blood-vascular sinuses in the medulla. Their chief function is the phagocytosis and lysosomal digestion of soluble and particulate antigens that arrive in lymph nodes through the afferent lymphatics. Most of this foreign material is digested and never reaches immunogenic form. A very small percentage of this ingested antigen is somehow protected from lysosomal enzymes and remains "bound" to the cell membrane. It is this macrophage-processed antigen that is responsible for inducing an immune response.

The second type of macrophage, the dendritic macrophage, is found associated with germinal centers and lymphoid follicles in the cortex. The dendritic macrophage is distinguished from the medullary macrophage by numerous long cytoplasmic extensions, or dendrites, that are in intimate contact with developing B lymphocytes. These macrophages are responsible for providing the antigenic stimulus to developing cells in germinal centers. Specific antibody adsorbs to the dendritic surfaces by the Fc portions of the molecule (cytophilic antibody), and the antigen is thus trapped in an extracellular environment and is closely exposed to developing B and T cells. This form of antigen processing is more of an adjuvant effect (i.e., enhancing a previously-existing effect) than an inducing event.

Functions of phagocytic cells

Phagocytosis

The process of phagocytosis is an important innate defense mechanism (as discussed in Chapter 1). Both neutrophils and macrophages are capable of engulfing and killing bacteria and other

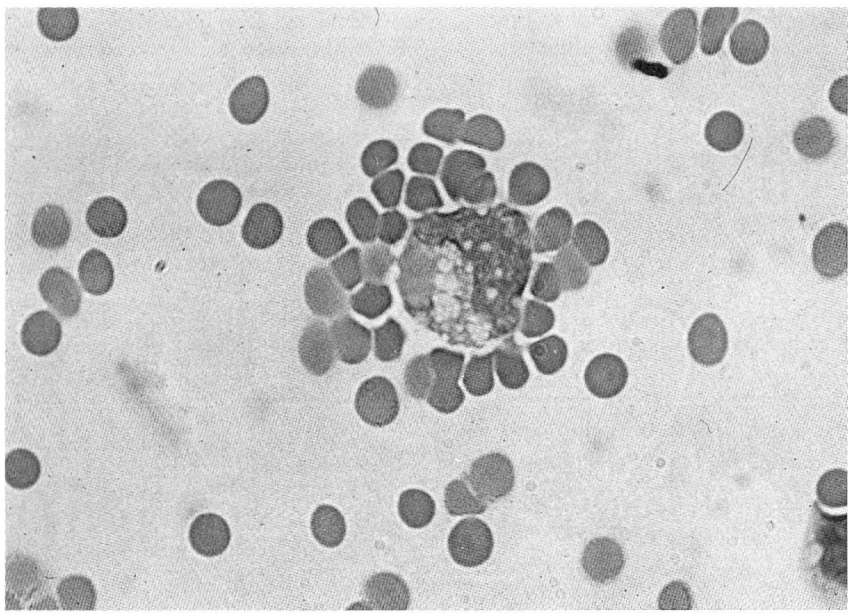

Figure 3-7 A canine peripheral blood monocyte/macrophage containing phagocytosed latex beads (clear cytoplasmic particles) and forming nonimmune rosettes with ovine erythrocyte (E), canine anti E, IgM (A) murine complement (C) complexes. Note the intracellular location of some EAC.

infectious particulates. The role of phagocytosis in obtaining processed antigens for presentation to T lymphocytes is an important macrophage function of the macrophage. Phagocytosis by neutrophils is a singular event that serves to eliminate the engulfed organism.

Macrophages recognize, bind to, and ingest foreign material coated with serum protein, IgG, and compliment (chiefly C3b) (see Figure 3-7). Tumor cells, N-acetyl glucosamine (possessed by many bacteria), lactoferrin, alpha^2-macroglobulin, and transferrin also bind macrophages with specific cell-membrane receptors for these substances. Macrophages also express cellular receptors for regulatory substances such as colony-stimulating factor, interferon and the T-cell lymphokines, macrophage inhibition factor (MIF) and a macrophage-activating factor (MAF). Macrophages are actively ameboid and respond to a variety of chemotactic stimuli of pathogen or host (C3a, C5a, C567) origin. Secretory products of macrophages facilitate digestion (see Chapter 1).

Antigen-Presenting Function

Induction of an immune response requires that antigen be presented to helper T lymphocytes and to B lymphocytes. Macrophages have historically been recognized as the chief APC. Antigen is taken in by phagocytosis and appropriate parts are expressed on the surface in conjunction with MHC Class II determinants. This occurs by intracellular binding of antigenic peptides with the MHC Class II molecule and the subsequent expression of this complex on the cell membrane. The binding of the antigen-Class II complex by the T lymphocyte, along with secretion of interleukin 1 (IL-1) by the macrophage, stimulates lymphocytes to begin the proliferation and differentiation process. Both the phagocytic and APC role of macrophages are regulated by pharmacologic substances and lymphokines (chiefly gamma interferon [γIFN]). It is important to point out that cells other than the macrophages can be induced to express MHC Class II and can function as APCs. Astrocytes of the brain, vascular endothelium, and a variety of ephithelia can, under certain circumstances, function as APCs. B lymphocytes can act as APCs, using their high-affinity immunoglobulin receptors to bind exogenous peptides; after endocytosis and reexpression in association with MHC Class II antigen, APCs efficiently present the antigen to helper T cells.

Secretory functions

A number of biologically active substances are produced by macrophages/monocytes. During the process of phagocytosis, lysosomal granules fuse with pinocytotic and phagocytic vacuoles, releasing enzymes into the resultant phagolysosome. A portion of these products leak out into the surrounding tissue, resulting in local tissue destruction and/or enhanced inflammatory responses. Macrophage enzymes such as hydrolyses, lysozyme, neutral proteases, prostaglandin E, and reactive oxygen intermediates (O_2, H_2O_2, and OH) are all secreted by metabolically active macrophages.

In addition to enzymes, macrophages are known to produce numerous proteins of the complement system (see Chapter 6). These proteins are: Clq, C2, C4, C3, C5, factors B and D, properdin of the alternate pathway, and the inhibitors of C3b and B1H. Finally activated macrophages produce IL-1, essential to the initial activation of immunocompetant T cells during the inductive phases of the immune response, and interferon, chiefly of the gamma and beta types.

Lymphocytes

Lymphocytes are the cells ultimately responsible for antibody production and manifestation of cell-mediated immunity. In blood smears, lymphocytes are 6 to 10μ in diameter and possess an eccentric ovoid nucleus with a thin rim of slightly basophilic cytoplasm. A subpopulation of lymphocytes, referred to as large granular lymphocytes (LGL) or natural killer (NK) cells, contains azurophilic cytoplasmic granules. All lymphocytes ultimately arise from bone marrow. T lymphocytes differentiate during residence in the thymus whereas mammalian B lymphocytes differentiate in B-cell–dependent areas of secondary lymphoid tissues. Because lymphocytes, regardless of origin, are morphologically similar (Figure 3-8), determination of origin is delineated by functional analysis, anatomical location in secondary lymphoid tissues, and expression of cell-surface marker proteins on resting or activated cellular populations.

T lymphocytes

T lymphocytes occupy paracortical regions of lymph nodes (Figure 3-9) and periarteriolar sheath regions in the spleen. They constitute the majority (65% to 85%) of lymphocytes in peripheral blood. Categories of T cells include those responsible for helper, cytotoxic/effector, suppressor, and memory functions. All murine, human, and canine T cells express the pan T-cell marker, originally designated as Thy-1 or theta antigen. Genetic analysis of murine lymphoid cells have shown that functional subsets express different lymphocyte glycoprotein alloantigens (Lyt). Helper T cells were identified by expression of murine Lyt1 using alloantisera. With the advent of monoclonal antibodies, recognition of more leukocyte cell-surface molecules (called antigens because they can be detected with antibodies) required a better system of nomenclature. The "cluster of differentiation" (CD) terminology was therefore adopted. CD indicates a particular leukocyte cell-surface molecule that is identified by a cluster of mono-

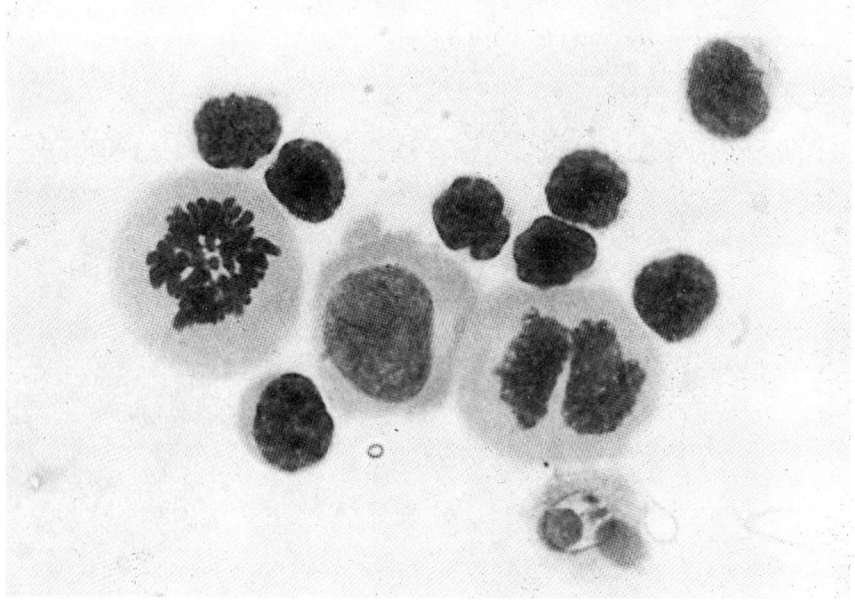

Figure 3-8 In vitro culture of lymphocytes with a phytomitogen. All morphologic stages of lymphocyte proliferation are apparent from resting (small cells with scanty cytoplasm), lymphoblast (large cells with prominent cytoplasm), and dividing mitotic forms.

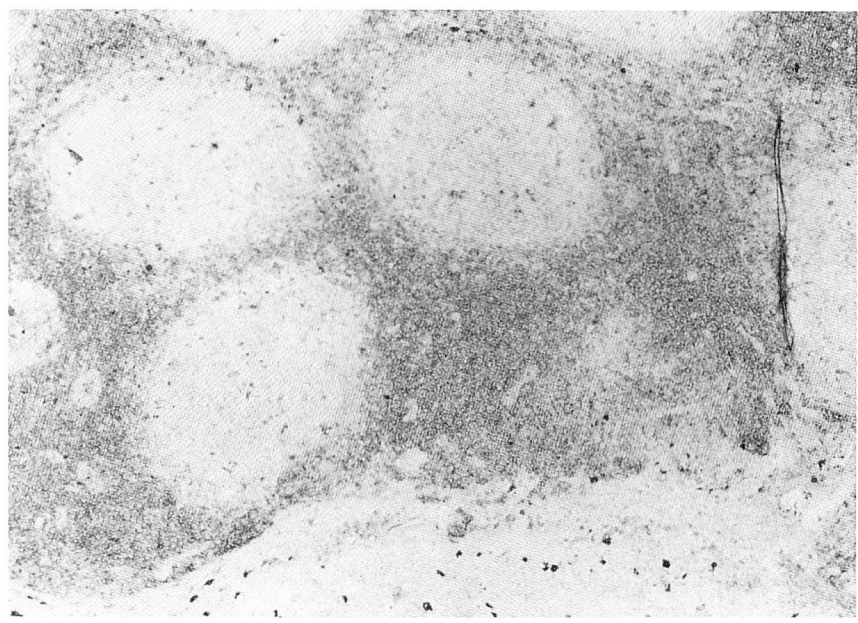

Figure 3-9 A frozen section of human lymphoid tissue stained with a horseradish peroxidase-conjugated monoclonal antibody to pan T lymphocytes. Note that germinal center areas are largely devoid of positive-staining cells.

clonal antibodies. In humans, the equivalent glycoprotein to murine Lyt1 is designated CD4. It is involved in antigen recognition in association with Class II MHC molecules. The CD8 molecule designates another T-cell subpopulation with suppressor/cytotoxic cell function. It is analogous to Lyt2 on murine cells.

The T-cell receptor (TCR) for antigen consists of two polypeptide chains, either alpha and beta or gamma and delta. They are members of the Ig gene superfamily, and each chain contains a variable region and a constant region, as well as a transmembrane segment. All T cells express CD5 (T1) and CD3, a five-chain complex that is responsible for signal transduction during interaction with antigen. Monoclonal antibody panels for human and murine lymphocyte subsets are commercially available and are routinely used in marker analysis. Antibodies have been developed for T cells and the major subsets of most domestic animal species. The exquisite specificity of human/murine monoclonals renders cross reactivity with animals unlikely. There are a few exceptions; for example, both polyclonal and monoclonal antisera to rat Thy-1 react with canine cells.

In addition to these T-cell lineage-specific glycoproteins, T cells also express more conventional cell-membrane receptors. Helper T cells possess Fc receptors for IgM, whereas suppressor/cytotoxic cells express Fc receptors for IgG. Both can be demonstrated by rosetting or fluorescence microscopy assays. As mentioned, inducible IL-2 receptors are characteristic of T lymphocytes. The CD designations for the low affinity Il-2 receptor (TAC) is CD25. Immature T cells contain a cytoplasmic enzyme, terminal deoxynucleotidyl transferase (TdT), which is detected by immunofluorescence assay. The TdT assay has been applied to the study of feline T cells. T lymphocytes, like monocytes, contain cytoplasmic serine esterase. Unlike the former, reaction product is punctate.

T cells will also form nonimmune rosettes with erythrocytes (E). In humans and primates, rosette formation with ovine erythrocytes was previously accepted as a T-cell marker before the availability of monoclonal antibody reagents. The cell-surface molecule responsible for this reaction is now recognized to be CD2, an adhesion molecule. The T11 antigen recognized by T11 and Leu5 monoclonal antibodies is specific for the E receptor on T cells and is synonymous with CD2. Rosette-forming assays in domestic animals are less definitive. Guinea pig E rosette formation by canine, feline, and equine T cells was formerly thought to be T-cell specific. B cells, platelets, neutrophils, and monocytes form rosettes with guinea pig E. Porcine T cells form nonimmune rosettes with neuroamidase-treated ovine E and this assay appears to be T-cell specific.

Recently an instrument has been developed that can screen and characterize a population of cells labeled with fluorescent marker–conjugated antisera. The fluorescence-activated cell scanner (FACSCAN) is a user-friendly adaptation of the fluorescence-activated cell sorter. The identification and quantification of CD4 and CD8 cells using the FACSCAN have important implications in evaluation of helper versus suppressor cell numbers. This methodology is currently being used to characterize lymphocyte populations in various diseases of the horse, cattle, dog, cat, and sheep species. The application of this technique to the demonstration of CD4 and CD8 cells in bovine lymph fluid is illustrated in Figure 3-10.

B lymphocytes

B lymphcytes are programmed to differentiate into antibody-producing mature cells and plasma cells. Unlike T cells, B lymphcytes are sessile and only a small proportion of peripheral blood lymphocytes (5% to 15%) are B-cell origin. Because of their function, the most widely accepted cellular marker is the presence of cell-surface bound immunoglobin. Resting, unstimulated B cells express IsD or IgM. The latter can be detected by fluorescence (IF) assays using anti-u chain specific or anti-light (kappa, lambda) chain-specific antisera. Since B cells also produce an Fc receptor for IgG, caution must be taken in interpretating IF results on freshly-isolated cells (which may con-

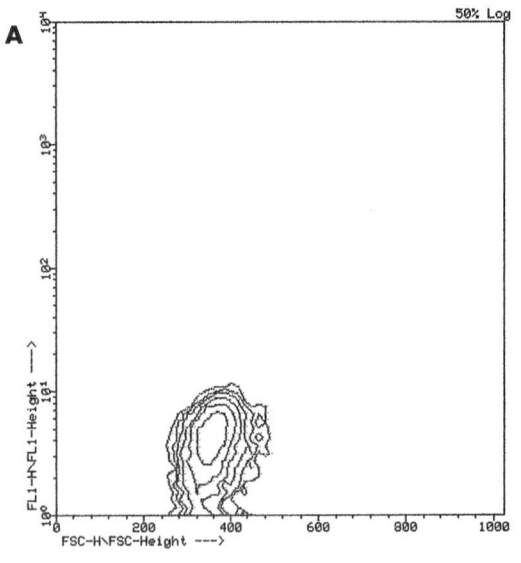

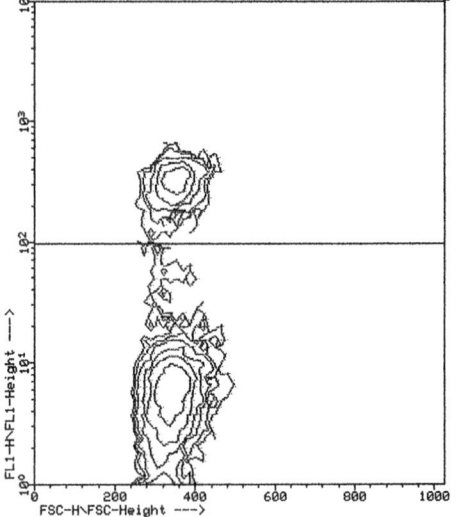

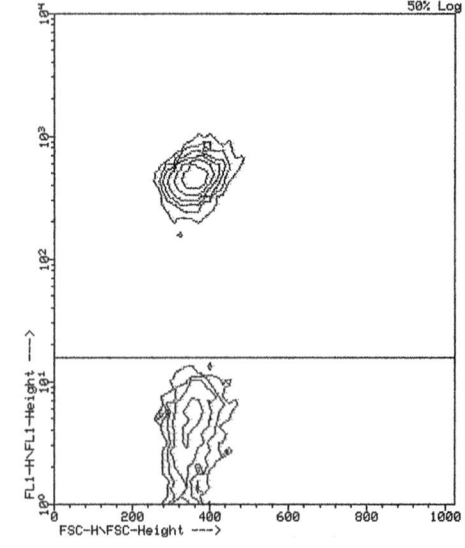

Figure 3-10 FACS analysis of bovine lymphocytes from mediastinal lymph. **A,** Unlabeled cells. **B,** Cells labeled with moab specific for CD4-FITC. **C,** Cells labeled with moab specific for CD8-FITC. Fluorescence intensity is measured on the Y axis. (FACS analysis courtesy of G. Boyle.)

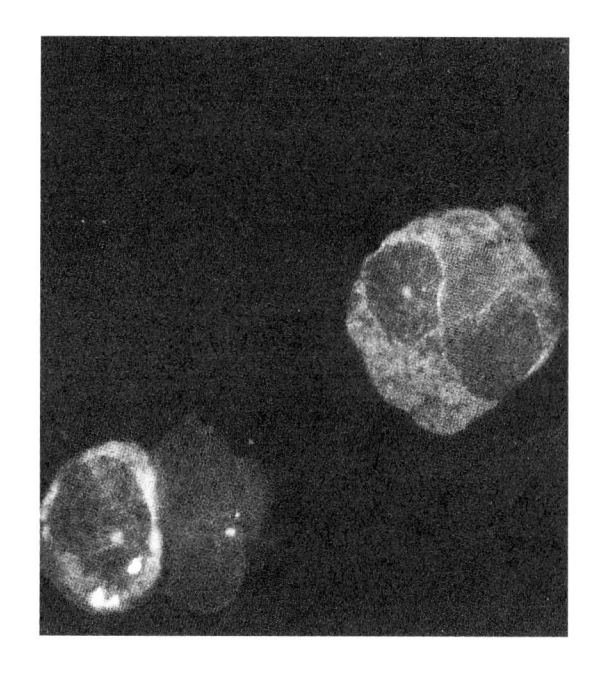

Figure 3-11 Pokeweed mitogen-induced canine B-lymphocyte differentiation in vitro. The cytospin smear is stained with polyclonal anticanine IgG conjugated to fluorescein isothiocyanate. Note the resting IgG-positive cell (*lower left*) and the dividing IgG-positive B cell (*center*).

tain passively-absorbed IgG), or if the secondary reagent contains aggregated IgG-FITC complexes.

Most B cells express Class I and Class II MHC antigens and the complement component receptors CR1 (for C3b) and CR2 (for C3d). A number of differentiation antigens have been recognized on B cells; more have been characterized in murine and human systems than in domestic animals. Mature B cells have a receptor for C3d (complement receptor) that is designated as CD21. B cells express CD40, a heterodimeric antigen that has a role in B-cell growth and the generation of immunologic memory. Certain other B cell CD antigens have been identified, but their function is still not known.

Plasma cells

Plasma cells are the end result of terminal antigen-driven B-cell differentiation. In vitro, culture of B cells with the phytomitogen, pokeweed mitogen, will result in differentiation into plasma cells (Figure 3-11). Plasma cells are short-lived (3 to 4 days) and do not migrate from their sites of production. They are rich in protein-producing rough endoplasmic reticulum (Figure 3-12) and produce and secrete prodigous amounts of immunoglobulin. In histologic sections, plasma cells have a distinct morphologic appearance. The nucleus is round and eccentrically placed, and nuclear chromatin is dense and arranged in a wheel-like fashion. The cytoplasm is darkly basophilic and may contain dense, homogeneous, cytoplasmic droplets of immunoglobulin, known as Russel bodies. In lymphoid tissues, plasma cells are abundant at the

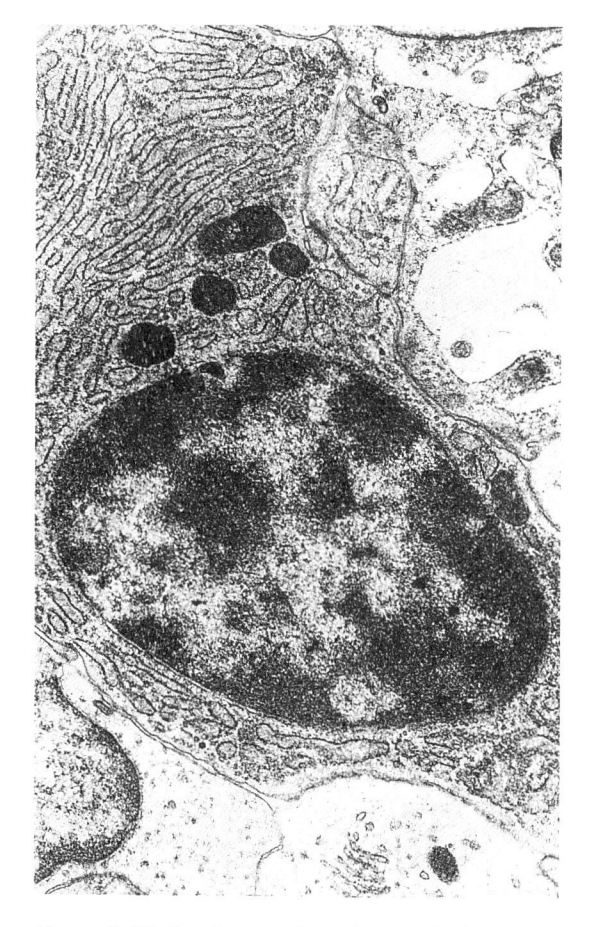

Figure 3-12 An electron photomicrograph of a feline plasma cell. Note the abundance of cytoplasmic rough endoplasmic reticulum ($\times$12,500).

margins of germinal centers and lining sinusoidal areas of the spleen and medullary cord regions of lymph nodes. Their appearance in tissues are characteristic of chronic inflammatory processes, and they occur commonly in the lamine propria of the genital and gastrointestinal tracts (Figure 3-13).

Natural killer cells

A subpopulation of cells derived from the bone marrow that appears as large granular lymphocytes are called natural killer (NK) cells. These cells lack markers characteristic of T cells (TCR, CD3, CD4, CD8) and B cells (surface lg). NK cells express the CD2 antigen. These cells are operationally defined by their ability to kill heterologous tumor cells and virus-infected cells independent of antibody and in a non–MHC-restricted fashion (Figure 3-14). NK-cell–mediated cytotoxicity is independent of requirements for the induction of immunity and so constitutes a part of the innate or natural system of bodily defenses. Body-compartmental distribution is somewhat species-dependent. For example, peripheral blood of rodents is devoid of NK cells yet rich in spleen and lymph nodes. NK cells have been identified in most domestic animal species. They express the Thy-1 cell-membrane antigen characteristic of T cells and can be activated by γ-IFN and induced to clonal proliferation by exogenous interleuken-2. They share common antigen(s) with macrophages (notably Mac-1). The majority of NK cells possess a low affinity Fc-receptor for IgG, CD16 (see Figure 3-14) yet are negative for CR1 and CR2 complement receptors. Antisera to a specific ganglioside (asialo-GM_1) appear to bind preferentially to NK cells. This reagent is commercially available and is a convenient NK-cell–specific marker.

Effector cells of anaphylaxis

Accesory cell types, uninvolved in induction of immune responses, are prime cellular effectors of immediate type hypersensitivity and anaphylaxis. Regarding immunity, the chief importance of effector cells is their tissue damage-inducing responses following interaction of antigen with cell membrane-bound IgG or IgE.

Basophils and mast cells

Mast cells (myeloid origin) and basophils (blood equivalents of mast cells) possess high-affinity cellular receptors for cytophylic IgG and reaginic (IgE) antibodies. They have a characteristic cytologic appearance in blood smears (basophils) or tissue sections (mast cells). Basophils have a multilobulated nucleus typical of myeloid series cells, whereas mast cells have a round, centrally-placed nucleus. The cytoplasm of both contain numerous

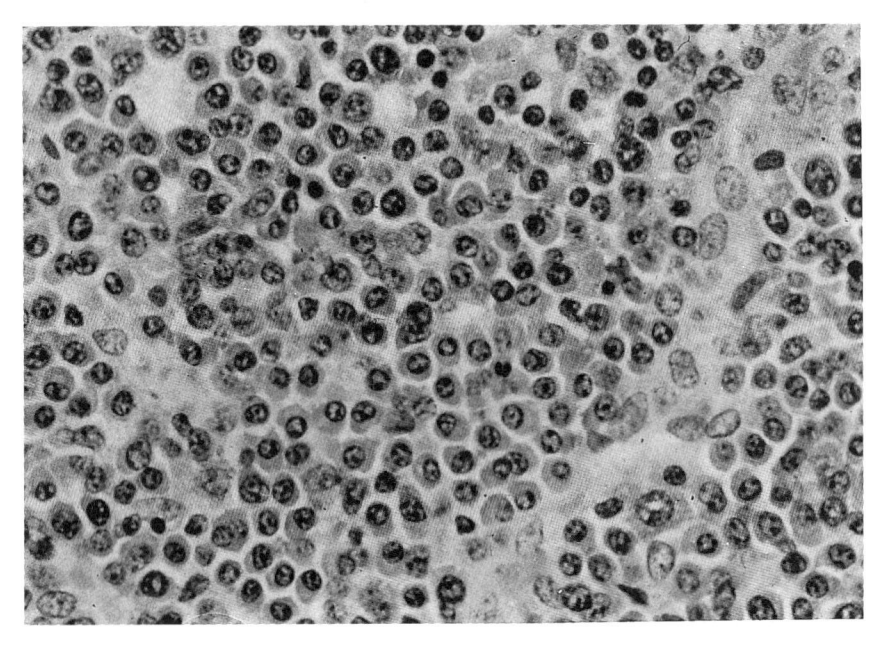

Figure 3-13 A collection of plasma cells along the margins of a chronic inflammatory focus (×168).

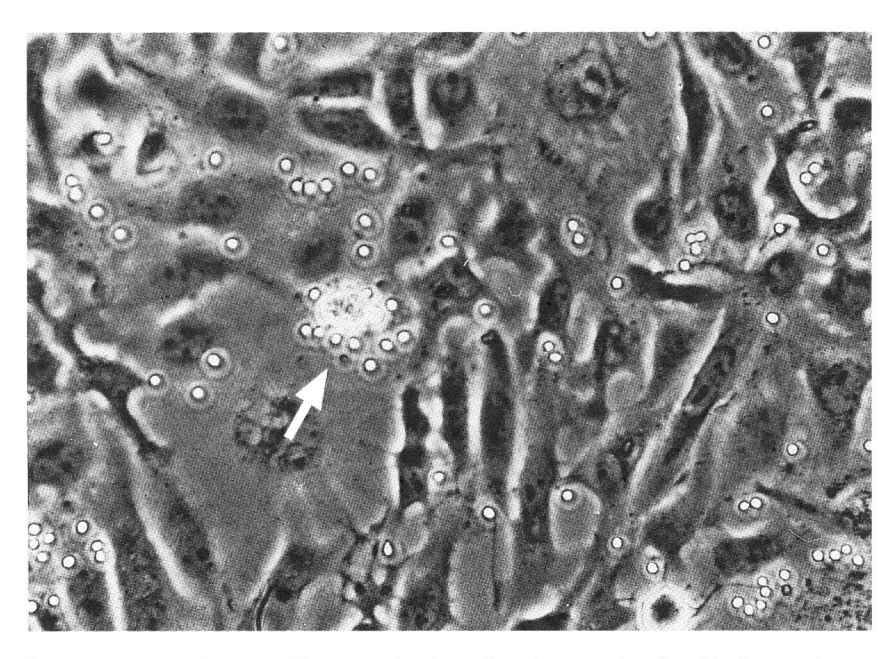

Figure 3-14 A canine NK cell (*arrow*) that has adhered to a canine thyroid adenocarcinoma target-cell monolayer forming nonimmune rosettes with IgG-coated ovine erythrocytes (EA complexes).

basophilic granules that stain metachromatically (purple) with aniline dyes such as toluidine blue.

There are two phenotypically different populations of mast cells present within the body: those present in the loose connective tissue and those present along mucosal surfaces. Mast cells in the connective tissue are a relatively stable population that are derived from bone marrow derived and that contain numerous granules with heparin and histamine as the predominant contents. The other population of mast cells lines the mucosal surface of the gastrointestinal tract. These mast cells proliferate in response to IL-3 and IL-4. It is interesting to note that IL-4 potentiates IgE production by B lymphocytes and has as another activity increasing the number of target cells for IgE binding. The granule contents of mucosal mast cells are different from that of connective tissue mast cells. Mucosal cells contain chondroitin sulfate as the major proteoglycan instead of heparin, and their histamine content is much lower. Much of the mast cell studies have been done in murine systems. Humans appear to have similar although not differentiation of mast cell populations. An overall conclusion regarding mast cell diversity is that there is variation in mediator content depending on the local environment of mast cells.

Tissues rich in mast cells include the skin, mucosa, and submucosa of the respiratory, genital, and gastrointestinal tracts (Figure 3-15). These granules are rich in preformed histamine, serotonin (rodents and horses), and the anticoagulent heparin. These pharmacologically active substances are released into the tissue milieu by a process of reversed endocytosis and are responsible for the clinical signs of anaphylaxis (e.g. smooth muscle contraction) and increased capillary permeability. The triggering stimulus is cross-linking of cell bound Ig with multivalent-specific antigen (allergen). Influx of calcium ions and activation of cyclic guanosine-mono-phosphate (GMP) induces microtubule polymerization and subsequent granule exocytosis. Leukotriene and prostaglandin production is also stimulated by activation of the lipooxygenase and cyclooxygenase pathways of arachidonic acid metabolism. Production of platelet-activating factor by mucosal mast cells increases mediator production by platelets. It is important to point out that granule exocytosis does not result in cellular death, so the potential for repeating the process (after a suitable resting period) is always present. In addition to Fc receptors for IgG and IgE, basophils and mast cells possess cell-membrane receptors for complement (CR1 and CR3) and other complement components (C3a and C5a). The CR3 molecule is also known as CD11b and is the alpha chain of the Mac-1 integrin.

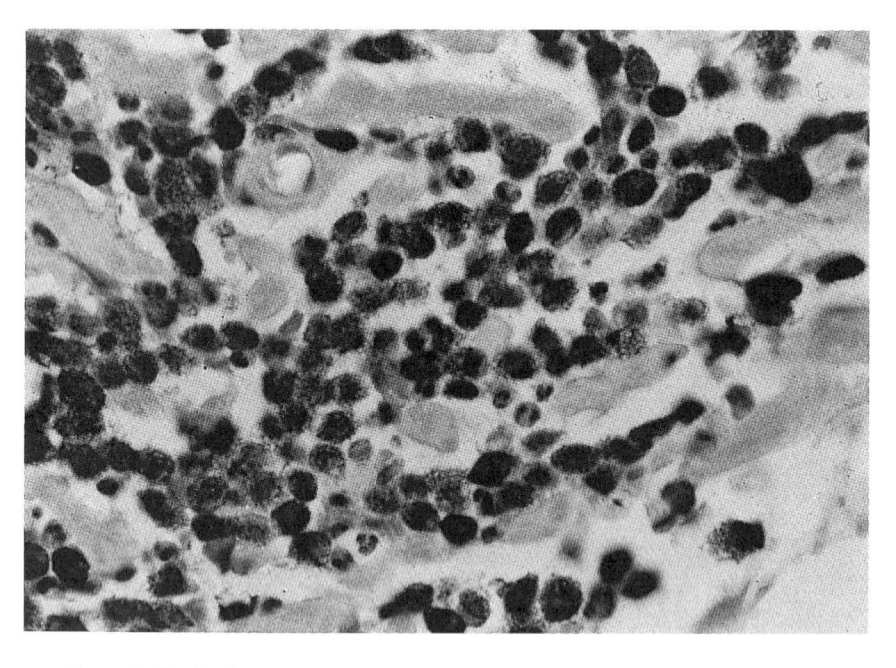

Figure 3-15 Canine cutaneous mast cell tumor. Neoplastic cells contain numerous cytoplasmic secretion granules (×168).

Eosinophils

Pathologists that have long noted that eosinophils accumulate in tissues rich in mast cells and their heightened appearance in blood (eosinophilia) or tissue is associated with certain parasitisms (Figure 3-16) and allergies. Eosinophils arise in the bone marrow and possess a lobated nucleus typical of myeloid series cells. The cytoplasm is rich in eosinophilic granules. The shape and size of these granules are species-dependent. In dogs and pigs, eosinophil granules are small and spherical. In horses, eosinophil granules are large and globular. Feline granules are cylindrical.

Eosinophils experience postmyeloid maturation on extramarrow sites such as the spleen. This event is mediated by factors under T-lymphocyte control and is crucial to full development of eosinophil function. Interleukin 5 (IL-5), produced by T lymphocytes, stimulates the growth and differentiation of eosinophils and activates mature eosinophils, enabling them to kill helminth parasites. Eosinophils are actively mobile and respond to various chemotactic stimuli, including eosinophil chemotactic factor (ECF) from T cells, mast cell degranulation products like histamine, allergen-IgE complexes, and various soluble products released from parasites. Eosinophil granules contain histaminase, arylsulfatase, peroxidases, and phospholipases, all of which antagonize the actions of mast cell materials. Two major proteins in the eosinophil granule are major basic protein and major cationic protein. These proteins are responsible for the toxic effect eosinophils can have on helminth parasites when they degranulate on the helminth cuticle (antibody-dependent cytotoxicity). In addition, eosinophils are potent sources of prostaglandins, which suppress mast cell degranulation. Like basophils, eosinophils possess cellular Fc receptors for IgG and IgE, CR1 and CR3 receptors for complement, and C3a and C5a component receptors. Thus eosinophils function to down-regulate mast cell activation and, for this teleologic reason, these cell types frequently occur together in tissues. The elaboration by mast cells of cytokines such as tumor necrosis factor (TNF) causes increased expression of endothelial leukocyte adhesion molecule-1 (ELAM-1) on endothelial cells. Binding to ELAM-1 by eosinophils expressing adhesin molecules facilitates their exit from the blood-vascular system to tissue. Thus the mast cell–eosinophil interaction appears to provide for its own regulation. Table 3-1 summarizes the important cell markers found on cells of the immune system.

LYMPHOCYTE CIRCULATION

It was demonstrated over three decades ago that lymphocytes circulate between the blood and the lymph. The initial observations were broadened to include a variety of species, including the mouse,

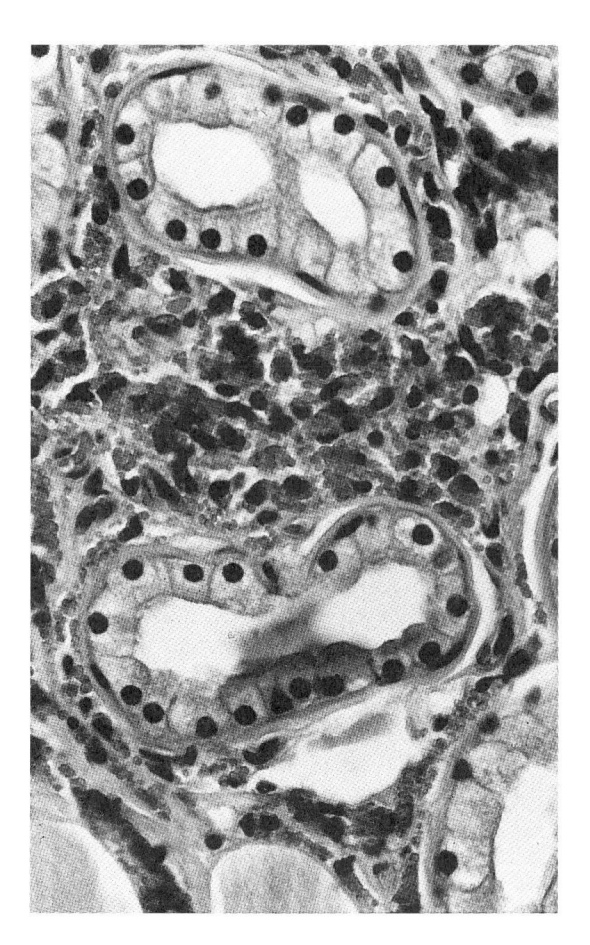

Figure 3-16 A collection of eosinophils in the skin and adenexal tissues of a horse with cutaneous habronemiasis.

human, and sheep species. In mammals the blood leaves the left ventricle of the heart and goes into the systemic circulation, where the newly-oxygenated blood delivers oxygen to the tissues. The blood then returns to the right ventricle and enters pulmonary circulation. Oxygenation occurs within the alveolar capillary system and the blood exits the pulmonary system through the pulmonary vein into the left ventricle, from where it is pumped again to the body. T and B lymphocytes enter the lymph node through postcapillary venules in the cortex of the node. The T cells circulate through the T-cell area and the B cells circulate through the B-cell area in the outer cortex. Lymphocytes that exit the node through the efferent lymphatic pathway eventually return to the blood-vascular system through the thoracic duct, which empties into the anterior vena cava and then into the right atrium.

Cell adhesion molecules, called integrins and selectins, allow lymphocytes to exit through the post capillary venule into the lymph node. Lymphocytes bind to high-endothelial cell venules by these homing receptors, or integrins. On the high-endothelial cells are ligands for the adhesin molecules on the lymphocytes. One such adhesin molecule found on lymphocytes that home to peripheral nodes is L-selectin. Another adhesin molecule found on cells that home to Peyer's patches is called VLA-4 (very late antigen). It is a member of the integrin family of adhesin molecules and is also expressed on other leukocytes. A third lymphocyte adhesin molecule is LFA-1 (lymphocyte function-associated antigen). It is also an integrin and does not cause tissue specificity for homing of the lymphocyte. LFA-1 is composed of two polypeptide chains, CD11a and CD18. It's ligand on the endothelial cell is a molecule called ICAM-1 (intracellular adhesin molecule-1). Genetic abnormalities associated with CD18 have been identified in humans, cattle, and dogs. Immunodeficiency syndromes caused by this deficiency are described in Chapter 12.

SUGGESTED READINGS

Adkins B, Mueller C, Okada CY and others: Early events in T-cell maturation, *Ann Rev Immun* 5:325-365, 1987.

Bhan AK, Bhan I: In situ characterization of human lymphoid cells using monoclonal antibodies. In Miyasaka M, Trinka Z: *Differention antigens in lymphohemopoietic tissues*, New York, 1988, M. Dekker.

Brand A, Gilmour DG, Goldstein G: Lymphocyte-differentiating hormone of bursa of Fabricius, *Science*, 193:319-321, 1976.

Blackman, M, Kappler J, Marrack P: The role of the T cell receptor in positive and negative selection of developing T cells, *Science* 248:1335-1341, 1990.

Copenhaver WM: *Bailey's textbook of histology*, Baltimore, 1964, Williams & Wilkins.

Dellman HD: *Veterinary histology: an Outline Atlas*, Philadelphia, 1971, Lea & Febiger.

Harlan JM, Liu DY: *Adhesion, its role in inflammatory disease*, New York, 1992, W.H. Freeman.

Nieuwenhuis P, Ford WL: Comparative migration of B and T-lymphocytes in the rat spleen and lymph nodes, *Cell Immunol*, 23:254-267, 1976.

Plaut MJ, Pierce H, Watson CJ, and others: Mast cell lines produce lymphokines in response to cross-linkage of FcE-R1 or to calcium ionophores, *Nature* 339:64-67, 1989.

Stamper HB, Woodruff JJ: Lymphocyte homing into lymph nodes: in vitro demonstration of the selective affinity of recirculating lymphocytes for high endothelial venules, *J Exp Med* 144:828-833, 1976.

Stevens RJL, Austin KF: Recent advances in the cellular and molecular biology of mast cells, *Immunol Today* 10:381-386, 1989.

Stites DP, Caldwell J, Carr MC and others: Ontogeny of immunity in humans, *Clin Immunol Immunopathol* 4:519-527, 1975.

van Ewijk W: T cell differentiation is influenced by thymic microenvironments, *Ann Rev Immunol* 9:591-615, 1991.

Weller PF: The immunobiology of eosinophils, *N Eng J Med* 324:1110-1118, 1991.

4 Immunoglobulins

Products of Activated B Lymphocytes

In 1890 Emil von Behring and Shibasaburo Kitasato discovered an effector substance in the blood of immune animals. They demonstrated that blood from an animal that survived tetanus, when injected into a nonimmune host, protected the recipient animal from tetanus. These substances in blood were called antibodies or immunoglobulins (Ig). Antibody is defined by its ability to specifically bind to the antigen that induced its formation. This family of serum glycoproteins (immunoglobulins) are unusual in that they possess antigenic specificity of individual antibody molecules yet, as a group, share common structural and functional features.

CELLULAR ORIGIN OF ANTIBODY

The source of antibodies is plasma cells, which are the differentiated progeny of B cells (Figure 4-1). These cells are found most often in the white pulp of the spleen, the medulla of peripheral node, the secondary lymphatic tissues, and in the submucosa or lamina propria of the respiratory, gastrointestinal, and genitourinary tracts (see Chapter 3). Plasma cells are characterized by abundant, cytoplasmic, rough, endoplasmic reticulum indicative of active protein synthesis, strongly basophilic cytoplasm, and marginated nuclear chromatin.

STRUCTURAL FEATURES OF IMMUNOGLOBULIN

The heterogeneous nature of Ig molecules was recognized by the differences in electrophoretic mobility and sedimentation coefficients obtained by ultracentrifugation. Although the majority of antibody activity takes place within the gamma globulin fraction of serum, there is also antibody activity in the beta fraction. Sizes range from a 900,000 dalton (D) (19S) molecule to a 150,000 D (7S) molecule; clearly immunoglobulins are a heterogeneous group of molecules. A fundamental structure of an Ig molecule is a 4-polypeptide chain glycoprotein held together by both intra and interchain disulfide bonds (Figure 4-2). The molecule contains two identical heavy chains (50,000 to 55,000 D) and two light chains (20,000 to 25,000 D). The intact molecule has functions associated with each end. One portion (the N-terminal end) is concerned with binding to antigen (variable region) and the other (constant region) interacts with host cells and complement components (the carboxy terminal end). The composition of the heavy chains ultimately determines the class or subclass of the antibody protein in question. Differences in amino acid sequence (and hence differences in antigenicity and/or electrophoretic mobility) have been used to delineate these classes of immunoglobulin. IgG (γ heavy chain) is the most abundant immunoglobulin and is the model for Ig structure. IgM (μ heavy chain) exists as a large pentamer and is composed of five IgG-like subunits. IgA (α heavy chain) occurs as a monomer like IgG, but also as an 11S dimer. IgD (δ heavy chain) is a cell membrane-bound monomer, and IgE (ϵ heavy chain) is a cytophilic species of immunoglobulin containing abundant carbohydrate moieties. Within these five classes of immunoglobulin subclasses of proteins exist. For example, total canine IgG in a serum sample contains four distinct IgG subclasses, which are identified by their relative electrophoretic mobility in agarose gels.

The light chain segment of the Ig molecule shows less variation than do the heavy chains. Light chains are called lambda and kappa chains. Each given Ig class may contain either lambda or kappa light chains, but never both on the same molecule (see Figure 4-2). Like their heavy chain homologues, each light chain possesses an N-terminal variable region responsible for binding the antigen and a constant portion concerned with host tissue interactions.

Genetic and immunologic analysis of immunoglobulins has revealed that there are three basic variations in Ig structure. *Isotypic variation* refers to gene products (e.g., constant regions of both heavy and light chains) that all individuals in the population possess. Isotypes of immunoglobulin are another way of referring to class and subclass

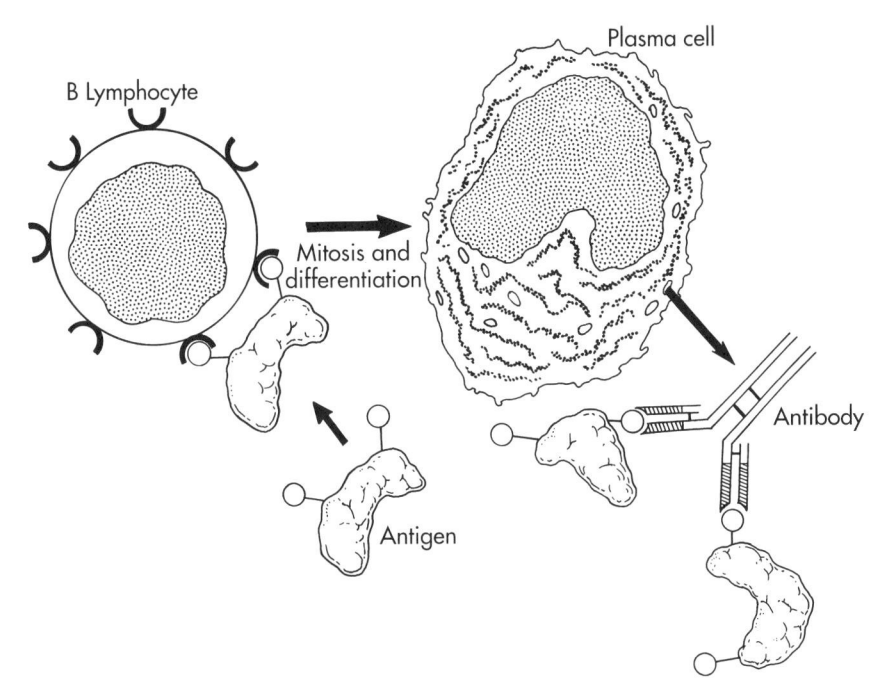

Figure 4-1 Antibodies are synthesized and secreted by plasma cells. Mature plasma cells are short-lived and release more than several thousand identical antibodies per second. Each antibody is capable of reacting specifically with the antigen that initiated the immune response.

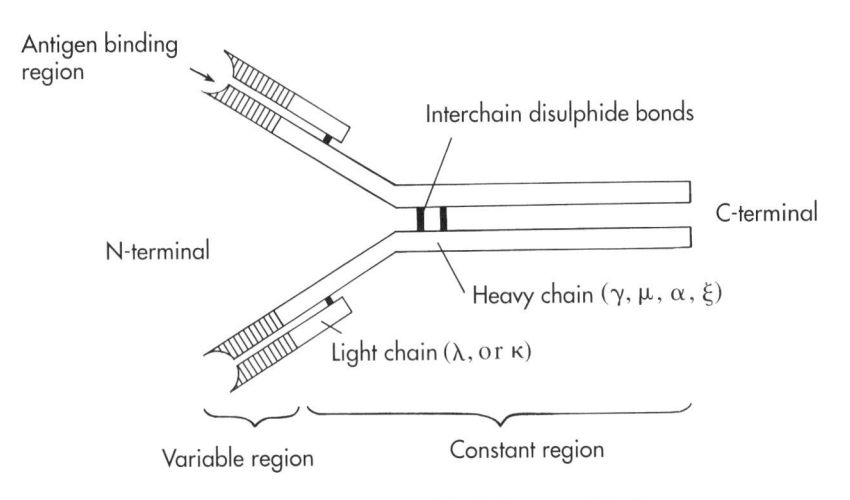

Figure 4-2 A schematic diagram of basic immunoglobulin structure.

distinctions noted earlier. In contrast, *allotypic* variants refer to gene products that are produced by different alleles at one gene locus, often a heavy chain determinant. Thus an individual within a population may express one, but not all, of the allotypes for that gene known to exist in the population. Therefore an allotype is a genetic variation on the otherwise constant region of an antibody molecule. *Idiotypic* variation is attributed to antigen specificity and is therefore located in the antigen-binding (variable) portion of the molecule, the hypervariable region. Idiotypes are identical for all Ig molecules that are produced by a clone of antigen-activated B cells. Except in the case of a specific genetic inability to produce antibody to that certain antigen, all individuals in the population have the capacity to produce identical idiotype responses.

Delineation of the structural-functional relationships of antibody molecules was first achieved by analyzing the results of limited proteolytic digestion of IgG by two enzymes, papain and pepsin. The results are summarized in Figure 4-3. Pepsin cleavage yields two fragments of immunoglobulin. The larger fragment (designated F[ab']$_2$) consists of a sulfide-bonded bifunctional molecule possessing antigen-binding capacity but devoid of the ability to interact with host tissues. The smaller crystallizable fragment (designated Fc) possesses no antibody activity yet can interact with host tissues. In contrast, papain digests yielded monomeric dipeptide with primary antigen-binding ability (the Fab) and a large crystallizable fragment (Fc). These data identified a hinge region that connects heavy chains to each other by disulfide bonds. Pepsin cleaved the Ig molecule distal (from the V region) to the hinge, whereas papain cleaved the molecule proximal to the hinge. The antibody products (F[ab']$_2$) and Fab are very useful immunologic reagents because they are small and possess antigenic specificity, yet they cannot interact with host cells or tissues.

The hinge region allows the immunoglobulin to unfold and subsequently permits the two antigen-binding sites to extend in opposite directions, facilitating the binding to antigen. The amino acid sequence of the hinge has a high proline content that permits the rotation of the Fab portion of the immunoglobulin.

As mentioned previously, the Ig polypeptide chains are joined together by disulfide bonds. For light chains, two intrachain disulfide bonds are found on the peptide—one bond near the variable region and one in the constant region. These intrachain bonds create loops in the proteins referred to as *domains*. Sequence analysis has revealed that these domains are homologous to each other. Like light chains, the heavy chains contain intrachain disulfide bonds that divide the protein into four domains. The variable region contains one domain (V_H) and the constant region contains three domains (CH_1, CH_2 and CH_3). Like their

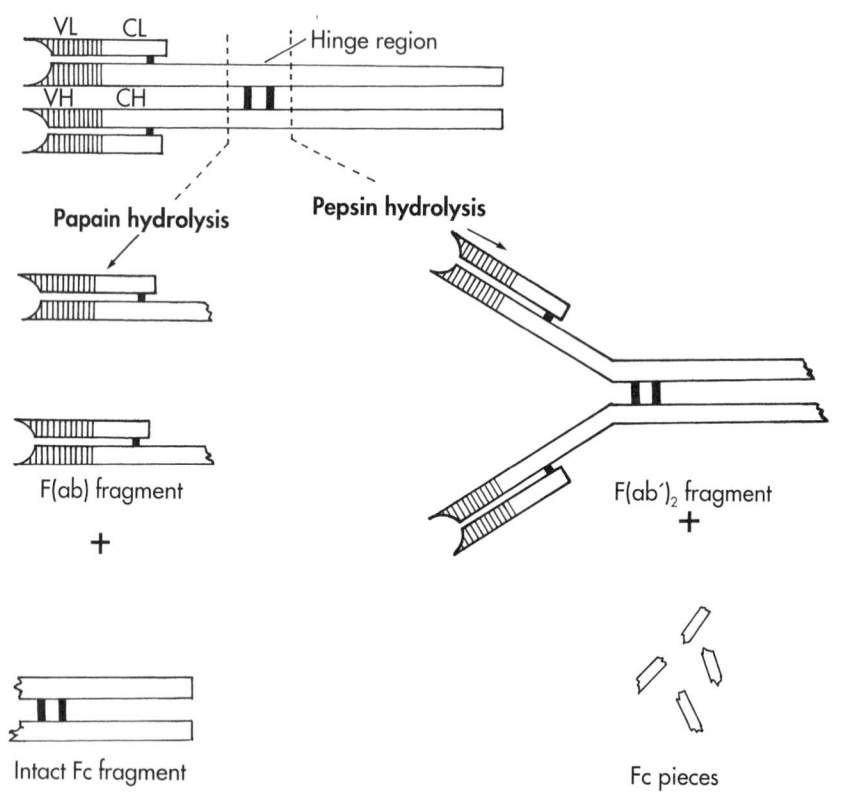

Figure 4-3 The basic IgG unit consists of two heavy chains and two light chains linked together by disulfide bonds. Enzymatic hydrolysis by papain produces monovalent antibody fragments (Fab) plus a crystallizable fragment (Fc) by cleavage proximal to the hinge region. Enzymatic hydrolysis by pepsin produces a bivalent antibody fragment, the F(ab)$_2$, and small fragments of the Fc region by cleavage distal to the hinge region.

light chain counterparts, domains are homologous to each other. These relationships are delineated in Figure 4-4.

Biologic activities have been associated with each of these domains. The first domain of the intact molecule contains variable-heavy (VH) and variable-light (VL) loops, which make up the antigen-binding site. The current theory regarding antigen-binding sites is that there are three hypervariable regions of amino acid substitution on each of the VH and VL areas. Moreover, these hypervariable areas are proximal to one another and make up the site of specific antigen binding. The binding site is approximately $(35) \times (10$ to $15) \times (6$ to $10)$ angstroms (Å) in size.

The CH_1 domain has been shown to bind the C4b fragment of complement and is responsible for antibody-associated activation of the alternate pathway. The CH_2 domain possesses the receptor for C1q and hence activates the classical complement pathway. The CH_3 domain binds to monocytes possessing an Fc receptor and hence is the Fc receptor portion of the molecule. The Fc receptor on neutrophils, platelets, and effectors cells, or antibody-directed cellular cytotoxicity (ADCC), binds to regions in both the CH_2 and CH_3 domains.

CHARACTERISTICS OF THE MAJOR IMMUNOGLOBULIN CLASSES

General features of the five Ig classes are well delineated (Figure 4-5). Table 4-1 delineates the important features of each Ig class. Table 4-2 summarizes general biologic properties of Ig classes; these properties apply to domestic animal species and humans. Differences in subclasses are described for dogs, horses, cattle, and other species. IgG subclasses often vary in their biologic functions, such that IgG1 in one species may not behave exactly as IgG1 in another species.

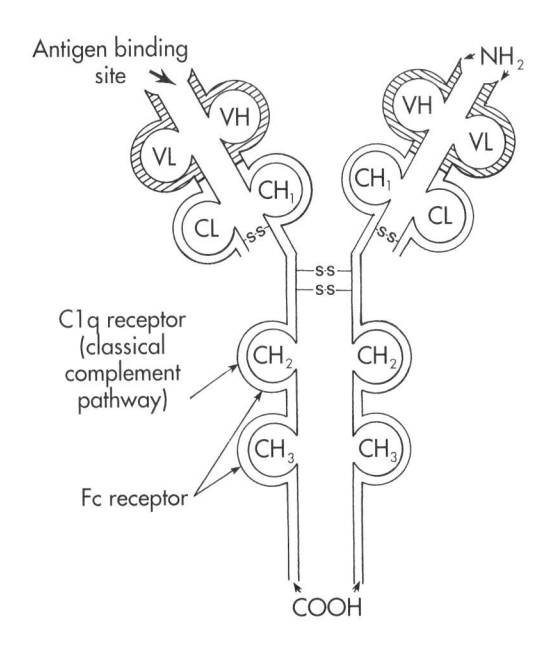

Figure 4-4 Immunoglobulin structure is arranged in domains. Each domain is an interchain loop held by disulfide bonds. Within the first domain is the antigen-binding site. The remaining domains possess close homologous amino acid sequences and are responsible for interaction of the molecule with complement and cells bearing Fc receptors.

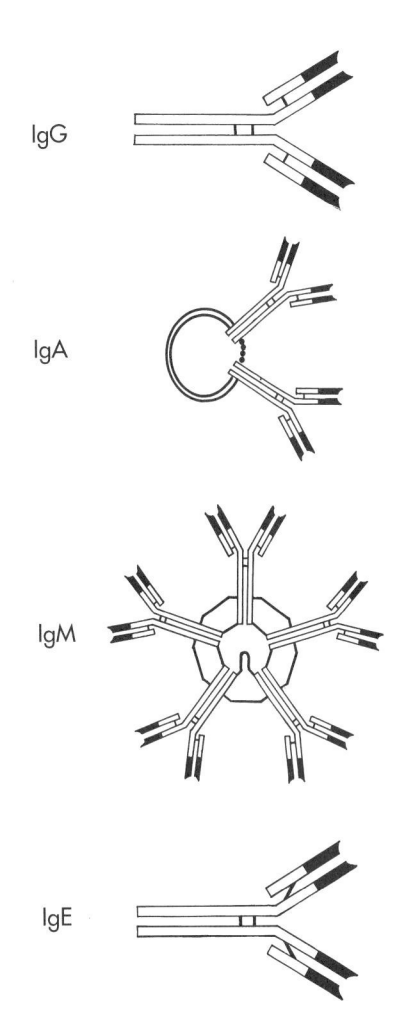

Figure 4-5 General structural features of four of the five main classes of immunoglobulin. IgG is a bivalent 7S monomer; IgA has four binding sites; IgM is a pentamer with 10 binding sites; IgE is a monomer with two binding sites. Secretory piece is found on IgG and monomeric IgM. The J chain is formed on IgA and IgM. The fifth class of IgD resembles IgG in configuration.

Table 4-1 General physicochemical properties of immunoglobulins

Property	IgG	IgM	IgA	IgE
Sedimentation coefficient(s)	7S	18S	7-11S	7-8S
Biologic form	Monomer	Pentomer	Monomer/dimer	Monomer
Molecular wt (daltons × 10³)	150-170	900	160-380	180
No. light chains	2	10	2-4	2
No. heavy chains	2	10	2-4	2
Carbohydrate content	Low (< 3%)	High (10%)	High (10%)	High (10%)
Valency	2	5	2-4	2
J-chain	No	Yes	Yes/no	No
Secretory component	No	Yes/no	Yes	No

Table 4-2 Biologic properties of various immunoglobulins

Property	IgG	IgM	IgA	IgE
Precipitation	+++	+	−	−
Complement activation classical	+++	+++	−	−
Alternate	++	−	+	+
Fc binding	+++	±	±	+

IgG

IgG is the most abundant Ig class in serum. It possesses two gamma heavy chains and two kappa or lambda light chains, has a molecular weight of approximately 150,000 D, and contains two antigen-binding sites. Various IgG subclasses exist, and their relative abundance and specific biologic properties also vary among the species (Table 4-3). For example, in humans, four subclasses have been described. Subclass variability is defined by antigenicity and is reflected chiefly in the number and distribution of intrachain and interchain disulfide bonds. IgG passes freely through most capillary beds (excluding the tight junctions of the brain) and consequently is found in abundance in interstitial tissues and all excretions and secretions. For most species IgG is the major protective immunoglobulin of the neonate, through either active placental transport in utero ("human") or with colostrum and milk. As a class, this Ig species is the one most effective in complement fixation, toxin and virus neutralization, particulate (e.g., bacterial) agglutination, and precipitation reactions. Certain subclasses are strongly cytophilic and bind to cells that possess Fc receptors in vivo.

IgM

IgM is the largest of the Ig classes and exists normally in serum as a pentamer with five functional bivalent units and a total of 10 antigen-binding regions. It is a circular protein comprised of 10 heavy chains and 10 light chains, with an approximate molecular weight of 950,000 D. In addition, a small polypeptide (J chain) is present in the interior of the molecule. Because of its relative size, it is largely restricted to the intravascular fluid compartments. IgM is often referred to as the "ancestral antibody" because it is the first antibody to appear in phylogeny and ontogeny, and the first antibody in a primary immune response to antigen. In most antibody-antigen reactions, IgM is the most efficient agglutinating and complement-fixing globulin. However, IgM plays a minor role in toxin neutralization and plays no role in immediate hypersensitivity reactions. A functional feature of IgM is its sensitivity to 2-mercaptoethanol reduction; 2-mercaptoethanol does not destroy the antigen-binding capability of IgM, but it destroys its capability to function as an agglutinin or a complement-fixing antibody. This sensitivity to 2-mercaptoethanol has been used historically as a means to distinguish between acute and chronic infections. For example, because IgM is the first immunoglobulin to appear during the immune response, destruction of serum-agglutinating capability by 2-mercaptoethanol indicates a current infection. If the animal has antibody activity not of IgM type (e.g., 2-mercaptoethanol–

Table 4-3 Immunoglobulin subclasses and nomenclature in domestic animal species

	Number of Ig subclasses			
Species	IgG	IgM	IgA	IgG(T)
Canine	4(1,2a,2b,2c)			
Equine	3(a,b,c)	2		2(a,b)
Bovine	2(1,2)			
Ovine	4(1,1a,2,3)		2(1,2)	
Porcine	4(1,2,3,4)		2(1,2)	
Human	4(1,2,3,4)		2(1,2)	
Avian				
Feline	2(1,2)			

resistant agglutinating activity), this is interpreted to mean that the animal had a previous exposure but is not currently infected. This property of IgM has been used for the identification of cattle that are actively infected with *Brucella abortus*. An indirect immunofluorescence test is performed in the clinical immunology laboratory that uses canine serum dilutions incubated with slides upon which are fixed canine distemper virus-infected cells. The test is performed in duplicate with a secondary antibody conjugated with fluorescein. By using an anticanine conjugate on one test and an anticanine gamma conjugate on a duplicate test, the relative amounts of virus-specific IgM and IgG can be determined. This assay is useful for differentiation of acute infection versus previous infection or previous vaccination titers.

IgA

IgA, or secretory immunoglobulin, is the third major Ig class involved in the immune response. It exists in both dimeric and monomeric forms. The former is largely found in secretions and excretions, whereas the latter is characteristic for serum. Like IgM, IgA possesses an additional fragment called the J chain, which, if secreted, is closely associated with secretory component. The dimeric form contains four antigen-binding sites and consequently contains four alpha heavy chains and four light chains. The monomer is similar in structure to IgG. In spite of basic biochemical similarities recent evidence suggests that serum and secretory IgA are produced by separate cellular compartments. Secretory IgA is produced by resident plasma cells/B cells in the lamina propria of the gut, respiratory, genitourinary, and mammary tracts. Because dimeric IgA is found on mucous membranes and in nearly all secretions (e.g., tears, saliva, trachea secretions), it plays a very important role in defense against invading pathogens. Thus secretory IgA is a major component of immune defense systems. In contrast, the precise junction of serum IgA is not delineated. It is deficient in complement activation (except by the alternate pathway) and is a poor opsonin, chiefly as a result of the paucity of Fc receptors for IgA on effector cells. In terms of classical serology, serum IgA does not agglutinate particulates or precipitate with soluble antigen. It is possible that serum IgA may facilitate the clearance of IgA-antigen immune complexes from serum through the hepatobiliary route, a pathway documented thus far only in rodents.

An important attribute of secretory IgA is its close association with secretory component. The secretory component is synthesized by glandular epithelium, whereas the Ig molecule itself is synthesized in adjacent lymphoid cells. Secretory component binds to dimeric IgA on the basal surface of the epithelial cell and functions by transporting the IgA through the cell, releasing it on the lumen side. A peptide is cleaved and remains with the IgA. This secretory piece is responsible for the resistance of IgA to digestive enzymes. Therefore IgA is one of the major antibodies in colostrum. The transport piece permits IgA to survive movement through the gut and allows for absorption into the newborn circulation. Selective inherited IgA deficiency is the most common genetic defect in human immunology; its estimated frequency is as high as 1 in 1000 individuals. While many IgA-deficient individuals are clinically asymptomatic, a portion of them suffer recurrent episodes of respiratory, gastrointestinal, and cutaneous infectious diseases. It is thought that secretory IgM and secreted IgG compensate for IgA deficiency at mucosal surfaces. Excluding combined immunodeficiency disease (CID) in Arabian foals, selective IgA deficiency has been recognized only in dogs. In German shepherds, a relative IgA deficiency occurs that is often clinically silent. In contrast, selective IgA deficiency in beagles and Shar Peis is associated with recurrent dermatitis and gastrointestinal disease.

IgD

IgD is presumed to be present in domestic animals and likely functions in a fashion analogous to that described for humans. In humans, IgD is found only in trace amounts in serum and has a structure similar to IgG. IgD is the cell-bound monomeric antigen-recognition unit of uncommitted B cells. During the inductive phase of the immune response, antigen-reactive IgD receptors are rapidly replaced by IgM and then IgG molecules.

IgE

IgE, or reaginic antibody, is also found in trace amounts in normal serum. Elevated levels are found in persons with allergic or atopic diseases and in heavily parasitized animals. It has a four-polypeptide chain structure analogous to IgG but is distinguished from the other Ig classes by a high proportion of carbohydrate residues on the molecule.

IgE does not agglutinate or precipitate antigen. It does not fix complement by the classical pathway or neutralize toxin. The cytophilic nature of IgE is dependent on its ability to bind to the Fc epsilon type-1 receptors on mast cells and basophils. This high-affinity receptor binding is responsible for allergic sensitization, which sets up an indivdiual for an anaphylactic type of reactivity (see Chapter 10).

Another type of receptor for IgE is the low-affinity receptor present on B lymphocytes, eosinophils, and macrophages. Also known as CD23, this receptor allows IgE to bind to eosinophils, thus facilitating cell-mediated cytotoxicity against parasite larvae (e.g., schistosomula). Presumably CD23 has a role in IgE regulation by binding to B cells that are expressing the low-affinity receptor.

Because of the very small amounts of circulating IgE and its lack of participation in complement fixation or prepititin-type reactions, quantitation of IgE has historically been done by an in vivo test called the *passive cutaneous anaphylaxis test*. In this test, serum from an animal suspected of being allergic (i.e., having IgE antibodies) to a particular antigen is injected intradermally into the skin of a normal animal of the same species. If there is any IgE in the injected serum, it will bind to the mast cells in the skin. When the animal is injected with the antigen by the intravenous route hours later, the IgE triggers the mast cells to degranulate, releasing their mediators and causing a wheal to appear at the injection site. More recently, in vitro tests have been developed to measure IgE. In humans, dogs, and cattle, enzyme-linked immunosorbent assays (ELISA) or radioimmunoassays (RIA) are finally available to measure IgE in serum. The availability of highly-specific antiserum to epsilon chains in the various species is a necessary prerequisite to the development of such tests. Several clinical studies have demonstrated a lack of specificity in ELISA type IgE assays as compared to intradermal testing. Two points should be considered when evaluating the usefulness of these in vitro correlates of allergic reactivity. An in vitro assay, such as ELISA or radioallergosorbent test (RAST), is only as specific as the anti-IgE reagent that is used in the assay, secondly, assays performed on a serum sample test for circulating IgE, whereas intradermal tests test for mast cell bound IgE.

IMMUNOGLOBULINS IN DOMESTIC ANIMALS

A considerable body of literature exists regarding the properties and levels of Ig classes in domestic animals. Specific antisera to many of these immunoglobulins exist and are commercially available. Table 4-4 and 4-5 summarize Ig levels in serum and colostrum/milk in domestic animals. However, a number of idiosyncracies exist, and these species-dependent phenomena frequently complicate knowledge about structure and function across species lines. For example, the major protective species of immunoglobulin in bovine colostrum is IgG1, not IgA. In contrast, piglets absorb all orally-administered immunoglobulin before intestinal closure, and serum Ig profiles of post-suckle piglets closely resemble that of the colostrum. The horse possesses a unique IgG species referred to as IgG(T). This immunoglobulin is a poor precipitin and activator of complement. In classic serology, IgG(T) antibody is referred to as a floccular protein. Horses that are hyperimmunized with various antigens, notably pneumococcus and diphtheria toxins, eventually produce specific antibodies largely of the IgG(T) class. IgG(T) is important in that it appears in serum during certain stages of equine infectious anemia (EIA) virus infection. Because IgG(T) does not activate complement, viral infection cannot be detected by complement fixation. EIA is detected by a precipitation test called Coggin's test.

ANTIGEN-ANTIBODY INTERACTIONS

The binding of an antibody to an antigenic determinant for which it is specific involves several noncovalent interactions. Such forces as hydrophobic interactions and Van der Waal's forces stabilize the bonding. There are several terms used to describe the strength with which antigen binds to antibody. *Affinity* refers to the strength of the attraction between the hypervariable region of the antibody molecule and the antigenic determinant.

Table 4-4 Serum immunoglobulin levels (mg/dl

Species	IgG	IgM	IgA	IgG(T)	IgE
Canine	1800	250	80	*	0.8-4.2
Equine	1200	150	200	800	trace**
Bovine	2200	300	30	*	trace
Ovine	1800	200	30	*	trace
Porcine	2300	300	250	*	trace
Human	1000	90	180	*	0.03
Avian	500	125	60	*	

*, Not present; **, detected in these species by passive cutaneous anaphylaxis (PCA) test.

Table 4-5 Immunoglobulin levels in colostrum and milk

	Colostrum			Milk		
Species	IgG	IgM	IgA	IgG	IgM	IgA
Canine	210	40	1100	2	25	400
Equine*	3000	200	1000	30	8	70
Bovine	6000	800	400	200	10	10
Ovine	4500	800	400	80	5	10
Porcine	5000	300	1000	200	50	500

*Equine IgG(T) level in colostrum is approximately 1500 mg/dl and 10 mg/dl in milk.

Avidity refers to the overall strength of the binding between antigen and antibody, taking into account the number of binding sites being used. Generally as an antibody response matures, antibody made later in the response is of higher affinity than that made earlier. IgM has a high avidity because of the potentially high number of determinants that can be bound by one antibody molecule.

THE MOLECULAR BASIS OF ANTIBODY DIVERSITY

As the knowledge about common structure and function of various immunoglobulin was accumulated, the dilemma it posed soon became apparent. How can a family of molecules resemble each other so closely yet contain exquisite specificity for a large number (at least 10^9) of antigens encountered during life? In the early part of this century, long before knowledge of protein structure and function existed, Paul Erlich proposed a theory to explain the occurrence of antibodies by a process of antigen-induced selection. Other researchers proposed instructive hypotheses.

Finally, in 1957, Sir McFarland Burnet proposed the clonal selection hypothesis. This theory states that every person has clonally-derived lymphocytes that come from a single precursor cell. These lymphocytes have Ig-like molecules as receptors and use their variable regions to recognize antigen. Antigen then selects the preexisting clone that recognizes it, and the clone is triggered to begin expansion. Therefore the DNA of each cell must contain all of the information to respond to all possible antigens. How, then, does one cell become specific for a single antigenic determinant?

To account for the occurrence of both variable and constant regions on the same molecule, Dreyer and Bennett suggested in 1965 that genes coding for these regions exist as distinct entities on chromosomes and that the hybrid Ig protein produced was accomplished by a combination mechanism. That is, two genes were responsible for coding the Ig molecule, one for the variable region and one for the constant region. Development of in vitro tumor cell lines that secreted only one type of immunoglobulin (myelomas), along with recombinant DNA technology, provided the framework for understanding the problem of antibody diversity. It was determined that the DNA coding for Ig molecules in those myeloma cells committed to making antibodies was different than the DNA from that of nonlymphoid tissues. This discovery confirmed that somatic DNA recombination occurs during B-cell differentiation into antibody-forming cells. It is now known that a number of separate genes exist that code for an unknown number of V-region domains. In addition, it has been determined that these V-region genes experience somatic mutation during the process of B-cell differentiation. These slight changes in the variable region can give rise to increased affinity of the antibody for the antigenic determinant to which it binds.

THE IMMUNOGLOBULIN SUPERFAMILY

The Ig superfamily includes a variety of cell surface proteins that share some structural homology with the heavy and light immunoglobulin chains. Members of this family are thought to have been derived from a common primordial gene. The domain structure, which utilizes disulfide bonding to form separate intrachain domains, is a common feature in members of the Ig superfamily. Some of these features include: T cell alpha/beta and gamma/delta receptors, major histocompatibility complement (MHC) Class I and Class II proteins, T-cell accessory proteins (such as CD2, CD4, CD8), and certain adhesin molecules (ICAM). The presence of these domains and the beta-pleated sheet structure characteristic of Ig molecules is thought to be important for cell-cell or receptor-receptor interaction. Several members of the Ig gene superfamily will be discussed in more detail in a later chapter.

MONOCLONAL ANTIBODIES

The occurrence of tumors in antibody-producing plasma cells provided a uniform source of immunoglobulin that facilitated studies to obtain much of our current information on the biochemical composition of antibody molecules. In 1975, Kohler and Milstein described the use of these myeloma cells as fusion partners for splenic lymphocytes, thereby introducing a now routine process that creates a heterokaryon called a *hybridoma*. A hybridoma is a cell that has the neoplastic growth characteristics of the myeloma partner and the antibody-producing characteristics of the lymphocyte, with which the myeloma cell was fused. By specifically immunizing mice with an antigen and using B cells from the spleen as fusion partners, a cell line is created that continuously produces a monoclonal antibody with defined specificity.

The production of monoclonal antibodies involves the following steps: the initial fusion; selection for hybrid cells; screening of supernatants of the cultured cells to identify hybridomas secreting the desired antibody specificity; cloning the cells; and mass propagation of the hybrid cells to produce large quantities of homogeneous antibody of the desired specificity. There are several important characteristics of the myeloma fusion partner that make this process work. First, the myeloma cell line used is no longer capable of secreting antibody itself. Secondly, the myeloma cells have a genetic mutation in the enzyme hypoxanthine phosphoribosyl transferase (HGPRT), which prevents them from using the salvage pathway for incorporation of nucleotides into DNA. In the presence of the chemical aminopterin, the cells cannot perform de novo synthesis of purines and pyrimidines and therefore must use the salvage pathway. Thus in the selection media hypoxanthine-aminopterin-thymidine (HAT)-myeloma cells will not grow. However, myeloma cells that have fused with B cells that still contain HGPRT are able to grow. This procedure allows selection of the myeloma-lymphocyte fusions and elimination of other cell-type fusions. Such antibodies have wide applications in diagnostics and many are used in test kits available for use by veterinary practitioners. The procedure is depicted in Figure 4-6.

The original hybridomas were produced with murine myeloma cells as the fusion partner and murine splenic B cells as the other partner. Subsequently there has been considerable interest in creating antibodies that are of human origin for potential therapeutic uses. Those interested in veterinary species have developed heterohybridomas, in which the murine myeloma cells have been fused with immune lymphocytes from another species. Although these hybrids are generally less stable, successful heterohybridomas secreting bovine and porcine immunoglobulins have been produced.

SUGGESTED READINGS

Allen PZ, Johnson JS: Studies on equine immunoglobulins. III. Antigenic interrelationships among horse and dog IgG, *Comp Biochem Physiol* 418:371-383, 1972.

Beh KJ: Immunoglobulin clan specificity of non-agglutinating antibody produced in cattle following *Brucella abortus* 45/20 vaccination, *Aust Vet J* 51:481-483, 1975.

Bourne FJ: Gamma globulins in pre-colostral piglet serum, *Res Vet Sci* 17:36-38, 1974.

Butler JE, Keddy CA, Pierce CS and others: Quantitative changes associated with calving in the levels of bovine immunoglobulins in selected body fluids, *Can J Comp Med* 36:234-242, 1972.

Dreyer WJ, Bennett JC: The molecular basis of antibody formation: a paradox, *Proc Natl Acad Sci USA* 54:864-869, 1965.

Fey H, Pfister H, Messerli J and others: Methods of isolation, purification and quantitation of bovine immunoglobulins, *Zentralbl Veterinaermed* 23:269-300, 1976.

Grant JA, Harrington, JT, Johnson, JS: Carboxy-terminal amino acid sequences of canine immunoglobulin G subclasses, *J Immunol* 108:165-168, 1972.

Halliwell REW, Schwartzman RM, Montgomery PC and others: Physiochemical properties of canine IgE, *Transpl Proc* 7:537-543, 1975.

Higgins DA: Fractionation of fowl immunoglobulins, *Res Vet Scie* 21:94-99, 1976.

Hudson L: Immunoglobulin-bearing lymphocytes of the chicken, *Eur J Immunol* 5:691-698, 1975.

Husband AJ, Lascelles AK: Antibody responses to neonatal immunization in calves, *Res Vet Sci* 18:201-207, 1975.

Ishazaka K, Ishizaka T: Immunoglobulin E, *Arch Pathol Lab Med* 100:289-292, 1976.

Johnson JS, Vaughn JH: Canine immunoglobulins. I. Evidence for six immunoglobulin classes, *J Immunol* 98:923-934, 1967.

Johnson JS, Vaughn JH, Swisher SN: Canine immunoglobu-

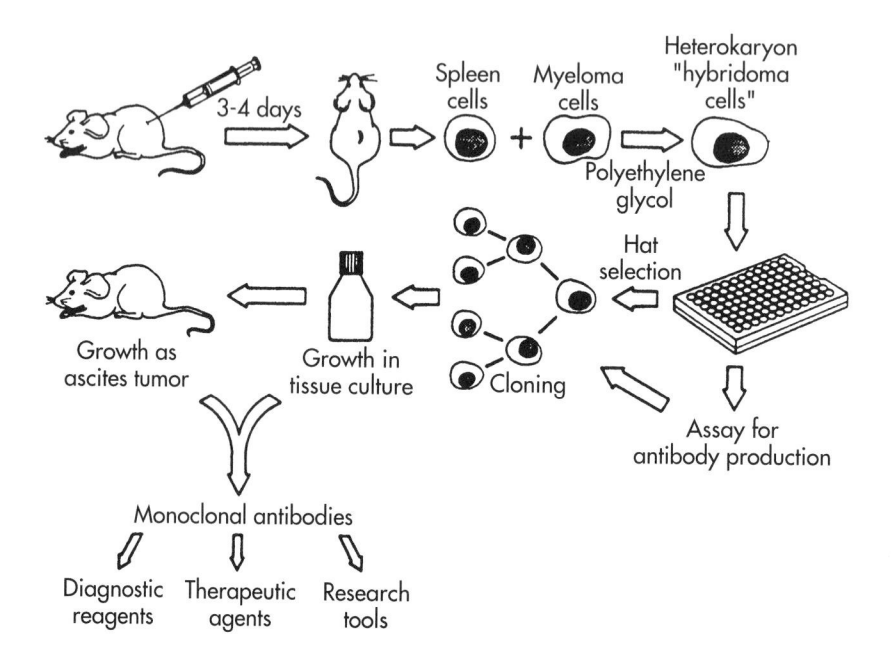

Figure 4-6 Schematic showing the production of monoclonal antibodies. From Gershwin LJ: California Veterinarian 10:31-33, 1981.

lins. II. Antibody activity in six immunoglobulin classes, *J Immunol* 98:935-940, 1967.

Kohler G, Milstein C: Continuous cultures of fused cells secreting antibody of predefined specificity, *Nature* 256:495-497, 1975.

Low TLK, Liu YV, Putnam FW: Structure, function, and evolutionary relationships of Fc domains of human immunoglobulins A, G, M, and E, *Science* 191:390-392, 1976.

Marx JL: Antibody structure, now in three dimensions, *Science* 189:1075-1076, 1975.

Micesan VV, Bordas HG: Preferential transport into colostrum of the fragment derived from serum IgG immunoglobulin in the goat, *Res Vet Sci* 21:150-154, 1976.

Nansen P: Selective immunoglobulin deficiency in cattle and susceptibility to infection, *Acta Microbiol Scand* 80:49-54, 1972.

Newby TJ, Bourne IJ: The nature of the local immune system of the bovine small intestine *Immunology* 31:475, 1976.

Nielsen K, Holmes W, Wilkie B and others: Bovine reaginic antibody, *Int Arch Allergy Appl* 51:441-450, 1976.

Poljak RJ: X-ray crystallographic studies of immunoglobulins. In Reisfeld RA, Mandy WJ editors: *Contemporary topics in molecular immunology,* New York and London, 1973, Plenum.

Rejnak J, Prokesova L: Immunoglobulins and antibodies in pigs. In Reisfeld RA, and Mandy WJ editors: *Contemporary topics in molecular immunology*, New York and London, 1973, Plenum.

Reynolds HY, Johnson JS: Quantitation of canine immunoglobulins, *J Immunol* 105:698-703, 1970.

Roitt I, Brostoff J, Male D: *Immunology* ed 3, C. St Louis, 1985, Mosby.

Schultz RD, Scott FW, Duncan JR and others: Feline immunoglobulins, *Infect Immun* 9:391-393, 1974.

Setcavage TM, Kun YB: Characterization of porcine serum immunoglobulins IgG, IgM, and IgA and the preparation of monospecific anti-chain sera, *Immunochemistry* 13:643-652, 1976.

Smith WD, Dawson AM, Wells PW and others: Immunoglobulin concentration in ovine body fluids, *Res Vet Sci* 19:189-194, 1975.

Thompson RE, Reynolds HY: Isolation and characterization of canine secretory immunoglobulin M, *J Immunol* 118:323-329, 1977.

Vaerman JP, Heremans JF: The immunoglobulins of the dog. II. The immunoglobulins of canine secretions. *Immunochemistry* 6:779-786, 1969.

Vaerman JP, Heremans JF, Kerckhoven GV: Identification and IgA in several mammalian species, *J Immunol* 103:1421-1423, 1969.

Varela-Diaz VM, Soulsby EJL: Immunoglobulin synthesis in sheep: IgG2 deficiency in neonatal lambs, *Res Vet Sci* 13:99-100, 1972.

Weir RC, Porter RR: Comparison of the structure of immunoglobulin from horse serum, *Biochem J* 100:63-68, 1962.

5 Cytokines

Soluble Factors of the Immune Response

James S. Cullor

The immune system is comprised of a complex series of cell types that are divided into two groups—those participating in antigen-specific recognition and those responsible for a broad-spectrum defensive role, thereby providing an antigen nonspecific response. This antigen-specific immune capability and the continuation of an innate resistance is finely controlled by molecular signals that are mediated through the release of *cytokines*. This general term denotes biologic mediators that participate in immune regulation. Cytokines form a network of communication signals between cells of the immune system and the immune system and other organs. When these molecules are produced by lymphocytes, they are referred to as *lymphokines*. When they are produced by monocytes or macrophages, they are referred to as *monokines*. The term *interleukin* is applied to the molecules that function as communicators between leukocytes. Thus interleukins and lymphokines are cytokines. The term cytokines includes interleukins as well as molecules that act on cells other than leukocytes. The primary groups of molecules classified as cytokines are proteins or glycoproteins of a molecular weight less than 80 kilodaltons (kD) and include: all of the interleukins (IL1 to IL12), the interferons, colony-stimulating factors, tumor necrosis factors, the transforming growth factor beta family, and other growth factors that include erythropoietin, nerve growth factor, epidermal growth factor, fibroblast growth factors, insulin-like growth factors, and platelet-derived growth factor.

BIOLOGIC PROPERTIES OF CYTOKINES

Cytokines play a role in the development and maintenance of immunity and inflammatory processes, regulate the amplitude and duration of the response, and act as potent modulators of cell behavior. Cytokines mediate their effects by binding to specific receptors on their target cells. They can be functionally classified as factors that promote proliferation and/or differentiation of various cell types, chemotactic for inflammatory cells, and cytotoxic factors that kill allogenic, neoplastic, or microbe-infected cells. Cellular activation is essential for cytokine production and release. This feature is exemplified during hematopoiesis, in which cells mature from multipotential bone marrow stem cells into progenitor cells for various blood cell types. This maturation process is characterized by the exposure of bone marrow cells, at different stages of development, to combinations of cytokines that will determine the fate of each particular cell.

There are numerous examples of cytokines acting in a multifunctional manner. Certain cytokines, including IL-1, IL-6, and granulocyte macrophage-colony stimulating factor (GM-CSF), possess a broad-target cell specificity. IL-1 and IL-6 stimulate acute phase protein production by hepatocytes. IL-1 produces diverse effects including: basophil and eosinophil activation, fibroblast proliferation and collagen production, the release of hypothalamic and pituitary peptides including ACTH, antiproliferative effects on some tumor cell lines, and an increase in the resistance of mice to gram-negative bacterial infection. In contrast, granulocyte-colony stimulating factor (G-CSF), macrophage-colony stimulating factor (M-CSF), IL-5, and erythropoietin have a more limited set of target-cell specificities. The mature cells that result from these proliferative and differentiating events include erythrocytes, granulocytes, lymphocytes, monocytes, macrophages, mast cells, and platelets.

MOLECULAR MESSENGERS

T lymphocytes, although they possess common ontogenic origins, differentiate into diverse subsets. Not only can T cells serve as the effector arm of the immune response through production of cytotoxic lymphokines, but they also can control proliferation and differentiation of B cells, T cells, and other hemopoietic cells. Lymphokines also regulate the immune system by producing soluble polypeptides that enhance or suppress various immune cell functions. These polypeptides function as either "helpers" or "suppressors" and serve to partially control the immune response. Thus the interleukins and other cytokines produced by cells of the immune system function as molecular messengers to activate and regulate immune function. Some of these functions are described below and listed in Table 5-1.

Interleukin

Interleukin 1 (IL-1), a 17-kD immunoregulatory hormone, was originally isolated from activated macrophages and is considered an important mediator of inflammation. IL-1 can be produced by virtually any cell, including monocytes, macrophages, endothelium, keratinocytes, and glial cells. This molecule promotes the differentiation of both T and B lymphocytes, activates macrophages, and stimulates the synthesis of other lymphokines (IL-2, IFN-γ). IL-1 has been reported to produce clinical signs of elevated body temperature, induce sleep, produce ACTH release, and result in other systemic acute-phase responses. Other biologic activities that are attributed to IL-1 include acting as a cofactor for other hematopoietic growth factors, producing collagenases, increasing bone resorption by osteoclasts, and rendering endothelial cells more adhesive for leukocytes (Table 5-2). Macrophage-origin IL-1 is a key factor in "switching on" T-lymphocyte proliferation and "up regulating" T-lymphocyte functions, such as IL-2 synthesis.

Interleukin 2

Interleukin 2 (IL-2) is a protein of 19 to 22 kD that is produced by activated T cells (T-helper lymphocytes: T_h). This molecule induces proliferation or differentiation of T lymphocytes (activated T and B cells) and other cell types (i.e., it activates and promotes the growth of natural killer [NK] cells, activates monocytes) that participate in the immune response (see Table 5-2). IL-2 is produced by T-helper lymphocytes upon recognition of the appropriate antigen-Class II MHC signal from antigen-processing cells. The subsequent release of IL-2 promotes the proliferation of IL-2 receptor bearing positive cells. Only cells that bear a specific receptor for IL-2 respond to its immunoregulatory effects.

IL-2 is both a growth factor and a differentiation factor. For example, IL-2 may cause T cells to release a variety of other lymphokines such as

Table 5-1 Major cytokines produced by activated lymphocytes

Cytokine	Function
Interleukin 2	Stimulates growth of T cells
	Stimulates B-cell differentiation
Interleukin 3	Stimulates mast cell growth
	Multipotential hemopoietic cell growth factor
Interleukin 4	Stimulates B-cell proliferation
	Stimulates T-cell growth
	With IL-3, stimulates IL-3 mast cell growth
	Enhances IgE and IgG production
	Stimulates MHC Class II antigen expression on B cells and macrophages
Interleukin 5	Enhances IgG production
	B-cell growth factor
	Eosinophil differential factor
Interleukin 6	Interferon beta (B-cell differentiation)
Interleukin 7	Pre–B-cell growth factor
Interleukin 8	Neutrophil activation protein
Interleukin 9	Autocrine T-cell growth factor in absence of antigen
Interleukin 10	Inhibits cytokine production by T_{H1} cells
Gamma interferon	Inhibits viral replication
	Induces MHC Class II antigen expression on macrophage
	Antagonist of IL-4 on B cells
Tumor necrosis factor alpha	Monocyte origin general cytotoxin
Tumor necrosis factor beta	T-lymphocyte origin general cytotoxin
Macrophage inhibitor factor	Inhibits macrophage inhibition

Table 5-2 Interleukin 1: biologic properties

Source	Antigen-presenting cells, including macrophages, dendritic cells, and B lymphocytes after stimulation with lysopolysaccharide, PMN cells, glia and glioma cells, epithelial cells of skin keratocytes, glomerular mesangial cells, Langhan's cells
Biochemical properties	Glycoprotein, molecular weight 175 kD
Functions	T-lymphocyte proliferation
	Endogenous pyrogen
	Causes neutrophil release from bone marrow
	Fibroblast proliferation
	Leukocyte adhesion to endothelial cells
	Acts on monocytes directly to induce tumor cytotoxicity
	Enhances bone reabsorption and cartilage degradation
	Stimulates prostagland E_2 synthesis by chondrocytes and synoviocytes
	Regulates IL-2 receptor expression

gamma interferon (IFN-γ). The promotion of INF-γ in turn enhances NK cell differentiation, generation of cytolytic T cells (Tc), and induction of macrophage activation; it also influences expression of both IL-2 receptors on T cells as well as the expression of MHC antigens. IL-2 induces T cells to secrete B-cell–stimulating factors (IL-4 or IL-5) which, in turn, influence B-cell growth and subsequent differentiation to antibody producing and secreting cells. Independent of interferon, IL-2 activates NK cells and lymphocyte-activated killer cells (LAK). Recent studies demonstrate that some B cells express IL-2 receptors. In the presence of IL-2, these cells increase in antibody secretion. It is evident that IL-2, a product of T-lymphocyte activation, is central to the activation and maintenance of the various cell types that participate in the immune response.

Interleukins three through ten

Interleukin 3 (IL-3) is secreted by antigen- or mitogen-activated T lymphocytes and induces growth and differentiation of hematopoietic precursor cells and mast cells. Murine keratinocytes produce a cytokine similar to IL-3, that also enhances the activity of NK cells and stimulates the release of oxygen radicals by granulocytes. Consequently, keratinocytes may participate in regulating the activity of different hematopoietic cells and thereby turn nonspecific host defense mechanisms against transformed cells and various harmful microbial organisms.

Interleukin 4 (IL-4), which is also secreted by T lymphocytes, is a growth factor for B lymphocytes (formerly called B-cell stimulatory factor), certain subsets of helper T cells, and mast cells. IL-4 also enhances IgE and IgG production. IL-4 differs from IL-2 in that the former stimulates proliferation only of certain helper T cells. Two types of helper T cells have been categorized based on their secretion of interleukins. Type 1 helper T cells secrete IL-2, IFN-γ, lymphotoxin, IL-3, and GM-CSF. Type 2 helper T cells produce and secrete IL-4 and IL-5, which enhance IgE and IgA synthesis respectively. This molecule has also been described as possessing the ability to increase expression of HLA Class II antigens on B cells. Many cell types, primarily of hematologic origin, express receptors for IL-4. Accordingly, effects of IL-4 have been described on T and B lymphocytes, NK cells, mononuclear phagocytes, mast cells, fibroblasts, and hematopoietic progenitor cells. IL-4 appears to play an important role in regulation of B-cell growth and of antibody isotype expression, stimulation of T-cell growth and generation of cytotoxic T lymphocytes, and indect regulation of the growth and differentiation of hematopoietic bone marrow stem cells.

Interleukin 5 (IL-5) is produced by activated T cells. It induces differentiation of activated B cells into IgA antibody-producing plasma cells and induces eosinophil differentiation.

Interleukin 6 (IL-6) has been described as a secretory product of activated T cells, fibroblasts, and monocytes. This molecule has been previously known as B-cell stimulatory factor (BSF-2), interferon-beta (IFN-β2), 26-kD protein, and hepatocyte stimulating factor (HSF). The cytokine IL-6 has emerged as a major "systemic alarm signal" that appears to be produced by essentially every injured tissue. IL-6 gene regulation is initiated by inflammation-associated cytokines, bacterial products, viral infection, and activation of any of the three major signal transduction pathways (diacylglycerol-, CAMP-, and Ca^{++}-activated). Injured skin (keratinocytes) is a major site of IL-6 production. This molecular messenger enhances maturation of activated T and B cells, stimulates growth of hematopoietic progenitor cells, and inhibits the growth of fibroblasts. The antiviral activity of IL-6 appears to be negligible. It is clear that IL-6 elicits major changes in the biochemical, physiologic, and immunologic status of the host. The biologic effects now associated with IL-6 include: stimulation of immunoglobulin secretion by mature B lymphocytes, growth stimulation of plasmacytomas and hybridomas, activation of T cells, stimulation of hepatic acute-phase protein synthesis, stimulation of hematopoiesis, cell differentiation, inhibition of tumor cell growth activity, and other INF-like effects.

Interleukin 7 (IL-7) is a cytokine that was initially referred to as pre–B-cell growth factor. Subsequent investigations found IL-7 to influence the activity of cells in the T lineage. In addition to its effects on cells from long-term marrow cultures, IL-7 stimulates growth of cells in cultures of fresh bone marrow.

Interleukin 8 (IL-8), also known as neutrophil activation protein-1 (NAP-1), is an 8,400 D protein that is a chemoattractant and granule release stimulus for neutrophils. NAP-1 has been isolated from culture fluids of LPS-stimulated peripheral blood monocytes, LPS-stimulated lung macrophages, mitogen-stimulated lymphocytes, and virus-infected fibroblasts. IL-1 or TNF induces IL-8 mRNA in many cells, including monocytes, fibroblasts, and endothelial cells. IL-8 belongs to a family of host defense small proteins that have a degree of sequence and structural similarity. IL-8 does not appear to serve as a chemoattractant for monocytes. The wide spectrum of cell sources and production stimuli suggests that IL-8 mediates neutrophil recruitment in host defense and disease.

Interleukin 9 (IL-9) is an autocrine growth factor that supports proliferation of murine T-cell clones in the absence of antigen. It is a glycoprotein that is secreted by helper T-2 lymphocytes.

Interleukin 10 (IL-10), cytokine synthesis inhibitory factor (CSIF), is an important regulator of humoral and cellular immunity. It is produced by the helper T-2 subpopulation of T cells and suppresses cytokine production of helper T-1 cells. The helper T-1 response favors INFN-γ and IL-2 production, which is important for cell-mediated immunity. Helper T-2 subpopulations secrete IL-4 and IL-5, which favor humoral responses, particularly IgE and IgA.

TUMOR NECROSIS FACTOR (TNF-α/CACHECTIN)

Tumor necrosis factor (TNF) was first discovered in the serum of mice after they were injected with bacterial cell wall products. Sera from these mice were cytotoxic to certain tumor cells. The TNF-α was subsequently found to be produced by activated macrophages, activated T cells and NK cells; it is similar to lymphotoxin, T-lymphocyte cytokine, or TNF-β. TNF-α has been cloned; it has been reported to have a molecular weight of 17,000 D and to contain approximately 157 amino acids in its active form. Although there are similarities to lymphotoxin, which is produced by mitogen-stimulated lymphocytes, and to IL-1, which is also produced by macrophages, TNF possesses distinctive differences, primarily in its antiproliferative effects. TNF-α is one of the major signals regulating the production of IL-1 in rheumatoid arthritis, but not in the osteoarthritic joint. To date, tumor necrosis factor is the only cytokine that has been demonstrated to fulfill Koch's postulates and, thus, to be causally related to host responses.

The mechanisms of action and biologic properties of TNF are diverse. This soluble mediator mimics many actions of IL-1 on T cells, B cells, macrophages, and endothelial cells. TNF induces fragmentation of targeted cell DNA. However, TNF also results in synthesis of prostaglandins, producing the generation of cytocidal free-oxygen radicals, and is responsible for inducing other acute-phase reactions. Cytotoxic properties resulting from TNF release include the induction of lysosomal enzymes in target cells and some tumor cell destruction. Other inhibitory properties associated with TNF are those described on the hematopoietic stem cells and inhibition of lipoprotein lipase in fat cells; thus, a state of "cellular cachexia" in enzyme synthesis is created in vitro. Persistent TNF-α/Cachectin production by the body occurs in chronic infection and malignancy. Chronic exposure to TNF-α induces a cachexia syndrome characterized by anorexia, weight loss, and anemia. Acute systemic appearance of cachectin/ TNF-α is capable of inducing a state of lethal shock, disseminated hemorrhagic necrosis, catabolic hormone release, and multiple organ injury. Thus TNF can be a growth factor, cytotoxin, cytostatic agent, or an inducer of differentiation. This cytokine is also an important inflammatory mediator, regulating the activity of neutrophils, eosinophils, and T and B lymphocytes and modulating the properties of the vascular endothelium. TNF-α, whether a natural or recombinant product, offers an interesting area of research in veterinary medicine as a treatment for neoplastic diseases and as a tool in understanding the pathophysiology of certain infectious diseases.

INTERFERONS

Issacs and Lindenmann discovered that cells infected with a virus produce a protein that renders uninfected cells resistant to subsequent viral infection. This interference factor was called an interferon (IFN). IFNs are a group of proteins produced by diverse cell types. They all have the ability to inhibit viral replication by degradation of viral mRNA and by blocking the initiation of protein synthesis. IFNs perform a variety of other cellular activities, including antipoliferative effects on tumor cells and enhancement of expression of histocompatibility antigens. IFNs have been reported to induce the up-regulation of Fc receptors and increase the phagocytic capabilities of immune cells. By prompting macrophage activation, IFNs are responsible for enhanced cellular metabolic activity, therefore enhancing phagocyte microbicidal and cytotoxic activity. Conclusions reached by various scientific experiments indicate that IFNs can boost, as well as inhibit, inflammation. Thus the IFN system is emerging as a broad-based host defense system that is involved in both the primary nonspecific resistance to a variety of microorganisms and in specific immune responses. The several types of IFN and their cell origin are listed in Table 5-3.

GAMMA INTERFERON

IFN-γ may be classified as an interferon because of its viral interference properties, but it also func-

Table 5-3 Interferons

Category	Origin	Primary Induction
Alpha interferon	Leukocytes	Viruses; polynucleotides
Beta interferon	Fibroblasts	Viruses; polynucleotides
Gamma interferon	Lymphocytes	Mitogens; antigens

tions as a lymphokine. As a lymphokine, IFN-γ augments the cytotoxic functions of T cells, NK cells, K cells, and macrophages, resulting in increased phagocytosis of bacteria.

The reported sources for this molecule are activated T cells and NK cells. IFN-γ activates macrophages and induces expression of HLA Class II molecules on macrophages and many other cells. Additional biologic properties attributed to IFN-γ include the suppression of hematopoietic progenitor cells, the activation of endothelial cells, and in vitro antiviral activity. Cellular immunity is the major mechanism in host defense against viral and intracellular parasitic diseases. Selective immaturity in certain functions of T lymphocytes appears to be a major factor in the neonate's susceptibility to infection. Particularly striking is the deficiency in production of IFN-γ.

MACROPHAGE INHIBITION FACTOR

Inhibition of macrophage migration from spleen explants cultured in the presence of specific antigens was first described in 1932. In the early 1960s, this phenomenon was reinvestigated and shown to be a good in vitro correlate of developing cell-mediated immunity.

Two basic approaches to the study of macrophage inhibition factor (MIF) have been devised. In the first method, a cell suspension of peritoneal exudate cells is packed into capillary tubes, centrifuged, and then submerged in a medium that contains specific antigen or MIF materials. The migration of macrophages from these tubes is then measured and calculated as migration indices compared to antigen-free controls. Lymphocytes and macrophages from different species can be mixed in this assay.

MIF is secreted by T lymphocytes after antigenic or mitogenic stimulation. It is a nondialyzable macromolecule of about 40,000 kD with biochemical properties of an acidic glycoprotein. MIF production is dependent on protein, not DNA synthesis.

In addition to MIF, a number of different substances affecting macrophage functions have been described. These materials are named after the assay designated to measure their presence. Included in this list are an activating factor, an aggregating factor, a factor that causes the disappearance of macrophages from the peritoneal cavity, and a factor that inhibits spreading of macrophages on glass. It is likely that these mediators are similar to MIF.

COLONY-STIMULATING FACTORS

A more precise understanding of the steady replacement and renewal of hematopoietic cells is of extreme interest when considered in the context of infectious disease. These control mechanisms can increase the production of various cell types in response to specific demands (e.g., erythrocytes in cases of acute blood loss or leukocytes in response to inflammation and especially bacterial infection). Throughout life, this continuous replacement of mature hematopoietic cells and bone marrow production of these cells is closely regulated by colony-stimulating factors.

Colony-stimulating factors are a class of growth factors required for the survival, clonal proliferation, and differentiation of hemopoietic progenitor cells in vitro. The development of in vitro culture techniques for bone marrow cells led to the discovery that there must be continuous stimulation for successful growth and proliferation of these cells. These colony-stimulating factors have been isolated from a variety of cells, including fibroblasts, macrophages, endothelial cells, and T lymphocytes (Table 5-4). At least five human hematopoietic growth factors have been identified and their genes cloned, including GM-CSF, G-CSF, M-CSF, IL-3, and erythropoietin (EPO). These factors interact with separate but overlapping progenitor cells. Progenitor cells that give rise to megakaryocytes, erythrocytes, and granulocytes are stimulated by granulocyte/macrophage colony-stimulating factor (GM-GCSF) and IL-2 (multi-FCSF). Late progenitor cells of the neutrophilic series are stimulated by granulocyte colony-stimulating factor (G-CSF). A monocyte colony-stimulating factor (M-CSF) stimulates the late progenitor cells of the monocytic cell line. The release of colony-stimulating factors from these cells is orchestrated in a complex manner. For instance, two substances produced and released by monocytes, IL-1 and TNF, have been reported to stimulate the release of colony-stimulating factor from endothelial cells in vitro.

Table 5-4 Colony-stimulating factors

Name	Cellular Origin	Primary Progeny
G-CSF	Monocytes Fibroblasts	Granulocytes
GM-CSF	T cells Endothelial cells Fibroblasts	Granulocytes Macrophages
M-CSF	Monocytes Fibroblasts Endothelial cells	Macrophages
IL-3	T cells	Granulocytes, Macrophages, RBCs, eosinophils Mast cells, stem cells Megakaryocytes
IL-7	Bone marrow stromal cells	Pre–B-cell growth factor

CHEMOTACTIC FACTORS PRODUCED BY LYMPHOCYTES

An essential feature of delayed-type hypersensitivity (DTH) reactions in vivo is the accumulation of inflammatory cells in the area of antigen deposition. The chief infiltrating cell is a macrophage that is derived from circulating blood monocytes. T lymphocytes possess the ability to secrete a macrophage chemotactic factor following antigenic or mitogenic stimulation. The substance is distinguishable from MIF by virtue of its lower molecular weight of 12 to 15 kD. Other chemotactic factors for neutrophils and fibroblasts are initially being described as secretory products of activated lymphocytes. DTH reactions are the setting in which these investigations are centered, with particular emphasis on delineating pathophysiologic events.

LYMPHOTOXIN

Lymphotoxin (LT) was one of the first lymphokines to be described and has been one of the most difficult to fit into a conceptual framework. Twenty years after its discovery, the structure, genetic organization, and linkage are well understood in the mouse and human, and insight has been gained into its biologic role. It is a T-cell derived glycoprotein of 25 kD coded by a gene within the MHC. It is somewhat (35%) structurally homologous to the macrophage product TNF. The genes for LT and TNF are tightly linked, and the proteins share most biologic activities and compete for the same cell-surface receptor. LT is induced in an antigen-specific MHC-restricted fashion from Class I and Class II restricted T cells. Viral infection is also associated with LT production by lymphoid cells. LT has several effects on target cells, including killing, growth stimulation, and induction of differentiation. The mechanism of LT's effects involves receptor binding, internalization, and several sequelae, including changes in prostaglandins and chromosome integrity. LT probably plays several biologic roles. It can contribute to immunoregulation, defense against viruses, parasitic infections, and rejection of tumors. Understanding the role of LT in the pathogenesis of diseases involving autoimmunity and immune dysregulation will be an important key to devising effective regimens for prophylaxis and treatment.

The number of cytokines identified, cloned, and investigated for structure-function relationships increases each month. As with all new information, the cytokine literature will take some time to become clear. For instance, the current nomenclature for cytokines may be misleading. The name is often derived from the first biologic property of the cytokine observed in vitro, and in many cases these are not the most important properties of the molecule. Additionally, laboratory investigations using pure preparations have provided evidence that single cytokine molecules (e.g., IL-1) may act on a wide variety of target cells, whereas other cytokines (e.g., G-CSF) act on a more restricted target cell population. Interactions between members of the cytokine families may serve to amplify or down-regulate various host defense activities. These interactions are not well defined at the present time. The stimulation of a cell by a cytokine may have several outcomes that are dependent on the target cell type, the presence of other coexisting cytokines, and the variance in the repertoire of cytokine activities between species, although there is a significant degree of homology.

CYTOKINE THERAPY

Cytokines play a decisive role in determining the immune status. The integrity of the immune system is controlled by efficient cellular responses to cytokine stimulation. The body's natural defense system is maintained on heightened alert, and the specific immune response to foreign antigens can be efficiently mobilized as a consequence of cytokine activation. Consequently, it is reasonable to initiate investigations directed toward delineating the role of exogenous cytokine administration in prophylaxis or therapy for which stress- or pathogen-induced immunosuppression has been linked to disease susceptibility.

POTENTIAL APPLICATIONS OF CYTOKINES IN VETERINARY MEDICINE

Modulation of the immune response in various circumstances of infectious disease processes may be a fertile area to apply "biologic response modifiers" or "immunomodulators." There is evidence that stressors releasing glucocorticoids, in combination with viral or bacterial infections, may exert their immunosuppressive effects through interference with synthesis and/or action of cytokines. Therefore there is interest in combating these induced immunodeficiency states by stimulating production of intrinsic cytokines or by using recombinant DNA-derived cytokines as immunoprophylactic agents.

Recombinant DNA-derived human and bovine IL-2 is available for investigative purposes. Both are undergoing in vitro and in vivo testing for efficacy in restoring immune function in bovine cells infected with viruses. It is possible that extrinsic human or bovine IL-2 may have a role in the prevention or modulation of infectious diseases. IL-2 appears to play a central role in regulating B-cell activation, proliferation, and differentiation. These activities serve to facilitate the production of immunoglobulins of all isotypes. A wide array of additional cytokines can amplify antibody production, but none appear to be able to accomplish this task without IL-2. Presently there are insufficient data to come to any judgment concerning the real or potential therapeutic value of these compounds.

IFNs are reported to possess extensive antiviral, antiproliferative, and immunoregulatory activities. IFNs exhibit a wide range of activity against the replication of both DNA and RNA viruses. Pertinent literature contains reports of IFNs inhibiting the replication of bacteria, fungi, protozoa, and both tumor and normal cells. Immunoregulatory activities that influence humoral and cell-mediated immunity, enhance the cytotoxic activity of NK cells, and stimulate the phagocytic activity of macrophages stimulates interest in IFNs for therapeutic considerations. A potential drawback is that IFNs usually exhibit a limited host range; therefore species-specific applications become an important factor in planning for potential clinical applications.

A study was implemented to assess the hematologic changes in lactating dairy cattle induced by two dosage regimes of human recombinant colony-stimulating factor (Hr-GCSF) as a prelude to mammary gland challenge experiments. The study documents the capability of the human recombinant colony-stimulating factor to produce hematologic changes in both a time- and dose-dependent manner when administered to the adult lactating bovine. A "screening dose" of 1 μ/kg of Hr-GCSF administered to three study subjects produced a threefold to fourfold increase in peripheral blood mature neutrophil counts by day 12 of the trial. The "priming dose" (3 μg/kg of Hr-GCSF) treatment group of four lactating cows exhibited a threefold to fivefold increase in peripheral blood mature neutrophil counts and twofold to threefold increase in white blood cell counts by day five of the trial. Hematologic examinations of the control group ($n = 4$; no Hr-GCSF administration) did not detect significant changes in their neutrophil counts over baseline values. The milk-somatic cell counts did not statistically shift over baseline values in any of the control or Hr-GCSF treatment groups. When attempting to alter the course of infectious disease processes, potential applications of colony-stimulating factors provide interesting speculations about new therapeutic modalities.

SUGGESTED READINGS

Balkwill FR, Burke F: The cytokine network, *Immunol Today* 10(9):299, 1989.

Blecha F: Cytokines: applications in domestic food animals, *J Dairy Sci* 74(1):329-339, 1991.

Cullor JS, Fairley N, Smith WL and others: Hemogram changes in lactating dairy cows given human recombinant granulocyte colony stimulating factor (r-MethuG-CSF), *Vet Pathol* 27:311, 1990.

Farrar WL, Ferris DK, Harel-Bellan A: The molecular basis of immune cytokine action, *Crit Rev Ther Drug Carrier Sys* 5(4):229, 1989.

Fong Y, Moldawar LL, Shires GT and others: The biologic characteristics of cytokines and their implication in surgical injury, *Surg Gyn Obst* 170(4):363, 1990.

Kehril ME, Cullor JS, Nickerson SC: Immunobiology of hematopoietic colony-stimulating factors: application to disease prevention in the bovine, *J Dairy Sci* 74:2448-2458, 1991.

Lipsky PE: The control of antibody production by immunomodulatory molecules, *Arth Rheum* 32(11):1345, 1989.

Moore MA, Muench MO, Warren DJ and others: Cytokine networks involved in the regulation of haemopoietic stem cell proliferation and differentiation, *Ciba Found Sym* 148:43, 1990.

6 Complement System

Over eighty years ago Bordet discovered a serum factor that if present with antibodies and specific antigens such as bacteria, caused bacterial lysis. It was clearly distinguishable from bacterial agglutins in that heating the serum destroyed its lytic abilities without affecting its agglutinating properties. Further, lytic potency could be restored if serum from animals lacking agglutins was added to mixtures of previously heat-inactivated serum and bacteria. This property of fresh serum complemented specific bacterial agglutins, and the antibody-independent system mediating lysis was called the complement reaction.

For many years the relationship between complement and antibody was viewed solely as the prime effector mechanism for *in vivo* antigen-antibody reactions. In past decades, however, interrelationships between complement, the clotting system, and other factors associated with inflammation have broadened the role of complement as an integral part of the body's defenses against disease processes. Today complement is involved as an effector of cell membrane damage, as an integral part of the inflammatory response, and in the promotion of blood coagulation. Not only do complement-lysed cells activate the clotting cascade through the Hageman factor, but C3b directly promotes thrombus formation by causing platelet aggregation. The major contribution of the complement system to the inflammatory process is by chemotactically attracting leukocytes to sites of complement activation.

The proteins of the complement system form two interrelated enzyme cascades, providing two routes for the cleavage of C3, the central protein of the cascade. A third set of plasma proteins (membrane attack complex) becomes assembled into the structures that are responsible for the lytic lesions in the lipid bilayers of cells or bacterial membranes. Thus the complement system functions in cellular activation, cytolysis, and opsonization.

CLASSICAL COMPLEMENT ACTIVATION SEQUENCE

The complement (C) reaction involves the sequential actions of nine discrete serum proteins, the first of which consists of three distinct subunits.

In 1968 a standard nomenclature was adapted to facilitate research in this area. In the model system used to study the reaction, a sheep erythrocyte (E) antibody (A) complex (EA) initiates the reaction. The order of the reaction sequence is C1, C4, C2, C3, C5, C6, C7, C8, and C9. Intermediate complexes generated during the reaction sequence are written as EAC142. Enzymatically activated forms are designated by a bar above the symbol used (e.g., C1). Complement fragments generated during the course of the reaction by enzymatic attack on various complement components are indicated by a lowercase letter along with symbol for the parent molecule (e.g., C3a, C3b, C3c, and C3d). Inactivated fragments are designated with a lowercase i (e.g., C3bi). Some immunologists designate the larger fragment as "b" and the smaller one as "a", but others continue to use a more arbitrary, albeit historic, designation. This results in some confusion.

The general outline of the sequence of events in the classical complement activation cascade is given in Figure 6-1. Conceptually, the complement reaction is viewed as a series of enzymatic events in which amplification of the initial activation of C1 is attained. The reaction is controlled by internal mechanisms such as a rapid decay of several components to inactive forms and by the enzymatic action of various distinct inactivators on several biologically active components in the sequence. In addition, a number of by-products of complement activation possess potent biologic activity independent of their contributions to cellular lysis.

C1

The sequence is initiated by interaction of the trimolecular complex of C1 with a specific portion of the immunoglobulin (Ig) molecule located on the Fc region. This region is exposed to C1 following unfolding of the antibody molecule (A) produced as a consequence of binding to E. A single molecule of IgM is sufficient to activate the classical pathway, but aggregates of IgG are required for efficient activation. *C1 is composed of three subunits (C1q, C1r, C1s)* held together by calcium ions and sediments at 18S. C1q contains the

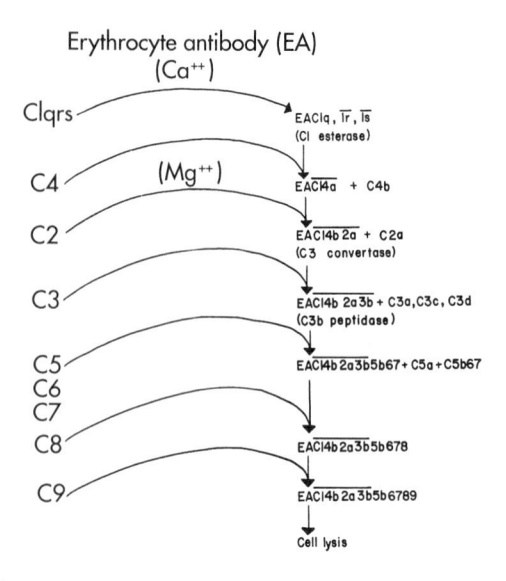

Figure 6-1 The classical pathway of complement activation.

recognition unit that causes the complex to bind to Ig immunoglobulin. C1q is multivalent and has a unique structure that is half globular and half collagen-like. The other two subcomponents, C1r and C1s, do not bind to the immunoglobulin but are involved in the subsequent classical pathway activation. The third subunit, C1s, contains esterase activity necessary for activation of the next C component, C4. C1 has been produced by epithelial cells of the colon, bladder, and renal pelvis, all of common endodermal origin.

C4

Binding of C4 to EAC1 occurs next and is independent of calcium ions. C1s esterase cleaves C4 into two fragments, *C4a and C4b*. This process activates C4b by exposing a thioester bond and allowing it to bind not only to the EAC1 complex but also to multiple sites on the adjacent red blood cell membrane. C4 has an approximate molecular weight of 290,000 daltons (D) and consists of two subunits held together by disulfide bridges. Macrophages, chiefly in the liver, are the sites of synthesis of C4. The smaller fragment, C4a, is an anaphylatoxin; it induces mediator release from mast cells. The next component of the reaction, C2, requires the presence of magnesium ions before it can react with EAC14.

C2

C2, the third complement component involved in the sequence, is a beta globulin of 117,000 to 130,000 D. Macrophages are the sites of C2 synthesis. In the presence of magnesium, C2 binds with cell membrane-bound C4 and is then split into two fragments by the action of C1 esterase. One fragment (35 kD) is released from the site of the reaction (C2b), and the other fragment 75kD, C2a in combination with membrane-bound C4b, has enzymatic activity for the next component in the sequence (C3) and is called C3 convertase. Thus *C3 convertase of the classical pathway is C4b2a*. Those authors who use the newer designation of fragment size would consider C4b2b to be correct.

C3

C3 is a major serum protein that migrates as a beta globulin and has been shown to be composed of two polypeptide chains linked by disulfide bridges. C3 is a pivotal serum protein in the reaction sequence, since it constitutes a common pathway for involvement of the clotting system. Macrophages and hepatocytes synthesize C3.

C3 convertase acts on C3 and generates at least four separate subunits (C3a, C3b, C3c, and C3d). C3a is released from the reaction site, whereas C3b is bound to the cell surface, resulting in the intermediate EAC14b2a3b. C3b is not bound to the enzyme C3 convertase but instead binds to other sites on the cell surface. There is little doubt that the generation of C3b coating on target cells is the major biologic function of complement. Bound C3b immediately adjacent to C14b2a has peptidase activity necessary for binding of the next three complement components, C5, C6, and C7.

Opsonic fragments of C3 that are created include C3b, C3bi, C3d, and C3i. These opsonins have an important role in host defense; their function and that of the receptors to which they bind are discussed later in this chapter.

Membrane attack complex

Completion of the complement activation sequence occurs via activation of C5 through C9. This complex is referred to as the *membrane attack complex (MAC)* and can be described by the general formula $C5b_1$, $C6_1$, $C7_1$, $C8_1$, and $C9_n$ wherein 1 to 20 molecules of C9 are activated and deposited on the cell membranes. The MAC represents a multimolecular assembly and constitutes the only known mechanism of blood origin enzymes that is capable of impairing biologic membranes.

The reaction sequence is initiated by action of C5 convertase on C5 with subsequent generation of activated C5b. C5 is beta globulin produced by macrophages. Two C5 convertases exist: the *classical C5 convertase (C4b2a3b)* is generated via the classical pathway. The *C5 convertase of the alternate pathway* is *C3bBb* (see Alternate Pathway of Complement Activation). Cleavage of C5 produces two distinct C5 fragments. One small fragment, *C5a*, remains in the fluid phase and acts as a mediator of inflammation. *C5b*, with a molecular weight of 170,000 D, does two things. It remains attached to the red blood cell membrane and forms a membrane-bound complex with C6 and C7, or it combines with C6 as a fluid phase C5b6 complex. In serum, C5, C6, and C7 are closely associated with one another, so that activation of C5 is usually associated with activation of C6 and C7. There is no proteolytic cleavage associated with the binding of C6 or C7. The C5b67 complex transfers from the site of generation to a different site on the cell membrane, and the first phase of cell membrane attack is initiated.

The activated *C5b67* complex is stable and strongly amphiphilic, and once attached to any lipid bilayer, including cell membranes, it interacts sequentially with C8 and C9.

At the cell membrane surface, *C8* combines with the C5b67 fragment, and C9 then combines with C8. At this point, cell lysis is initiated. Lysis appears to be mediated directly by the action of C9 on the membrane, since EAC1 through EAC8 complexes are relatively stable to lysis. The lytic attack mechanism acts on the lipid matrix of the cell membrane, not on its membrane proteins.

Characteristically, the MAC contains *multiple C9 molecules* that spontaneously polymerize to form tubular structures on cell surfaces. Studies have indicated that for each C5-8 complex there are 12 to 15 associated C9 molecules. The functional membrane lesions (channels) caused by the MAC are the result of phospholipid reorganization caused by highly complex protein-protein and protein-phospholipid interactions. The MAC acts by forming hydrophilic protein channels and hydrophilic lipid channels, called a "donut" and "leaky patch" models, respectively.

Actual holes (about 100 Å in diameter) on the cell membrane have been observed by electron microscopy. Disruption of the membrane allows free exchange of water and salts; the cell first swells and then bursts. The holes are envisioned as donuts, lined by hydrophilic lipids or complement components through which fluids leak.

Analogous mechanisms between the MAC and lymphocyte-mediated cytotoxicity

There appears to be a striking homology between MAC-mediated cell pore formation and target cell damage elicited by killer lymphocytes. Target cell-bound killer cells (cytotoxic T, NK, and K cells) produce a cylindric protein called membrane attack protein (MAP), cytolysin, lymphopore, or *perforin*. Perforin is a C9-related protein found in cytoplasmic granules of these effector cells that can form membrane pores in the presence of calcium ions. The microtubule system and the Golgi apparatus of natural killer (NK) cells and cytotoxic lymphocytes (CTL) are repositioned to face the contact area with the target cell. This arrangement serves to direct the secretory granules toward a contact site, thus allowing granule exocytosis.

ALTERNATE PATHWAY OF COMPLEMENT ACTIVATION

In the 1950s, Pillemer and colleagues described a pathway of complement activation that bypassed early complement proteins (C1, C4, C2) and was initiated by activation of C3. This pathway was independent of antibodies and resulted in lysis of some targets alone, without consumption of C1, C4, and C2. This pathway has great pathogenic importance, since it explains complement consumption in bacterial sepsis or endotoxin shock and provides a common link between the clotting and complement systems through involvement of Hageman factor XII.

It is important to point out that at low levels C3, the pivotal complement protein for both the classical and alternate pathways, is continually and spontaneously activated to C3b. Normally inactivation of C3b occurs by binding of C3b to *factor H*. However, when certain surfaces are present (bacterial cell wall, yeast, some virus-infected cells, and other foreign substances)—surfaces that have in common a lack of sialic acid-factor H is inhibited from binding to C3b; instead, *factor B* binds to C3b. Factor B is a 90 kilodalton (KD) serum globulin that is cleaved by *factor D* into Ba and Bb. Thus a new enzyme is created in the presence of the appropriate type of activating surface. This new enzyme is *C3bBb, a C3 convertase of the alternate pathway*. Like the classical pathway convertase, C3bBb is unstable and decays. Increased stability is provided by the binding of an additional protein of the alternate pathway, *preperdin (P)*, in the presence of magnesium ions. The sequence of events for activation of the alternate pathway of complement activation is shown in Figure 6-2.

Terms such as alternate, C3 activator, and C3 shunt system have been used to designate attack of C3 by pathways other than those of C3 convertase (EAC14b2a). The alternate pathway provides a mechanism of innate or nonimmune opsonization of offending particles and, in phytogenetic terms, is probably older than the recently evolved classical pathway.

Certain species of Ig, though not complement activating through the classical pathway described earlier, can initiate the complement cascade via

Activators

Some gram negative bacteria/LPS
Some gram positive bacteria/teichoic acid
Zymosan (fungi, yeasts cell wall origin)
Some viruses
Some parasites
Some tumors

} These surfaces do not degrade C3b because they have low sialic acid content

1. C3 → C3a + C3b   (occurs naturally at low rate)
2. Factor B + Mg → Bb + (Factor D facilitates)
3. C3bBb (stabilized by Properdin) = C3 convertase of alternate pathway

Figure 6-2 The alternate pathway of complement activation.

the alternate route. For example, the guinea pig possesses two distinct IgG subclasses, IgG1 and IgG2. IgG2 activates complement through the C14b2a pathway. In contrast, IgG1 activates complement through the alternate system only. Furthermore, sites of complement attachment on these antibodies are different. IgG2 possessses an activation site for C1 on the Fc portion of the molecule, whereas IgG1 does not. Both IgG1 and IgG2 possess a second site of activation located on the $F(ab')_2$ fragment and use the alternate pathway.

Other control mechanisms in the complement cascade

Complement activation, if allowed to continue unchecked *in vivo*, would have disastrous consequences. Thus various controls exist to minimize damage to the host's own tissues. These are of two general types. In the first type of control, many of the complement fragments, once activated, undergo rapid spontaneous decay and thus have short half-lives. The second type of control consists of normal serum inhibitors and destructive enzymes. Control mechanisms are less well understood than is the reaction sequence. Table 6-1 lists the various recognized inhibitors of the complement sequence.

In humans a genetic disorder of C1 inhibitor has been described in which C1 esterase activity is allowed to proceed unchecked. This disease, angioneurotic edema, is due to C1-mediated increases in vascular permeability, as well as to inappropriate activation of the remaining complement components.

Recently a group of structurally, functionally, and genetically-related plasma and membrane glycoproteins that control amplification of complement at the C3 step have been recognized. These are referred to as the regulators of complement activation (RCAs). Included in these are CR1 and CR2 (see Complement Receptors), C4-binding protein, factor H, and membrane cofactor protein (MCP or CD46).

BIOLOGIC ACTIVITIES OF COMPLEMENT COMPONENTS
Complement fragments with biologic activities

Various complement fragments generated during the course of complement activation have potent biologic activities. Generally, they fall into three separate categories: opsonic factors, chemotactic factors, and anaphylatoxins. Particulate activators of complement, such as bacteria, are more efficiently engulfed by neutrophils and macrophages, because the presence of C3b on the cell membrane binds to a C3b receptor on the phagocyte, thereby allowing the phagocyte to "grip" the particle strongly, thereby allowing phagocytosis to

Table 6-1 Soluble and membrane-bound inhibitors of complement activation

Substance	Site of activity
C1 inhibitor	Blocks C1 esterase activity on C4 and C2
C3 inactivator	Blocks action of C3b on C5 by converting C3b to soluble C3 and Cd
C4bp (soluble)	Accelerates decay of C4b2a
C6 inactivator	Blocks action of C6 or C7
Factor H (soluble)	Competes with factor B for binding sites on C3b
Factor I (soluble)	Inactivates C3b and C4b
CR1 (CD35)	Accelerates decay of C3 convertase
MCP (CD46)	Functions as cofactor in factor I–mediated cleavage of C3b and C4b
HRF[*]	Blocks binding of C8 to C9; inhibits bystander cell lysis
MIRL (CD59)[+]	Blocks binding of C7 and C8; inhibits bystander cell lysis

[*]Homologous restriction factor.
[+]Membrane inhibitor of reactive lysis.

proceed. Several complement components possess potent chemotactic activity for both neutrophils and monocytes. For example, C5a creates a chemotactic gradient that attracts neutrophils and stimulates their movement to the site of the inflammatory reaction. Finally, complement intermediates may incite pharmacologic events associated with anaphylaxis by causing mast cell degranulation in the absence of an IgE response. For biologic effects to occur, the complement fragments that are active must bind to cells; this is accomplished through complement receptors in the cell membrane of macrophages and other target cells.

Opsonins

The word *opsonin* is derived from the Greek word *opsono*, which means "to prepare food for." With or without immunoglobulin, passively absorbed tissue, and serum protein, including those of the coagulation scheme, complement fragments are the prime opsonins of tissue fluids. Fragments C3b, C3bi, C3d, and C3di, along with Clq, C4b, C5, and C5b, have been shown to exhibit opsonic activity for phagocytic cells (Table 6-2). Of these, solid-phase C3b is dominant. Neutrophils, monocytes, and B lymphocytes possess cell-surface CR1 receptors for C3b. Interaction of complement-coated particles with phagocytic cells provides a mechanism that promotes phagocytosis. This opsonic activity can be independent of specific antibody if C3b is generated via the alternate pathway. Bovine serum contains a substance called conglutinin, a heat-stable, calcium-dependent protein that agglutinates antibody-coated particles. This appears to be an activity of C3 that is unique to ruminants.

Chemotactic factors

The predominant chemotactic factor produced during complement activation is C5a. It stimulates directed movement of neutrophils along a concentration gradient. C567 complexes are generated by the action of EAC14b2b3b on C5. A portion of C567 is bound to the reaction site, whereas the remainder freely diffuses into adjacent tissues. C567 cannot be generated from heat-inactivated serum. This trimolecular complex is a potent attractant for neutrophils and has been found in synovial fluids of patients suffering from rheumatoid arthritis. C567 is not produced by proteolytic enzymes and is observed only following sequential interaction of the complement sequence. Thus this substance is probably the most active chemoattractant produced as a consequence of complement activation.

Vasoactive factors

Uncontrolled generation of C1 esterase results in increased vascular permeability. Animals intradermally injected with C1 show a wheal/flare reaction at the site of injection.

A major fragment of C3, fluid-phase C3a, along with C5a, is an anaphylatoxin that when injected into laboratory animals, produces an anaphylactic reaction indistinguishable from that observed when antigen is injected intravenously into a sensitized individual.

C3a, C4a, and C5a cause smooth muscle contraction and release of histamine from mast cells. The physiologic sequela to mast cell degranulation is similar to that seen when an IgE-antigen reaction triggers mediator release from mast cells (see Chapter 13). It is likely that C3a and C5a play a major role as mediators of anaphylactoid reactions, which mimic an IgE-mediated reaction but occur in the absence of antigen-specific IgE.

Complement receptors

Complement component receptors on cells of the immune and inflammatory systems are thought to play diverse roles in immunity and inflammation, respectively. The CR1 receptor binds the C3b fragment, thereby indirectly limiting the activity of C3 convertase and thus decreasing the consequences of complement activation. As mentioned, the opsonic role is well recognized. In addition, immune complexes can be transported from their site(s) of formation via binding to Fc receptors on circulating cells. In conjunction with fibronectin, complement receptors facilitate adhesion of phagocytic cells to pathogens and/or connective tissue.

Complement receptors have been grouped into four types. These cell-surface molecules are important in the mediation of the biologic functions of complement, such as opsonization and chemotaxis, and some have a role in regulation of the complement cascade.

Table 6-2 Biologic activies of complement intermediates

Complement component or fragment	Biologic activity
C3b, C3bi, C3d, C3di, Clq, C4b, C5, and C5b	Opsonin
C1 (C1 esterase) and C3 proteolytic fragment	Increased vascular permeability
C5a proteolytic fragment and fluid-phase C567	Neutrophil chemotaxis
C3a and C5a	Monocyte chemotaxis
C3a, C4a, and C5a	Anaphylatoxin

Complement receptor type 1 (CR1) is glycoprotein found in the cell membrane of several cell types, including neutrophils, monocytes/macrophages, B cells, T cells, eosinophils, erythrocytes, and follicular dendritic cells. CR1 receptors are cross-linked by bound C3b and become associated with the cytoskeletal machinery of the cell. Since most effector cells lack receptors for IgM, C3b fixation to target particles is probably the critical opsonizing event during the early IgM phase of primary immune response. Although CR1 binds C3b with the highest affinity, these receptors can also bind to C3bi, C4b, and C4bi, albeit with lower affinity. Expression of the CR1 receptor is regulated by a variety of stimuli, including lymphokines and C5a.

Complement receptor type 2 (CR2) is also an integral membrane glycoprotein, with expression limited to B cells and some T cells; it is designated as CD21. The ligand for CR2 is degradation products of C3b including C3d and C3bi. The role of CR1 is not yet fully elucidated; however, it is thought to be involved in B-cell activation.

A third C3 receptor (CR3) has a higher affinity for C3bi than for C3b. Along with the fourth complement receptor (CR4), CR3 is a member of the integrin family of receptors. They both have an alpha chain that is unique and a common beta chain. The integrin family of receptors is important in cell-cell adhesion. CR3 and CR4 are present on phagocytes, NK cells, and subpopulations of T cells, and they bind to the C3 degradation product, C3bi. The adhesion function of these receptors may facilitate neutrophil egress from blood vessels during inflammation.

Resting neutrophils and monocytes bind but do not phagocytize C3b-coated sheep erythrocytes. The particles form rosettes on the surface of the phagocytic cell. If the cell is triggered by a second signal, phagocytosis will proceed; the second signal may be provided by a few molecules of IgG antibody on the particle to be phagocytized.

Anaphylatoxins (C3a, C4a) produced during complement activation bind to receptors on mast cells, basophils, and granulocytes to facilitate their activity. The most potent chemotactic factor, C5a, has receptors on those cells, as well as on platelets, endothelial cells, and monocytes/macrophages.

COMPLEMENT AND IMMUNE RESPONSES

Experimentally, cobra venom factor (CoVF)–treated mice depleted of C3 through C9 are deficient in IgG, but not IgM, responses to thymus-dependent antigens. Immunized C4-deficient guinea pigs produce less antibody than do C4-normal animals and are unable to maintain serum titers over time. Memory responses, chiefly a function if IgG-secreting B cells, are also absent in C4-deficient animals. This in vivo immune deficiency can be completely reversed by administration of small amounts of normal guinea pig serum.

Complement and defense against bacteria

Complement serves a major protective role in limiting damage or invasion by bacterial pathogens. Bacteria-specific antibody activates the classical sequence through the C142 pathway. In the absence of antibody, the alternate pathway is activated by binding of bacterial cell wall components such as the polysaccharide component of lipopolysaccharide (LPS), teichoic acid, and/or peptidoglycan. Complement activation leads to deposition of the opsonic complement fragments, as well as the bacteriolytic MAC.

All gram-positive cell walls appear to activate the alternate pathway efficiently in nonimmune serum, leading to the deposition of C3b on the bacterial wall. C-reactive protein (CRP) is a 115-kD protein that binds specifically and with high affinity to phosphorylcholine, a major component of cell wall teichoic acid. This binding site for CRP is exposed only in gram-positive organisms. Gram-negative bacteria, unlike gram-positive organisms, can activate complement by both the alternate and classical pathways.

It is clear that intact bacteria possessing rough LPS can activate the classical pathway in an antibody-independent fashion, although noncomplement factors may be required for completion of complement activation. Most types of LPS directly bind Clq or C1. LPS in the absence of antibody is, however, the prototypic activator of the alternate pathway.

For both gram-positive and gram-negative bacteria, the presence of a capsule is a major determinant of the ability of complement to opsonize the bacterium effectively. Encapsulation of bacteria interferes with the process of C3 fixation in normal serum, rendering organisms resistant to subsequent phagocytosis by neutrophils. In addition, complement with or without antibody may directly kill organisms by generation of the MAC on the cytoplasmic cell membranes. Not all bacteria are killed by complement deposition on their surfaces. The following three distinct avoidance mechanisms have been identified for these resistant bacteria: (1) shedding of the completed MAC from the bacterial surface, (2) the formation of noncovalent interactions that prevent the MAC from inserting into the bacterial outer membrane, and (3) the presence of a thick peptidoglycan layer that shields the vulnerable inner membrane from attack.

Complement and defense against viruses

Complement can neutralize virus infectivity by several mechanisms. When complement is fixed by binding of antibody to virus capsid or envelope proteins, complement infection of cells can be prevented by (1) interference with the ability of the virus to adsorb to or penetrate the cell; (2) disruption of the viral envelope by C^1 lysis, causing loss of infectivity; or (3) attachment of opsonized virus to phagocytic cells with consequent intracellular destruction. For some viruses (e.g., retroviruses) the alternate complement pathway may be activated in the absence of antibody.

INHERITED COMPLEMENT DEFICIENCIES

A number of inherited complement deficiencies have been described in humans. In general, the mode of inheritance is autosomal recessive. In the main, there is a strong association between complement deficiency and immune complex-like or lupus-like disorders and a strong association between C5, C6, C7, and C8 deficiencies and disseminated gonococcal and meningococcal infection. C2 deficiency is the most common, whereas absence of C3 is the most life threatening. Hereditary angioneurotic edema is an autosomal dominant condition in which little or no C1 inhibitor is produced. Patients suffer from continuous and uncontrolled C1 activation and its biologic consequences.

A genetically determined deficiency of the third component of complement has been identified in Brittany spaniels. Immunochemical methods show no detectable C3 in the serum of the affected dogs, and there is no evidence of an inhibitor of C3 in the serum. The C3 deficiency is transmitted as an autosomal recessive trait. Affected animals suffer recurrent episodes of life-threatening bacterial septicemias and, even when treated aggressively with appropriate chemotherapeutic regimens, suffer shortened life span due chiefly to the development of immune complex-type renal glomerular disease. Three allotypes (F, FS, and S) of canine C3 have been described. Known genetically determined complement deficiencies in laboratory animals are listed in Table 6-3.

Complement levels in domestic animal species

Except for guinea pigs and humans, very few detailed studies of complement systems in domestic animal species are available. Titrations for total hemolytic complement levels have been performed (see Chapter 8), and the optimal conditions as well as the amount of complement measured by this method vary widely with each species (Table 6-4).

Complement levels are depressed in newborns and young animals, patients exhibiting endotoxic shock, and in horses with clinically apparent equine infectious anemia. They are increased during neutropenic episodes in grey Collie dogs affected with cyclic *hematopoiesis*. Experimentally, malnutrition reduces the levels of many complement components but does not decrease total classical or alternate complement activity.

GENERAL METHODS FOR TITRATING COMPLEMENT

In theory, levels of individual complements could be measured by application of commercially available human or murine monoclonal reagents. Success of this approach has not been reported for domestic animal species. Except for avians, biologic activities of each component appear to be phylogenetically conserved. This fact makes titration of individual components in diseased or normal serum possible by construction of reactive intermediates (e.g., EAC142) using commercially available isolated human complement components.

Chelating substances such as 10 mM EDTA will remove ionized calcium and hence inhibit classical pathway activation without affecting the magnesium-independent alternate pathway. Two

Table 6-3 Recognized inherited complement deficiencies in animals

Deficiency	Species
C2	Guinea pig
C4	Guinea pig
C3	Brittany spaniels
C5	Mouse (B10D2)
C6	Rabbit

Table 6-4 Complement levels per milliliter of fresh serum in various animal species

Species	CH_{50} units/ml	Approximate range
Human	40	25-50
Guinea pig	270	200-350
Dog	3	32-96
Cat	—	70-150
Goat	45	18-75
Sheep	—	32-64
Pig	90	75-210
Horse	30	8-32
Rat	32	19-50
Rabbit	9	7-12
Mouse	0.7	.04-1.5

different methods of complement titration are in use: total hemolytic (CH_{100}) and 50% end point method (CH_{50}). Of these, the CH_{50} method is most accurate. A simple technique for measuring CH_{100} uses agar gel containing sensitized erythrocytes (EA).

Agar-EA mixture is poured on a slide or Petri plate, and a series of holes is punched in the agar. Fresh serum or dilutions are placed in the holes, and the plates are incubated for several hours at 37° C. The diameter of the ring of hemolysis of EA around the well is then measured and compared with dilution of a complement standard of known hemolytic potency. The method is similar to the Mancini technique for quantitation of immunoglobulin (see Chapter 9).

SUGGESTED READINGS

Abbas AK, Lichtman AH, Pober JS: *Complement In Cellular and molecular immunology*, Philadelphia, 1991, WB Saunders, pp 259-282.

Ahern JM, Feron DT: Structure and function of complement receptors, CR1 (CD35) and CR2 (CD21), *Adv Immunol* 46:183-219, 1989.

Barta O, Barta V: Canine hemolytic complement: optimal conditions for its titration, *Am J Vet Res* 34:653-657, 1973.

Barta O, Barta V, Shirley, RA, and others: Haemolytic assay of sheep serum complement, *Zbl Vet Med* 22:254-262, 1975.

Barta O, Oyekan PP: Feline (cat) hemolytic complement optimal testing conditions, *Am J Vet Res* 42:378-381, 1981.

Blum JR, Cork LC, Morris JM, and others: The clinical manifestations of a genetically determined deficiency of the third component of complement in the dog, *Clin Immunol Immunopathol* 34:304-315, 1985.

Colten HR: Biosynthesis of complement, *Adv Immunol* 22:67-118, 1976.

Fearon DT, Ruddy S, Schur PH, and others: Activation of the properdin pathway in patients with gram-negative bacteremia, *N Engl J Med* 292:937-940, 1975.

Gorman NT, Hobart MJ, and Lachmann PJ: Polymorphism of the third component of canine complement, *Vet Immunol Immunolpathol* 2:301-307, 1981.

Gotze O, Muller-Eberhard HJ: Thr C-3-activator system: an alternate pathway of complement activation, *J Exp Med* 134:90s-108s, 1971.

Hourcade D, Holers VM, Atkinson JP: The regulators of complement activation (RCA) gene clusters, *Adv Immunol* 45:381-416, 1989.

Joiner KA, Brown EJ, Frank MM: Complement and bacteria: chemistry and biology in host defense, *Ann Rev Immunol* 2:461-491, 1984.

Kolb W, Muller-Eberhard HJ: The membrane attack mechanism of complement: isolation and subunit composition of the C5b-9 complex, *J Exp Med* 141:724-735, 1975.

Liszewski MK, Post TW, Atkinson JP: Membrane cofactor protein (MCP or CD46): newest member of the regulators of complement activation gene cluster, *Ann Rev Immunol* 9:431-455, 1991.

Levy AL: Complement levels in mammals, *Proc Sci Exp Biol Med* 99:584-585, 1958.

Madewell BR: Serum complement level in dogs with neoplastic disease, *Am J Vet Res* 39:1373-1376, 1978.

Mayer MM: Membrane attack by complement (with comments on cell-mediated cytotoxicity). In Clark WR, Goldstein P, editors: *Mechanisms of cell-mediated cytotoxicity*, New York, 1982. Plenum Press, 193-216.

Morrison DC, Kline LF: Activation of the classical and properdin pathways of complement by bacterial lipopolysaccharides, *J Immunol* 118:362-369, 1977.

Movat HZ: *Inflammation, immunity and hypersensitivity*, New York, 1971, Harper and Row, pp 459-478.

Muller-Eberhard HJ: The membrane attack complex of complement, *Ann Rev Immunol* 4:503-528, 1986.

Ochs HD, Wedgewood RJ, Franks MM, and others: The role of complement in the induction of antibody responses, *Clin Exp Immunol* 53:208-216, 1983.

Osler AG, Sandberg AL: Alternate complement pathways, *Prog Allergy* 17:51-92, 1973.

Oyekan PP, Barta O,: Hemolytic assay for goat (caprine) and swine (porcine) complement, *Vet Immunol Immunopathol* 1:317-328, 1980.

Pang ASD, Aston WP: Alternate complement pathway in bovine serum: lysis of human erythrocytes, *Am J Vet Res* 38:355-357, 1977.

Podack ER, Esser AF, Biesecker G, and others: Membrane attack complex of complement: a structural analysis of its assembly, *J Exp Med* 151:301-313, 1980.

Porter RR, Reed KBM: The biochemistry of complement, *Nature* 275:699-704, 1978.

Roitt I, Brostoff J, Male D: Complement. In *Immunlogy*, St Louis, 1985, Mosby, pp 7.1-7.14.

Sakamoto M, Ishii S, Nishioka K, and others: Level of complement activity and components C1, C4, C2, and C3 in complement response to bacterial challenge in malnourished rats, *Infect Immun* 32:553-556, 1981.

Sandberg AL, Oliveira B, Osler AG: Two complement interaction sites in guinea pig immunoglobulins, *J Immunol*, 106:282-284, 1971.

Trail PA, Yang TJ, Cameron JA: Increase in the haemolytic complement activity of dogs affected with cyclic hematopoiesis, *Vet Immunol Immunopathol* 7:359-368, 1985.

Winkelstein JA, Cork LC, Griffin DE, and others: Genetically determined deficiency of the third component of complement in the dog, *Science* 212:1169-1170, 1981.

Wolfe JH, Halliwell REW: Total hemolytic complement values in normal and diseased dog populations, *Vet Immunol Immunopathol* 1:287-298, 1980.

7 Histocompatibility Antigens and Blood Group Antigens

MAJOR HISTOCOMPATIBLITY COMPLEX

Individual animals in each species, mammals and birds, are immunologically unique, which is the reason for incompatibility in tissue or organ transplants between anything other than identical twins. This uniqueness is governed by a series of genes called the major histocompatibility complex (MHC). This region of the chromosome codes for several proteins, which are expressed on body cells. The proteins, called histocompatibility antigens, are divided into three classes: I, II, and III. Class I and Class II proteins are associated with self/nonself discrimination and antigen recognition; Class III proteins are a somewhat more heterogeneous group of proteins, including complement components. Class I MHC antigens are expressed on the surface of all nucleated cells in the body; Class II antigens are expressed only on certain cells, such as macrophages, dendritic cells, bursal-derived (B) cells, and activated thymus-derived (T) cells—all immune system-related cells.

There is a large amount of polymorphism within the population of any given species as a result of the large number of genes coded for by the MHC complex. The most definitive work on the MHC has been performed in the murine system, where syngeneic strains (highly inbred mice, equivalent to identical twins) are available. The MHC in mice is referred to as the H-2 complex. It contains up to 50 genes on chromosome 17. These genes are organized into three loci, corresponding to the Class I, Class II, and Class III products for which they code. Within each locus are several regions; for example, the Class I MHC locus contains two regions: K and D. At each of these regions are a large number of potential alleles. In humans the MHC is referred to as the HLA (human leukocyte antigen) complex; it contains the same three loci for Class I, Class II, and Class III. The Class I loci contains three regions: A, B, and C; the Class II loci contains the D region.

Definition of haplotypes

The highly polymorphic nature of the MHC loci means that there are many different alleles, or alternate forms of a gene. Inheritance of the MHC alleles is codominant, so that the alleles from both maternal and paternal chromosomes are inherited, with the protein products expressed on the cells of the offspring. An individual is said to have a haplotype, which describes its own inherited set of alleles, from both parents. There will be expression of both maternal and paternal alleles on a single cell. In outbred populations, as occurs with most of our domestic animal species, each individual has a unique set of MHC alleles. The exception is identical twins (derived from a single embryo).

Protein products of the MHC

The MHC codes for proteins present on the cell membrane, as well as proteins that exist as soluble factors, are important in immune responses. Class I MHC molecules are coded for by genes within several loci. These are A, B, and C in humans, K and D/L in mice, and B through F in chickens. The Class I molecule consists of two polypeptide chains; the larger chain (alpha chain) is a 44-kilodalton (kD) glycoprotein, which has a transmembrane portion. It is present with a smaller chain, beta-2 microglobulin, which is invariant and is coded for on another chromosome. The polymorphism exists in the alpha chain, which is composed of three distinct domains. Two of the domains of the alpha chain interact to form a deep groove or cleft, which functions to bind peptides of 10 to 20 amino acids for presentation to CD8+ T lymphocytes (Figure 7-1).

Also coded for by the MHC complex is the Class II molecule. The Class II molecule consists of two chains, both transmembrane glycoproteins. These chains, 33 kD alpha and 28 kD beta, are associated in the cell membrane as a noncovalently bound heterodimer (Figure 7-1). Together they form an antigen-binding cleft for processed antigen. Class II molecules are expressed on B cells, macrophages, dendritic cells, activated T cells, and Langerhans cells. The function of Class II MHC molecules in antigen presentation in the immune response is discussed in Chapter 8.

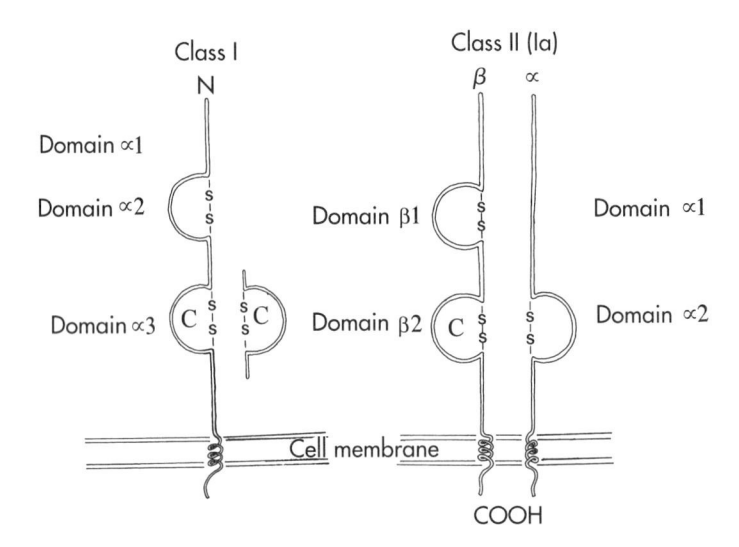

Figure 7-1 The MHC Class I antigen consists of two chains. The alpha (α) chain (approximately 45 kD) has three domains (α_1, α_2, and α_3) a short, hydrophobic transmembrane region, and a cytoplasmic region. The beta (β) chain is $beta_2$ microglobulin (12 kD). The MHC Class II antigen consists of two polypeptide chains, alpha (approximately 33 kD) and beta (approximately 28 kD). Both chains have two domains, a transmembrane segment, and a cytoplasmic region. An immunoglobulin-like region is present of both chains of the Class II and the alpha chain of Class I.

Detection of MHC polymorphism

The large array of alleles possible at each locus makes it very unlikely that the MHC molecules displayed on the surface of the cells of any two individuals would be identical. The practical significance of MHC type lies in several areas: (1) success of tissue transplantation relies on closely matched MHC type; (2) parentage disputes can be resolved by MHC typing of parents and siblings; and (3) genes on the MHC have an important role in immune response.

Serologic typing is performed for Class I MHC molecules. This test is a microcytotoxicity test, in which the cells to be typed are treated with a series of antibodies, each specific for a given MHC determinant, and then complement is added. Cells present in the wells that received an antibody that bound to MHC determinants will be lysed by the complement and will take up a blue dye that is added. The presence of stained cells indicates that the determinant specified by the particular typing serum put into that well is present on the cell. Performance of this test relies on the availability of a battery of typing sera. Originally these were obtained from several sources: multiparous females and individuals who have had numerous blood transfusions. With the advent of monoclonal antibodies, an additional source of antisera has become available.

Class II MHC molecules are typed using a cell-mediated assay, the mixed lymphocyte reaction. In this test the patient's cells are placed into a tissue culture well with typing cells that have been made metabolically inert by treatment with mitomycin C or irradiation. These typing cells have known MHC Class II molecules. When the responder cells (from the animal to be typed) come into contact with the MHC molecules that they do not express, they will undergo a blastogenic response, which involves increasing DNA synthesis in preparation for dividing. Addition of tritiated thymidine to the culture media at this time results in incorporation into the actively dividing cells. The amount of incorporated radioactive nucleotide is then measured and used to determine the reactivity of the responder cells to the typing cells. When a battery of typing cells is used, the specificities of the patient's cells can be determined.

Although these typing techniques are used clinically to determine the compatibility of tissue or organ grafts in patients, additional means are available to evaluate MHC polymorphism. The use of restriction fragment length polymorphisms (RFLPs) in determining differences in the DNA is being examined and employed with increased frequency in research and diagnostic laboratories.

Appropriate DNA probes are becoming available for use in detecting these polymorphisms.

MHC of domestic animal species

In recent years there have been many advances in our knowledge about the MHC of domestic animals. Although much work has been done in characterization of the MHC loci, there is still much left to be worked out. The immense clinical application of organ transplantation has driven the development of knowledge about human MHC, there is some application for these techniques in small animal medicine and as a model system for biomedical research. Of greater interest to the veterinary profession is the potential for determining disease associations with MHC. In veterinary medicine the potential of selective breeding to eliminate certain disease predispositions is a real possibility.

Bovine MHC

The MHC in cattle is called the bovine lymphocyte antigen complex and is abbreviated BoLA; Class I, Class II, and Class III loci have been identified. The BoLA region has been mapped to chromosome 23. Within the BoLA are two distinct subregions. The Class II region is designated BoLA-D and had been found to control the mixed lymphocyte reaction. The bovine Class II contains the DY, DR, and DQ (alpha and beta) loci. The BoLA Class II genes DQ and DR are organized similar to the Class II genes in humans and other species and are closely linked to the Class I genes. There is a subgroup of bovine Class II genes that is not closely linked to the Class I genes; it consists of a series of genes that are closely linked to each other. These are DOB, DYA, DYB, and Tcpb1. DYA appears to be a distinct bovine Class II gene. Another gene closely linked to DOB is DIB. This gene is also present in the Cervidae and Giraffidae families. Studies have been shown that there is little if any expression of BoLA-DIB and DOB on peripheral bovine lymphocytes.

The Class III locus is called Bf and codes for complement factor B, as in other species. Also present on the BoLA is a gene for cytochrome P450 steroid 21-hydroxylase (CYP21). Polymorphism has been demonstrated for CYP21.

Various methods are currently used to define polymorphism of the BoLA. Three typing methods have been applied: serology, RFLP, and isoelectric focusing (IEF). At the Fifth International Workshop on Bovine Lymphocyte Antigens held in 1992, 27 specificities were assigned to the Class I A locus. The remaining 26 specificities studied are still undecided and are designated as workshop specificities. Newly reported from this workshop are 13 Class II antigens defined serologically and 16 Class II specificities defined using IEF. RFLP has been used to study Class II specificities, and at least 32 different alleles are recognized using this technique.

Ovine MHC

The sheep MHC is referred to as OLA (ovine lymphocyte antigen). Class I, Class II, and Class III antigens have been identified. Using human cDNA probes on a Southern blot, Class I, alpha-DC, beta-DR, and C4 genes were identified. Polymorphism was demonstrated in Class I and Class II genes but not in Class III genes. Recently, genetic cloned material from sheep has been used to define sheep Class II genes by restriction mapping and hybridization with Class II probes. There appear to be both DQ and DR homologues in the sheep, but the existence of a DP homologue is still uncertain.

Goat MHC

The major lymphocyte antigen of goats (goat lymphocyte antigen), designated GLA, is incompletely understood. In the goat, two linked loci code for up to 10 serologically defined antigens.

Canine MHC

The dog has been used as an animal model for transplantation studies, and for this reason canine immunogenetics has received more attention than immunogenetics of some of the other domestic animal species. The canine MCH is called DLA (dog leukocyte antigen system). Three Class I loci have been identified by serologic testing: DLA-A, DLA-B and DLA-C. A single Class II locus, DLA-D, is also reported, originally defined by mixed lymphocyte culture reactivity. Genetic hybridization studies have revealed that the DLA-D locus contains at least five alpha genes (DRA, two DQA, DPA and DNA) and at least seven beta genes (two DRB, two DQB, two DPB, and DOB). There appears to be a single functional DQA gene, which has four alleles. Much of the polymorphism present in the D region is within the DRB region. At least ten alleles have been identified: DLA-DRB1, DW1, DW3, DW4, DW8, D4, D6, D7, D8 and D9. Unlike most other species, in which Class II determinants are expressed on a limited population of cells (B cells, monocytes, dendritic cells, endothelial cells, and activated T cells), there is evidence that DLA-B antigens are actually Class II gene products. It is unclear whether these gene products function as Class I or Class II molecules, Class III, coding for complement components, has also been identified and linked to the MHC in dogs.

Equine MHC

The horse is reported to have two Class I loci and one Class II locus. The A locus of Class I consists of at least nineteen alleles, whereas only a few alleles are identified for the second locus. The equine lymphocyte antigen (ELA) Class II molecules are similiar to those in other species, with an alpha chain and a beta chain expressed on the cell surface. Polymorphism has been demonstrated by serologic assays, mixed lymphocyte reaction, and RFLP. Polymorphism has been extensively studied in the DQB locus because of associations with certain equine diseases, such as sarcoids. Five allelic Class II specificities have been determined serologically in horses. Equine MHC Class II appears to be expressed on T lymphocytes. Experimental data suggest that Class II-positive equine T cells represent a memory cell population and that the presence of Class II can serve as a factor for differentiation of naive from memory cells.

Feline MHC

Definition of the MHC of the cat (FLA) has lagged behind that of other species because it has been difficult to obtain cytotoxic antibodies for serologic typing. Serum from multiparous females or from cats immunized with allogeneic cells has not yielded typing reagents. Recently investigators used a technique of multiple skin grafting to develop alloantisera against specificities present on a panel of outbred cat cells. With molecular analysis the feline MHC has been mapped to chromosome B2. Class II reactivity has been demonstrated using the mixed lymphocyte reaction. A single Class I and a single Class II locus are reported at this time. A Class III locus has not yet been mapped to the FLA.

Avian MHC

The MHC genes of chickens are cell-surface glycoproteins, identified as Class I (B through F), Class II (B through L), and Class IV (B through G). The B through G molecules were first identified as erythrocyte alloantigens within the B blood group of the chicken. They have since been identified on many cells other than erythrocytes, such as caecal tonsils.

Porcine MHC

The swine lymphocyte antigen (SLA) appears to contain 3 loci that code for Class I antigens (SLA-A, SLA-B AND SLA-C). Twenty-six Class I alleles have been defined. One genetic locus appears to control the mixed lymphocyte culture (MHC Class II) reaction.

Function of MHC antigens

The significance of Class I antigen became evident when it was discovered that viral-specific cytotoxic T cells (CD8+) would kill only virus-infected target cells that possessed the same Class I antigen as the immune T lymphocyte. This phenomenon is called histocompatibility restriction. Immune CD8+ lymphocytes recognize two factors on virus-infected cells. One factor recognized is the viral antigen expressed on the infected cell plasma membrane, and the second factor recognized is the Class I antigen.

Helper T lymphocytes (CD4+) also recognize two signals on the antigen-processing cells; one is antigen and the other is the Class II MHC molecule. Helper T cells are histocompatibility restricted by the Class II antigen. Table 7-1 summarizes the structure and function of Class I and Class II MHC antigens.

Generally, Class I restriction pertains to endogenous antigen, such as virus or other intracytoplasmic propagating agents, whereas Class II restriction pertains to exogenous antigen, such as bacteria that are engulfed by phagocytic cells and processed in phagosomes before presentation on the cell surface. More detail on the involvement

Table 7-1 Characteristics of antigens produced by the major histocompatibility complex

Characteristics	Class I	Class II
Physical properties	Alpha chain: 45 kD glycoprotein Beta$_2$—microglobulin	Alpha chain: 33 kD Beta chain: 28 kD Heterodimer
Tissue distribution	All nucleated cells	Antigen-presenting cells: macrophages, Langerhans' cells, dendritic cells, activated T cells (species differences)
Function	Restricts CD8+ T-cell antigen recognition	Restricts CD4+ T-cell antigen recognition
Detection	Serologic: microcytotoxicity	Mixed lymphocyte culture Restriction fragment length polymorphism (RFLP)

of histocompatibility antigens in the immune response is presented in Chapter 8.

Disease resistance and MHC

The MHC Class II gene is referred to as the immune response (Ir) gene. As stated, the MHC molecules function in immune response. Over 25 years ago it was discovered that MHC Class II genes were "immune response" genes in mice and guinea pigs. The incidence for associating the Ir gene with the MHC was obtained from studies testing the ability of inbred mice and inbred guinea pigs to produce antibody to certain synthetic antigens. For example, it was found that a certain strain of guinea pig (strain 13) failed to produce antibody to dinitrophenyl-poly-L-lysine homopolymer. Other inbred strains of guinea pig could produce antibody to this synthetic peptide. Subsequent experiments showed that the Ir gene that regulates the antibody response to this synthetic peptide was inherited as a single dominant allele. These studies suggest that the immune response to any one of 10^6 to 10^9 antigens is under genetic control. Furthermore, the overt susceptibility of given animals to certain diseases may be explained by the inadequacy of Ir gene functions. In cattle the ability of Norwegian Red cattle to respond to human serum albumin was shown to be associated with BoLA-W16 and BoLA-W6. High responders to human serum albumin were also shown to be more susceptible to mastitis. In studies on enzootic bovine leukosis, cattle with BoLA-W14 had a negative correlation with the presence of antibodies to bovine leukemia virus, BLV-gp51.

In the human species there are at least forty diseases that have some association with a particular HLA haplotype. Many of these are hormonal, or neurologic or chronic diseases resulting from an autoimmune or viral etiology. In domestic animals some of the earliest discovered associations were found in the avian species: B2 complex of chickens with susceptibility to the Rous sarcoma virus and Marek's disease. An association has also been found between scrapie in sheep and antigens of the OLA. In sheep there is a gene called Scr, which governs resistance/susceptibility to scrapie; this gene is linked to the OLA complex. In cattle there are several diseases associated with BoLA antigens: susceptibility to theileriasis, bovine leukemia, and mastitis. Resistance to ticks has also been linked to BoLA. As mentioned earlier, in horses ELA is linked to susceptibility to the development of a retroviral-induced fibroblastic tumor (sarcoid). Resistance to the development of abscess after infection with *Corynebacterium pseudotuberculosis* has been associated with OLA in sheep. The SLA in swine has been linked to increased resistance to encystment of the larval *Trichinella spiralis* parasite.

BLOOD GROUPS AND TRANSFUSION

Human blood group systems: background

In 1900 Landsteiner demonstrated that human erythrocyte antigens are not identical in all people. His work was initiated by the observation that a transfusion of donor blood to recipient was sometimes followed by a serious transfusion reaction. Using cross-matching procedures i.e., mixing donor erythrocytes with recipient serum, he was able to delineate four different categories of reaction. Although no comparable system exists in animals, discussion of his findings is helpful in illustrating the principle of isoantibody formation. Persons of type A possess the blood group antigen A on the red blood cell surfaces. Similarly, type B individuals possess antigenically distinct blood group B substances. Persons with AB blood type have both antigens, whereas type O individuals lack both antigens.

Incompatible blood transfusions, such as infusion of type A blood into a type B recipient, result in a type II hypersensitivity reaction. Anti-A antibodies in recipient plasma recognize the A antigen as foreign and bind to the offending erythrocytes. Complexing of antibody and antigen in the circulation activates the complement sequence, and a donor erythrocyte hemolytic episode follows. In addition, agglutinated erythrocytes form microthrombi in the bloodstream, which results in circulatory embarrassment. Patients show respiratory distress, disorientation, and cardiovascular collapse that can be fatal. Thus, any beneficial effects of transfusion are obviated by this reaction.

Blood group antigens have been isolated and biochemically characterized. Blood group substances are not unique to erythrocytes; that is, they have been identified in mucous secretions, saliva, gastrointestinal fluids, and ovarian cyst fluids. All antigens studied are water-soluble, large molecular weight complexes consisting of long-chain polysaccharides and polypeptides. Antigenic specificity resides in the spatial configuration of sugar components at the end of the carbohydrate chain.

Previous immunogenic exposure to foreign blood group antigens results in the generation of antibodies to them; yet, in humans isoantibodies are present in the absence of an initial transfusion of incompatible blood. Abundant experimental evidence indicates that the antigenic determinants of the ABO system are shared by many bacterial cell walls and plant cells. It is likely that natural exposure to these antigens during the neonatal period is responsible for immunogenic stimulation. Thus the ordinarily beneficial production of bacterial agglutinins is likely to be responsible for the iatrogenic transfusion reactions.

The ABO blood groups are the dominant antigenic system on human erythrocytes. However, many other minor blood group systems, including allelic differences of A and B antigens, are described.

Canine blood groups

In the old nomenclature, the canine blood group antigens were designated A1, A2, B, C, D, F, Tr, and HE. These original seven groups have been expanded to eleven blood group systems. Now blood group antigens include J, K, L, M, and N. Blood typing in dogs is done using agglutination, hemolysis, and antiglobulin testing, depending on the antigen-antibody system being identified. Blood typing of dogs is usually done before blood is used for transfusion because of the Tr antigen, for which many dogs have a naturally occurring antibody (similiar to the ABO system of humans). The A antigen is important because it is highly immunogenic, and an A-negative dog, once transfused with A-positive blood, will usually have anti-A antibodies present. Rarely, an A-negative dog will have naturally occurring anti-A antibodies present. CEA-1 and CEA-2 are alleles corresponding to A1 and A2. CEA-1 is inherited as an autosomal dominant characteristic over CEA-2. Recently a third allele, A3, has been identified. Most of the remaining erythrocyte antigens are inherited as simple mendelian dominant traits.

Bovine blood groups

The bovine species possesses the most complex of the blood groups of domestic animals. So far, at least eleven blood groups have been identified: A, B, C, F, J, L, M, R', S, Z, and T. The B group in cattle was originally described in the 1950s, and the polymorphism of its alleles has been used extensively by breed registries for parentage confirmation. The B group alone has at least 600 alleles. The B group is complex in that some of the antigens are inherited as a phenogroup. The J group is actually a soluble lipid that adsorbs onto the surface of the erythrocytes. Cattle have either high or low levels of the J substance on their erythrocytes; when an animal has low amounts of the J substance, it very often has circulating anti-J antibodies. Occasionally a J-negative animal receiving J-positive blood will undergo transfusion reaction. However, as a general rule, transfusion reactions are of minor consequence in this species. An interesting exception was a problem induced by veterinarians. Formerly, anaplasmosis vaccines consisted of formalin-treated whole dried blood obtained from anaplasmosis-carrier animals. Immunization of cattle with this vaccine preparation resulted in the production of antibody to red blood cell antigens contained in the vaccine. This was of little consequence to the animal itself; however, it often produced disastrous consequences in suckling calves. A calf born to a mother previously immunized with the vaccine could have the same blood type as the blood type contained in the vaccine. Accordingly, the isoantibody produced as a result of vaccination was passively transferred to the calf during the suckling period. This resulted in a neonatal isoerythrolysis syndrome similar to that observed in the horse. The A and F systems were most frequently implicated in this phenomenon. Following recognition of this problem, the source of the vaccine was changed.

Equine blood groups

Eight separate blood groups have been identified in the equine species. As with other species, single transfusions of incompatible blood are usually without consequence. The internationally recognized blood groups of the horse are A, C, D, K, P, Q, and U.

Blood-grouping information is of a major value in predicting the likelihood that a disease known as hemolytic disease of newborn foals, or neonatal isoerythrolysis, will occur. The syndrome is initiated by the inheritance and expression of stallion-derived erythrocyte antigens in the foal *in utero*. The pregnant mare, lacking these antigens, thus produces isoantibodies to these antigens. The first pregnancy is usually without adverse effect on the foal. However, during the birth process mares are exposed to foal erythrocyte antigens. Subsequent pregnancies involving the same stallion or an antigenically similar sire predisposes the newborn to isoerythrolysis. The foal acquires the isoantibodies by absorbtion in the alimentary tract in the neonatal period. A type II hypersensitivity reaction ensues with resultant erythrocyte destruction. Approximately six to forty-eight hours after birth, the foal is anemic, depressed, weak, and unable to suckle, with slow, shallow respiration. If the foal survives several days, icterus is observed. Postmortem examination of affected foals shows anemia and icterus. The spleen and liver are enlarged.

The blood group antigens most often associated with neonatal isoerythrolysis are A and Q. Blood typing of mare and stallion can predict the occurrence of sensitization. In subsequent matings the development of high titers specific to foreign blood group antigen can be monitored by Coombs' antiglobulin test.

Rapid diagnosis of neonatal isoerythrolysis can be performed by mixing foal or stallion erythrocytes with mare serum or colostrum. Agglutination occurs if isoantibodies are present. Also, erythrocytes from affected foals may spontaneously agglutinate in vitro and are Coombs positive.

A mare with a history of neonatal isoerythrolysis should be monitored closely during gestation. A rising isoantibody titer indicates active *in utero* immunization and a high likelihood of disease induction in the foal. The disease can be completely prevented in newborn foals by preventing colostrum ingestion until intestinal closure has occurred, usually within forty-eight hours after birth. Horsemen often keep frozen isoantibody-free colostrum in the stable for use in these situations. In the event of accidental consumption of the mare's colostrum, the foal can receive the washed erythrocytes of the mare as a replacement for erythrocytes lost to lysis.

Swine blood groups

Fifteen separate blood group antigens (A to O) have been identified in the swine species. The A blood group system has a complex system for antigen expression. The two antigens, A and O, are under the control of another genetic locus, which has alleles for secretion (S) and nonsecretion (s). For the A or O allele to be expressed on the erythrocyte surface, the S allele must be present. Hemolytic disease of newborn pigs, like anaplasmosis in calves, is an iatrogenic disease. Isoantibodies were induced by the use of an old-fashioned crystal violet hog cholera vaccine containing swine erythrocyte and tissue antigens. As with cattle vaccinated against anaplasmosis, the isoantibodies induced are of importance only in suckling piglets. This disease is of historical significance, because this vaccine is no longer in use. Some reported alloantibodies have been the source of hemolytic disease in suckling pigs.

Recently, susceptibility to porcine stress syndrome, a disorder that it characterized by sudden death following stress or physical exertion, has been linked to the H system of blood groups in swine.

Feline blood groups

There are two systems recognized in the cat: A and B.

Caprine and ovine blood groups

Six genetic systems of goat erythrocyte antigens have been recognized: A, B, C, R, E, and F. The B system is most complex, with at least 21 different alleles identified. The E system has only 2 alleles, but four possible phenotypes as a result of codominance. In the sheep system A, B, C, M, R, and X are recognized. The A system is quite similar in the sheep and in the goat. The hemolytic test is used for goat and sheep red blood cell antigen identification.

SUGGESTED READINGS

Albert ED, Erickson VM, Graham TC and others: Serology and genetics of the DLA system. I. Establishment of specificities, *Tissue Antigens* 3:417-430, 1973.

Davies C, Joosten I, Andersson, L, and others: Polymorphism of bovine MHC class II genes: Joint Report of the Fifth International Bovine Lymphocyte Antigen (BoLA) Workshop, Interlaken, Switzerland, August 1, 1992, *Anim Genet* (in press).

Davies C, Joosten I, Andersson, L, and others: Polymorphism of bovine MHC class I genes: Joint Report of the Fifth International Bovine Lymphocyte Antigen (BoLA) Workshop, Interlaken, Switzerland, August 1, 1992, *Anim Genet* (in press).

Demmock CK, Clark IA, Hill MWM: The experimental production of haemolytic disease of the newborn in calves, *Res Vet Sci* 20:244-248, 1976.

Deverson EV, Wright H, Watson S, and others: Class II major histocompatibility complex genes of the sheep, *Anim Genet* 22:211-225, 1991.

Doxiadis I, Krumbacher AK, Neefjes JJ, and others: Biochemical evidence that the DLA-B locus codes for a Class II determinant expressed on all canine peripheral blood lymphocytes, *Exp Clin Immunogenet* 6:219-224, 1989.

Hruban V, Simon M, Hradecky J, and others: Linkage of the pig main histocompatibility complex and the J blood group system, *Tissue Antigens* 7:267-271, 1976.

Kaufman J: The B-G multigene family of the chicken major histocompatibility complex, *Crit Rev Immunol* 11:113-143, 1991.

Lamont SJ: Immunogenetics and the major histocompatibility complex, *Vet Immunol Immunopathol* 30:121-127, 1991.

Madden KB, Murrell KD, Lunney JK: *Trichinella spiralis*: major histocompatibility complex-associated elimination of encysted muscle larvae in swine, *Exp Parasit* 70:443-451, 1990.

Millot P, Chatelain J, Dautheville C, and other: Sheep major histocompatibility (OLA) complex: linkage between a scrapie susceptibility/resistance locus and the OLA complex in Ile-de-France sheep progenies, *Immunogenetics* 27:1-11, 1988.

Monos DS, Wolf B, Radka SF, and others: Equine class II MHC antigens: identification of two sets of epitopes using anti-human monoclonal antibodies, *Tissue Antigens* 34: 111-120, 1989.

Nguyen TC: Genetic systems of red cell blood groups in goats, *Anim Genet* 21:233-245, 1990.

Ostrand-Rosenberg S: Topology of bovine red cell antigens as a function of the organization of their genes, *Immunogenetics* 3:53-64, 1976.

Sarmiento UM, DeRose S, Sarmiento JI, and others: Allelic variation in the DQ subregion of the canine major histocompatibility complex: II DBQ, *Immunogenetics* 37(2):148-152, 1993.

Sarmiento UM, Sarmiento JI, Storb, R: Allelic variation in the DR subregion of the canine major histocompatibility complex, *Immunogenetics* 32:13-19, 1990.

Sarmienio UM, Storb RF: RFLP analysis of DLA class I genes in the dog, *Tissue Antigens* 34:158-163, 1989.

Symons M, Bell K: Canine blood groups: description of 20 specificities, *Anim Genet* 23:509-515, 1992.

Van der Poel JJ, Groenen MAM, Dijkhof RJM, and others: The nucleotide sequence of the bovine MHC class II alpha genes: DRA, DQA, and DYA, *Immunogenetics* 31:29-36, 1990.

Winkler C, Schultz A, Cevario S, and others: Genetic characterization of FLA, the cat major histocompatibility complex, *Proc Natl Acad Sci* 86:943-947, 1989.

8 Immune Response

The ability of the immune system to respond specifically to antigen forms the basis for acquired immunity, the foundation on which vaccination strategies are formed. Initial exposure to antigen (virus, bacteria, parasite, or other) calls forth a primary immune response, which serves to prime the immune system and to create a system of immunologic memory, such that subsequent exposure to the same antigen will elicit a greater and longer-lasting immune response than the initial exposure, and will do so in a much more rapid time frame.

For years immunologists have debated over a variety of hypotheses to describe how the immune system is able to retain specificity when there is such an immense array of diverse antigenic specificities in nature. The hypothesis that was finally accepted was that of clonal selection proposed by Sir McFarland Burnet in 1957. According to the clonal selection hypothesis, each individual has a complete array of progenitor B lymphocytes, each with surface receptors capable of reacting with a single specificity present in nature, thereby providing a cumulative ability to detect all possible specificities. When introduced into a host species, antigen selects a specific clone of lymphocytes and, by reacting with it, stimulates division and an increase in cell numbers (clonal expansion). This explains why the secondary immune response is more rapid than the primary response; there are more antigen-reactive cells present to react, and these cells are further differentiated from those present in the antigen-naive animal.

This chapter explores the immune response, from processing of antigen-presenting cells to interaction with thymus-derived (T) and bursal derived (B) lymphocytes, as well as the importance and role of cytokines in these cellular interactions. The immune response is discussed in three major phases: the cognitive phase (antigen recognition), the activation phase (responses of lymphocytes after specific reaction with antigen), and the effector phase (functional elimination of antigen by antigen-stimulated cells).

ANTIGEN RECOGNITION AND PRESENTATION

T lymphocytes

Presentation of antigen to lymphocytes involves processing of the antigen by antigen-presenting cells and presentation of that antigen to surface receptors on B and T lymphocytes. Antigen presentation is different for B and T lymphocytes. B lymphocytes need only bind the appropriate epitope with the hypervariable region of the antibody molecule that serves as membrane receptor. However, T lymphocytes recognize antigen in the context of a major histocompatibility complex (MHC) molecule. The CD4+ T lymphocyte (helper T cell) requires presentation of antigen, along with recognition of an MHC Class II molecule on the antigen-presenting cell. The importance of MHC Class II identity between the antigen-presenting cell and the antigen-specific T cell was recognized in the 1970s and is termed MHC restriction. This simply means that for a helper T cell to respond to antigen, that antigen must be present on the cell membrane of another cell in association with an MHC Class II molecule that is identical to its own. Under normal circumstances this would be the natural course of events in vivo. However, in experiments using different inbred strains of mice as sources of antigen-presenting cells and T lymphocytes, it was clearly demonstrated that antigen-primed T cells from one strain of mice will not react with antigen-primed cells from a strain of mice with different MHC Class II antigens, even though the cells are sensitized to the specific antigen.

There are several cell types that can function as antigen-presenting cells. These cells have the ability to process antigen after taking it inside the cell and to display MHC Class II molecules on their surface membrane—two essential criteria for antigen presentation. Antigen-presenting cells include macrophages (mononuclear phagocytic cells), B lymphocytes, Langerhans' cells in the skin, and dendritic cells in the spleen and lymph nodes.

Antigen presentation begins with endocytosis of the antigen. Large antigens, such as bacteria or parasitic organisms, are dealt with by the macrophages. These cells often use Fc receptors and/or C3b receptors to attach to the opsonized antigen. B lymphocytes appear to be particularly efficient at presentation of protein antigens that are present in very small amounts, because the immunoglobulin receptors have a high affinity for the antigen and serve to concentrate it to the cell. Entry of the antigen into the cell follows attachment; this occurs by phagocytosis in the case of the macrophage and by endocytosis of receptors with bound protein antigen in the case of the B lymphocytes. Antigen processing proceeds readily in the low pH environment until a processed form of the antigen has been created. The peptide fragments so created bind to the MHC Class II molecules in the peptide cleft of the molecule (Figure 8-1), which accommodates from 10 to 20 amino acids. Binding of the peptide to the MHC molecule appears to occur within the cytoplasm by some interaction of vesicles containing newly synthesized MHC molecules with endosomes containing the peptides. Exactly how this interaction occurs is not completely understood.

Recognition of the antigenic peptide on the surface of the antigen-presenting cell involves interaction of receptors. The CD4+ helper T cell has an antigen receptor that is specific for the peptide. This T-cell receptor is a heterodimer of two polypeptide chains, alpha and beta. These chains each contain a variable and a constant regional domain, held together by disulfide bonds (Figure 8-2). Elucidation of the nature of the T-cell receptor for antigen has been relatively recent, although immunologists were reasonably sure that it had some similarity to the immunoglobulin molecule in that it must have a variable region to allow for diversity and specificity of the immune response. The N terminal of each chain sticks out from the cell, and the C terminal is embedded in the cytoplasm. This T-cell receptor provides for antigen peptide binding.

Another series of cell-surface molecules assists in antigen recognition. The CD3 complex consists of five separate integral membrane molecules that associate with each other and with the T-cell re-

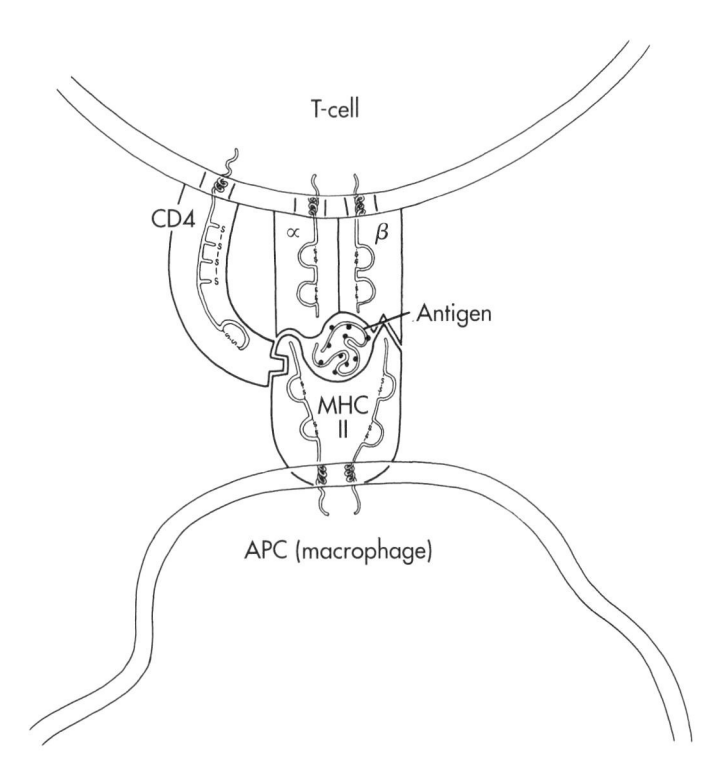

Figure 8-1 The interaction between the antigen-presenting cell (APC) and the T cell involves presentation of antigenic peptide held in the cleft formed by the alpha (α) and beta (β) chains of the MHC Class II molecule on the APC to the alpha and beta chains of the T-cell receptor. The CD4 molecule on the membrane of the helper T cell stabilizes this interaction and assists in signal transduction by binding to the MHC Class II molecule.

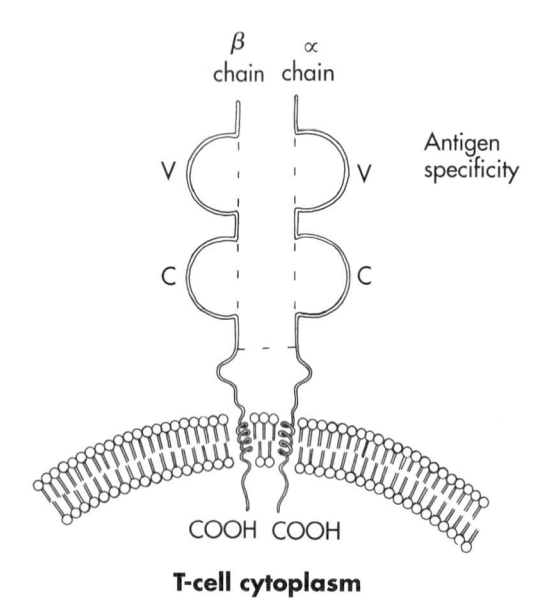

Figure 8-2 The alpha-beta T-cell receptor for antigen consists of two polypeptide chains with the transmembrane segments and variable (V) and constant (C) regions. The specificity for antigen is determined by the amino acids in the variable regions.

ceptor noncovalently. The CD3 complex is thought to function in signal transduction for the alpha/beta chains. The CD3 complex is also present on a small population of lymphocytes that does not express the alpha/beta chains but does express a related receptor, gamma and delta chains. The role of gamma/delta T cells in the immune system is currently being studied.

Recognition of the MHC Class II molecule is brought about through binding of the Class II molecule to the CD4 molecule on the helper T-cell membrane. The CD4 molecule is a monomer, consisting of a single polypeptide chain with a hydrophobic transmembrane portion. It has no variable region and hence does not bind directly to antigen. The CD4 molecule functions in cell adhesion. It has a high affinity for the Class II molecule and hence is important in stabilizing the binding of the antigen/MHC Class II to the T cell. It is also thought to play a role in signal transduction.

In summary, the alpha/beta T-cell receptor binds to the antigenic peptide lying in a groove of the MHC Class II molecule, which itself is bound and stabilized by the CD4 molecule. This binding initiates a signal that is transmitted throughout the cell membrane by the CD3 complex. It is thought that the positive charge of the transmembrane lysine-rich portion of the alpha/beta chains interacts with the negatively charged (aspartic acid rich) transmembrane portions of the CD3 complex to instigate this signal transduction.

For many years T cells were differentiated from B cells in vitro by their ability to bind sheep red blood cells, thereby producing rosette formations. The development of monoclonal antibodies as reagents has now made T-cell rosettes a curiosity of the past. However, it is now known that the T-cell molecule that binds sheep erythrocytes is called CD2. This cell-surface glycoprotein is present on more than 90% of T lymphocytes and serves nicely as a pan T-cell marker. The CD2 molecule is thought to function in cell adhesion because of its ability to bind to LFA-3 (leukocyte function antigen), which is present on a variety of cells.

B lymphocytes

Mature B lymphocytes express membrane-bound mu and delta immunoglobulin molecules. They are capable of reacting with antigen. When multivalent antigen binds to these receptors, a process is initiated in which the receptors are cross-linked and then begin to coalesce, finally forming a cap at one pole of the cell. This process is easily understood when Singer's fluid mosaic model of the phospholipid cell membrane with proteins floating freely is remembered. After capping, the antigen-bound surface immunoglobulins are endocytosed. Peptide fragments are generated as described earlier for antigen-presenting cells, and they are expressed along with MHC Class II molecules on the cell surface. This process serves two purposes: it presents antigen to helper T cells and begins the activation process for the B cells. The activated T cells, through their production of cytokines, send further activation and differentiation signals to the B cells.

A few antigens, primarily nonprotein in composition (e.g., lipopolysaccharide), do not require T-cell help and are called T-cell–independent antigens. These antigens generally induce only an IgM response, because helper T-cell cytokines are necessary for the process of B-cell differentiation into cells that produce other isotypes. Bacterial lipopolysaccharide is a polyclonal B-cell activator. It is able to induce B-cell proliferation without T-cell help. It is reasonable to assume that this is an important early defense mechanism against bacterial disease, leading to activation of B cells early in infection before clones of reactive T cells have been expanded.

T-cell help consists of the secretion of cytokines and is an important cell-cell interaction between the T cells and B cells. This cognate interaction between the T cells and B cells is most important in the primary immune response or in a response that has been dormant for a long time and in which the B cells are in a resting state.

T-cell–derived cytokines are important in several stages of development of humoral immune responses. B-cell stimulation and entry into the cycle of cell division (G0 to G1) is dependent on the action of interleukin (Il)-4. Proliferation of these cells is then further mediated by Il-4, Il-5, and Il-2. It is thought that during the primary immune response, when numbers of clonally expanded helper T cells are fewer, macrophage-derived cytokines, such as Il-1 and Il-6, play a role in stimulation of B-cell proliferation. The differentiation of B cells into antibody-producing plasma cells is further dependent on cytokines (Figure 8-3).

In the human and murine systems two subsets of CD4+ helper T lymphocytes are recognized: Th1 and Th2. These cells produce either predominantly Il-2 and gamma interferon (Th1) or Il-4 and Il-5 (Th2). These cytokines have different effects on B-cell proliferation: gamma interferon favors IgG2a production, whereas Il-4 favors IgE and IgG1 production, and Il-5 favors IgA production. The relative abundance of these cytokine signals is thought to play a crucial role in the final differentiation of antibody-producing plasma cells. These data are primarily from studies performed on cloned murine T cells. However, the cloning and expression of interleukins from domestic animal species is well underway. Homologues for Il-2, gamma interferon, Il-4, etc., have been reported for several domestic species. This work will facilitate development of an understanding of the role of cytokines in immune responses of interest to veterinary medicine.

LYMPHOCYTE ACTIVATION
T lymphocytes

Binding of antigen/MHC by the appropriate T cell is one initiating factor in the process of lymphocyte activation. Costimulation by appropriate cytokines is another important step in the activation process. Il-1 is produced by the mononuclear cell and binds to a receptor on the T lymphocyte. The activation interleukin (Il-2) gene transcription occurs within an hour of T-cell receptor stimulation, and Il-2 is both produced by and stimulates T lymphocytes. Il-2, an autocrine growth factor, binds to Il-2 receptors that are induced on the membrane of the T cell after binding of the T-cell receptor to antigen. Thus there is an increase of

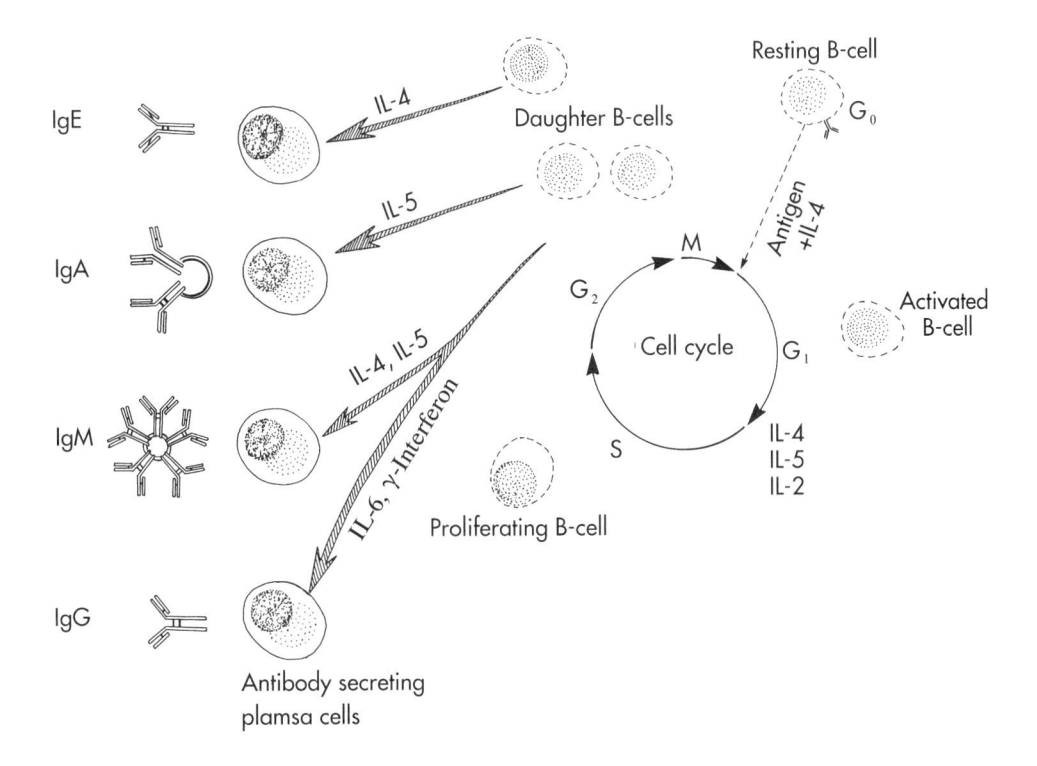

Figure 8-3 Stimulation of B-cell differentiation requires antigen and T-cell-derived cytokines. A resting B cell in the G_0 phase will be moved into the G_1 phase of the cell cycle after interaction with antigen and binding interleukin 4 (IL-4). Under the continued influence of cytokines, daughter B cells further differentiate into plasma cells producing IgM, IgG, IgA, and IgE. The type of interleukin produced influences the predominant isotype of antibody produced (e.g., IL-4 elicits IgE; IL-5 elicits IgA).

Il-2 receptors, which bind the newly secreted Il-2. The Il-2 receptor consists of two integral membrane proteins, each of which has a high affinity for Il-2.

These activation signals for T cells result in mitotic division and expansion of the clone of T cells reactive with the specific antigen used in stimulation. This expanded clone of T cells produces additional lymphokines, which influence the development and proliferation of B cells.

B lymphocytes

The end result of B-cell activation is the production of plasma cells that secrete immunoglobulins. The process of B-cell differentiation begins with the binding of antigen to the immunoglobulin receptor molecules on the B-lymphocyte membrane. A second signal received from helper T lymphocytes is required for primary immune response to a protein antigen. These secreted interleukins are important for proliferation and differentiation to proceed. The secondary immune response generally requires only the binding of antigen to B-cell receptor molecules.

B-cell differentiation begins with the entry of the resting mature B cell into the cell cycle. The first trigger for this transition is the binding of antigen to the B-cell receptors. Resting cells are quiescent and begin to synthesize more RNA and become metabolically more active after binding to antigen. Il-4, produced by helper T cells, aids in this transition from G0 to the G1 stage of cell division. Entry into the S phase of the cell cycle, proliferation, is dependent on the action of several T-cell cytokines (Il-2, Il-4, Il-5 [Figure 8-3], and probably to some degree Il-6) and on macrophage-derived factors, tumor necrosis factor (TNF), and Il-1.

The development of B cells into antibody-producing plasma cells occurs after the events just described. A characteristic of the immune response is that a single plasma cell produces a single type of antibody (i.e., a single isotype and idiotype). Which isotype is produced depends on several factors. The nature of the antigen itself is important, since some antigens preferentially induce a particular type of immune response (e.g., parasite antigens elicit IgE). Isotype selection is based on the type of helper T cell that is stimulated, which determines which cytokines and their relative concentrations are produced.

EFFECTOR PHASE

The effector phase of the immune response is the end result of antigen recognition and lymphocyte activation. Humoral immune defense mechanisms include a wide variety of antibody functions. These include complement fixation with subsequent lysis or phagocytic uptake of the target, virus neutralization, toxin neutralization, opsonization, and antibody-dependent cellular cytotoxicity. Cellular effector mechanisms include T-cell cytotoxicity and macrophage activation.

T-cell cytotoxicity

T-cell effector mechanisms include cytotoxic T-cell activity. The cytotoxic T lymphocyte is a T cell that carries the CD8 surface molecule. These cells also carry the T-cell receptor for antigen. Recognition of antigen by the cytotoxic T cell requires concurrent recognition of a homologous MHC Class I determinant on the target cell surface. Most antigens that are targeted by cytotoxic T cells are synthesized within the cytoplasm of the target cell and then associate with the Class I molecule on the target-cell surface. A good example of such an antigen is viral peptide. Killing of virus-infected cells by cytotoxic T cells is an important defense mechanism.

Killing of a target cell by a cytotoxic T cell involves two signals: binding of specific antigen on the surface of a target cell and production of cytokines by antigen-specific CD4+ helper T cells. Cytokines that are important include Il-4, Il-6, and gamma interferon. Binding of the T-cell receptor to the antigen on the cell surface is accompanied by interaction of the accessory molecule CD8 on the T-cell surface with the MHC Class I molecule on the target cell surface. As described for helper T-cell–antigen interaction, the accessory molecules are thought to assist in signal transduction.

Once activated, the cytotoxic T cell secretes a pore-forming protein that is contained within intracellular granules. This pore-forming protein, perforin, polymerizes to form a channel in the cell membrane, quite similar to the formation of channels in the cell membrane after a complement-mediated cell lysis reaction. After release of the pore-forming protein, the cytotoxic cell may move away from the target, leaving it to undergo lysis. The cytotoxic cell remains viable and can kill other target cells.

Macrophage activation

Macrophages become activated and more efficient killers of phagocytosed organisms after they are acted on by T-cell–derived cytokines. One such cytokine, gamma interferon, augments the ability of macrophages to engulf bacteria by increasing the expression of Fc receptors for opsonizing antibody. Gamma interferon also increases the expression of oxidative enzymes that are important in intracellular killing. Some bacterial pathogens are able to grow and thrive within the cytoplasm of macrophages after engulfment. These organisms, called facultative intracellular bacteria, are readily killed by activated macrophages. Some examples of these bacteria are Listeria, Mycobacterium, Salmonella, and Brucella.

Humoral response

The production of antibodies of varied specificities and different isotypes provides for a variety of effector mechanisms. Antibodies of the IgG and IgM class are capable of binding to circulating antigen and forming immune complexes, which may be removed by the reticuloendothelial system. Occasionally the size and persistence of these complexes gives rise to pathologic sequelae (see Chapter 14). IgG and IgM can also fix complement or lyse or damage invading pathogens. When the antigen is a toxin, the binding of antibody can neutralize the toxicity and prevent clinical signs of toxicity. In cooperation with phagocytic cells, antibody can bind by the Fc portion to Fc receptors and can facilitate engulfment and eventual destruction of organisms bound by the Fab pieces of the antibody. This process of opsonization is important in antibacterial immunity.

The antibody response to virus antigens, when directed against surface proteins, can be an effective way to neutralize infectivity. This is brought about by binding of the neutralizing antibody to the surface protein responsible for adsorption of the virus to the target cell. IgA produced along mucosal surfaces is particularly effective at neutralization of viral infectivity at the portal of entry.

The induction of an IgE response, although thought to be important in immunity to some parasite infections, may cause adverse responses by eliciting a type 1 hypersensitivity response (see Chapter 13).

SUGGESTED READING

Abbas AK, Lichtman, AH, Rober JS: *Cellular and molecular immunology*, Philadelphia, 1991, W B Saunders, pp 113-137.
Kuby J: *Immunology*, New York, 1992, W H Freeman, pp 271-294.
Roitt I, Brostoff J, Male D: *Immunology*, ed 3, St Louis, 1993, Mosby, pp 7.1-8.11.
Weaver CT, Unanue ER: The costimulatory function of antigen presenting cells, *Immunol Today* 11:49-54, 1990.

PART TWO

Methods to Evaluate Immune Function

9 Assays for Innate Immune Defenses

Neutrophils and Complement

Protection of the host from infection by the myriad of potential pathogens present in the environment is initiated by the innate immune system. In the naive animal this may be the sole source of protection until acquired immune responses are stimulated. Thus adequate function of these defenses is imperative. Chapter 1 describes the components of the innate immune system in detail; this chapter will stress methods of evaluating its functional adequacy.

In the evaluation of patients with suspected immune defects, the humoral and cellular arms of the immune system are usually examined prior to undertaking some of the more time-consuming neutrophil function assays mentioned here. There may be a significant overlap between manifestations of humoral and neutrophil deficiencies.

EVALUATION OF PHAGOCYTE FUNCTION

Phagocytes, macrophages and neutrophils act as the first line of defense against bacterial pathogens. The killing of invading microorganisms by phagocytes involves a complex series of events; flaws in any one of these steps will result in an impaired response. To evaluate the efficiency of the phagocyte system, it is therefore necessary to examine the numbers of phagocytes, their adhesion, chemotaxis, phagocytosis, and intracellular killing mechanisms. A systematic method of performing this evaluation is detailed in the following section.

Neutrophils: natural history

Neutrophils are the first line of defense against extracellular pathogens, such as bacteria. They circulate in the blood-vascular system with a relatively short half life. They are produced in the bone marrow and released into the periphery where they circulate for approximately 12 hours. After this intravascular phase, they exit into the extravascular space for an additional 1 to 2 days. Normally a stimulus, such as bacterial infection, signals the bone marrow to produce and release more neutrophils, thus creating a peripheral neutrophilia. The individual cells respond locally with up-regulation of adhesion molecules, margination, and diapedesis through the vascular endothelium and along the concentration gradient (produced by chemotactic factors) by way of chemotaxis toward the site of bacterial infection. At the site, the neutrophil will engulf the bacterial cells by phagocytosis, using antibody and/or complement as opsonins. Within the phagosome there is the emptying of lysosomal contents and the formation of a phagolysosome. Within this vesicle the bacteria are killed. Operation of several oxygen-dependent and oxygen-independent killing mechanisms occurs during this killing process.

Deficiency or malfunction at any one stage of neutrophil function can severely impair the animal's ability to overcome bacterial infection. Specific conditions, usually inherited, are described in domestic animals where one or more of these neutrophil functions does not work effectively. Table 9-1 describes assay systems for the evaluation and identification of neutrophil dysfunction.

Monocyte macrophage: natural history

The monocyte/macrophage has a dual role; it is important in both innate and acquired immune responses. As a phagocyte the macrophage is usually a second line of defense following the neutrophil response. The macrophage often functions as a "clean up" cell, ridding the tissue of debris. For some bacterial infections, namely facultative intracellular organisms (Mycobacteria, Salmonella, Listeria, etc.), the macrophage is an important effector cell. Activation of macrophages by gamma interferon (IFN-γ) produced by stimulated T lymphocytes is required for the macrophage to kill the organism effectively; thus the response is one that requires an acquired immune response.

Isolation of neutrophils

In vitro assessment of neutrophil function is an important method to evaluate suspected neutrophil defects. Chemotactic substances are also conveniently assayed with purified populations of poly-

Table 9-1 Evaluation of neutrophil function

Neutrophil parameter	Assay Method	Disease example
Number	Total leukocyte count; differential	Cyclic neutropenia
		Congenital agranulocytosis
Adhesion	CD11/CD18 surface identification (FACS)	Bovine leukocyte adhesion deficiency
Chemotaxis	Migration under agarose; Boyden chamber	Lazy leukocyte syndrome
Phagocytosis	Phagocytic index	Secondary to C′ or Ig deficiency
Killing	Bactericidal assay; NTB reduction test	Chronic granulomatous disease
	Morphology	Chédiak-Higashi syndrome
Associated parameters		
Opsonization	Complement levels; C3b	Congenital C′ deficiency
	(In vivo decreased chemotaxis may also result from C′ deficiency)	
	Bactericidal test using normal serum	Inadequate humoral response

morphonuclear (PMN) leukocytes. In domestic animals, neutrophil dysfunctions have been identified in cattle, cats, and mink with Chédiak-Higashi syndrome, grey collies affected with cyclic neutropenia, Irish setters with granulocytopathy syndrome, and weimaraners with neutrophil dysfunction disease. Feline and canine PMN leukocytes are readily isolated in >99% purity using a modified Percoll gradient. The cells band at the 80% (v/v) interface. Alternatively, PMN leukocytes may be recovered from heparinized blood by first isolating leukocytes with dextran. For this, equal volumes of blood and 2.5% dextran sulphate (v/v) are mixed together in a syringe and incubated in a vertical position (needle up) for 20 to 40 minutes. The separated leukocyte-plasma fraction is decanted into a tube facilitated by a bent 1½ inch 200-22 gauge needle and washed prior to conventional Ficoll-Hypaque centrifugation (specific gravity 1.0805). The layer of cells beneath the mononuclear cell band is erythrocyte-free and ≥ 95% PMN leukocytes. Slight variation in technique is used when isolating equine and bovine neutrophils. More specific protocols are provided in the references at the end of this chapter.

Neutrophil quantitation

Neutropenia is an obvious cause of depressed neutrophil function. The absence of a sufficient number of neutrophils can be caused by a variety of problems—both acquired and intrinsic. Among the acquired causes of neutropenia are post-infectious neutropenia, drug-induced neutropenia, autoimmune neutropenia, and nutritional neutropenia. Among the intrinisic causes are cyclic neutropenia and Chédiak-Higashi syndrome. Although not all of these types have been identified in domestic animals, the existence of these defects in humans provides a basis for awareness of their occurrence in animals.

Evaluation of neutrophil numbers and morphology is readily accomplished by performing a standard leukocyte quantitation and differential from peripheral blood. In cases of cyclic neutropenia, it is necessary to follow the blood count through a cycle in order to confirm the cyclic nature of the leukopoiesis.

Adhesion

Inflammation as a response to bacterial invasion is characterized by the accumulation of leukocytes, particularly neutrophils, at the area of infection. This occurrence requires the mobilization of vascular pools of neutrophils into the extravascular tissue. The well-characterized steps of margination and diapedesis through the endothelium are necessary components of an inflammatory response. Margination, the lining up of neutrophils along the endothelial cell border, requires the presence of cell surface molecules on the neutrophils. These cell surface molecules are called *adhesions*.

The importance of cellular adhesions in bacterial immunity is best demonstrated by the clinical syndrome leukocyte adhesion deficiency (LAD) in humans and its counterpart, bovine leukocyte adhesion deficiency (BLAD) in cattle. Patients afflicted with this problem have extremely high peripheral neutrophil counts, yet they lack the characteristic purulent exudate at sites of bacterial infection. Biopsy of such areas show blood vessels packed full of neutrophils but an absence of neutrophils in the surrounding tissue spaces. The structures that are important in cell-cell adhesion are the adhesion molecules. The defect that occurs in LAD results from defective biosynthesis of the CD18 cell surface molecule, which is a part of the two chain integrin adhesion molecule. The absence of a functional CD18 molecule prevents adherence of the leukocyte to the endothelial cell.

In BLAD there is a clinical history of poor wound healing, absence of purulent exudate, and marked leukocytosis. Monoclonal antibodies specific to CD18 can be used to evaluate the expression of the adhesion molecule on the patient's leukocytes using the fluorescence activated cell scanner. Diagnosis of this defect in Holstein cattle is possible at the genetic level with the use of genetic primers and polymerase chain reaction.

Chemotaxis

Induction of the inflammatory response requires that leukocytes be able to recognize a chemotactic stimulus and that they respond by moving toward the stimulus. Defective chemotaxis can result in less effective innate immunity. The lack of appropriate chemotaxis may be caused by a neutrophil defect or by a complement defect, in which the appropriate chemotactic stimuli are not produced. The complement cascade (as described in Chapter 6) normally generates C3a, C5a, and C5b67. In a clinical condition referred to as the "lazy leukocyte syndrome," neutrophils do not demonstrate directed forward movement in response to a chemotactic stimulus.

The chemoctactic ability of leukocytes can be evaluated using one of the two available assay systems. These include chemotaxis under agarose or through millipore filters in a Boyden chamber and a multiwell Millipore filter assay block. As a source of chemotactic stimulus a synthetic tripeptide N-formyl-L-methionyl-L-leucyl-L-phenylalanine is commonly used. It is usually tested over a range of dosages from 10^{-7} to 10^{-10} M with incubation of cells and stimulus ranging from 15 minutes to 2 hours. When performing such an assay it is imperative that a source of normal neutrophils be used as a positive control. The assay is performed on the principle that neutrophils placed in the middle well of an agarose plate will migrate under agarose in response to the chemotactic gradient generated by the tripeptide that has been placed in the adjacent well. Migration patterns are visualized microscopically.

Phagocytosis

Once leukocytes have arrived at a site of bacterial invasion they do little good unless they can engulf and kill the organisms. Defects exist in which phagocytosis and/or killing is impaired or absent. Patients afflicted with such a condition will display chronic infections with extracellular bacterial pathogens; these conditions are often resolved with appropriate antibiotic therapy only to recur after discontinuation of therapy.

Phagocytosis can be impaired by an actual leukocyte defect or by the absence of opsonins, specifically C3b and antibodies. To evaluate phagocytosis the phagocytic index can be determined. This is a relatively simple procedure that involves harvesting leukocytes from the patient and incubating the washed cells with a source of bacteria (e.g., *Staphylococcus aureus*) in the presence of its own and a normal control serum. Slides are made from these mixtures and stained with Giemsa stain for microscopic counting of engulfed organisms. The phagocytic index is determined by the average number of organisms within a phagocyte. A parasitic index can also be determined; this value is the number of leukocytes that have participated in the phagocytic process.

Killing defects

The ability to kill engulfed organisms is of primary importance to an effective antibacterial response. A variety of killing defects have been recognized and described in humans and domestic animals. The mechanism for decreased killing varies from impaired phagosome-lysosome fusion to enzyme deficiencies (see Chapter 12). An excellent assay that detects impaired killing regardless of the mechanism is the bactericidal assay. In this assay patient cells are incubated with a source of organisms (as described in detail in the next paragraph). At timed intervals sampled aliquots are removed and antibiotic is added to kill any extracellular organisms. The leukocytes are then lysed and plated on bacteriologic media. Colony counts are performed to evaluate the numbers of viable bacteria remaining in the leukocytes at the time of lysis. Data obtained after 30 minutes, 1 hour, 90 minutes, and 2 hours of incubation are then graphed and compared to a normal control (Figure 9-1). The absence of a decrease in viable bacteria over time is indicative of poor to absent killing. Such a profile is seen in human patients with chronic granulomatous disease and in a similar syndrome described in Irish Setter dogs.

Assays to evaluate the ability of neutrophils to kill bacteria include bactericidal assay, neutrophil chemiluminescence, and the nitroblue tetrazolium reduction test. Performance of this test involves the growth of a *Staphylococcus aureus* culture in Mueller-Hinton broth for 18 hours at 37°C. The cells are washed and adjusted to a concentration of 2×10^9 CFU/ml by measuring the optical density. When evaluating the patient's cells for their ability to kill, a pooled normal serum is used to opsonize the bacteria. This is performed by adding 0.5 ml of the bacterial suspension to 0.5 ml of the

Live bacteria counted (log)

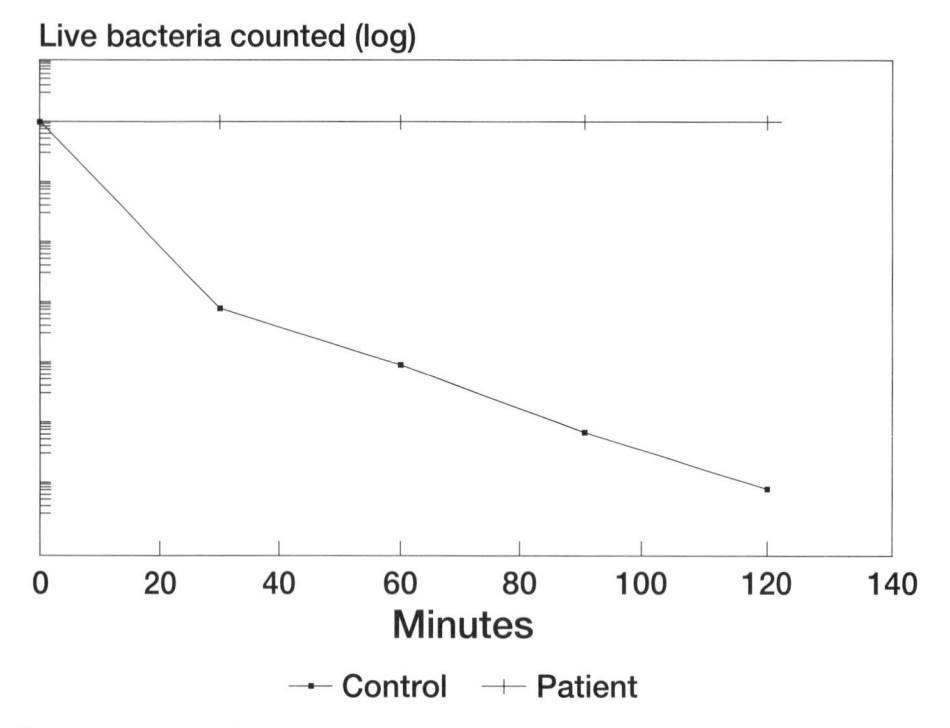

Figure 9-1 The bactericidal assay is performed by incubating the patient's neutrophils with live bacteria, and sampling and testing for live intracellular bacteria at 30-minute intervals. The control neutrophils engulf and kill the bacteria rapidly, losing several logs in the first 30 minutes. Patients whose neutrophils have a killing deficit are unable to kill, and the bacteria count remains high, even after 120 minutes.

serum pool and allowing opsonization to occur at 37° C for 30 minutes. After this time the bacterial cells are separated by centrifugation, washed, and resuspended at a concentration of 5×10^7 CPU/ml in a solution of Hank's balanced salt solution (HBSS) with 1% gelation. The patient's blood is taken in preservative-free heparin and the buffy coat cells are taken off and resuspended in HBSS at a concentration of 1×10^7 cells/ml. It is important that any neutrophil function tests be performed within several hours of the time blood is taken. A normal control cell sample should be assayed simultaneously with the patient's sample. To perform the assay, 0.5 ml of the bacterial mixture is added to 0.5 ml of the phagocyte mixture and the mixture is gently rotated at 37°C. Samples are taken from this phagocyte mixture at 0, 30, 60, and 120 minutes. Controls, consisting of normal phagocytes with bacteria and bacteria in HBSS without phagocytes, are treated and sampled in a similar fashion as test samples. The cells are lysed by addition of sterile distilled water to a sample aliquot and measured amounts are plated onto sheep red blood cell agar. After incubation for 24 hours, the number of colonies present on the agar are counted. Normally within the first 30 minutes as many as 90% of the bacteria are killed. In patients with a killing defect, this time is much more prolonged.

The nitroblue tetrazolium test (NBT) evaluates the respiratory burst in neutrophils. It is based on the principle that neutrophils will reduce the dye nitroblue tetrazolium to formazan during the stimulation of a respiratory burst. Since NBT is a soluble, colorless substance, its conversion to the dark, blue, granular formazan is an easily recognizable event. Some patients, humans with chronic granulomatous disease, lack the functional oxidase enzymes that are needed for production of the superoxide anions required in the oxidative burst. This enzyme deficiency makes the cells less efficient killers and is easily detectable by the lack of blue granules in the neutrophil cytoplasm in this test. Slides should be prepared with unstimulated neutrophils as well as with stimulated cells so that the quality of the reagent can be checked. As with other neutrophil function tests, the use of fresh cells is imperative.

Another method for evaluating the oxidative burst in neutrophils is the chemiluminescence assay. Stimulation of phagocytic cells with opsonized particles normally elicits an oxidative burst, which is coupled to a release of light. This released light can be detected using a beta scintillation counter or a special chemiluminometer. A defective oxidative reaction will be detected with this assay.

Cell quantification and morphology should not be overlooked when analyzing this arm of the immune system. One well-known example of compromised immunity as a result of inadequate phagocytic cell numbers is a cyclic neutropenia in grey collie dogs. In this syndrome, peripheral neutrophils are few or absent at certain times as a result of a recurrent bone marrow suppression. During this time, the dogs are affected with bacterial infection. In the Chédiak-Higashi syndrome of Persian cats and other species there is a defect that can be detected by examination of cell morphology; large granules are present in the neutrophils and lymphocytes.

Evaluation of complement

The presence of adequate amounts of functional complement is an important component of normal immune system function. The presence of complement is important in both innate and acquired immune responses. Specifically it is needed for opsonization, chemotaxis, and lysis of target cells (see Chapter 6). One test that is used as an indicator for total hemolytic complement activity is the CH50 assay. In this assay the patient's plasma is used as a source of complement, and its ability to lyse target-sensitized erythrocytes is measured. Interpretation of this test requires accumulation of normal values for the particular species as performed by the particular laboratory doing the assay.

Component quantitation, often performed by single, radial diffusion in human medicine, requires that there be purified complement components as well as specific antisera that recognizes that component available. These are available for several complement components in veterinary species, but generally we still lack the capacity to individually identify each complement component in our domestic animal species.

REFERENCES

Baehner RL, Nathan DG: Quantitative nitroblue tetrazolium test in chronic granulomatous disease, *N Engl J Med* 278:971-976, 1968.

Barta O: *Laboratory techniques of veterinary clinical immunology*, Springfield, Ill, 1984, Charles C Thomas.

Coates TD, Beyer LL, Baehner RL: Laboratory evaluation of neutropenia and neutrophil dysfunction. In Rose NR, DeMacario EC, Fahey JL, and others, editors: *Manual of clinical laboratory immunology*, Washington, D.C., ed 4, 1992, ASM Press, pp 419-420.

Dutta SK, Bumgardener MK, Scott JC, Myrup MS: Separation and identification of equine leukocyte populations and subpopulations, *Am J Vet Res* 42:1037-1039, 1981.

Metcalf JA, Gallin JI, Nauseef WM, Root RK: *Laboratory manual of neutrophil function*, New York, 1986, Raven.

Quie PG, Herron J: Neutrophil assessment: bacterial assay and chemiluminesence. In Rose NR, DeMacario EC, Fahey JL, and others, editors: *Manual of clinical laboratory immunology*, Washington, D.C., ed 4, 1992, ASM Press, pp 419-420.

Roth JA, Daeberle ML: Evaluation of Bovine polymorphonuclear leukocyte function, *Vet Immun Immunopath* 2:57-174, 1981.

10 Assays for Humoral Immunity, Including Serology

The subdiscipline of serology is based on the methods used to detect antigen-antibody reactions in vitro. The most convenient source of specific antibody is serum. Serologic reactions and patterns of antibody production identified in sera of individuals or in animal populations have tremendous practical importance. Identification of an antibody reactive with an antigen of interest (rabies, for example) implies that the individual has had immunogenic exposure to rabies antigen(s). Further, the kinetics and immunoglobulin class response characteristics of the antibody (usually determined on comparison of antibody levels in paired serum samples) will tell the investigator whether the exposure to rabies occurred recently. Conversely, because most disease-causing entities (viruses, bacteria, etc.) are immunogenic, antibodies collected from unrelated third-party individuals can be used to demonstrate these agents in tissues, secretions, or excretions of infected individuals. Finally, many substances of biologic importance such as hormones and drugs can now be assayed with serologic methods.

To quantitate the union between antigen and antibody, serologists must take into account several different phenomena relating to the antigen-antibody interaction. Serologists are interested in defining the total amount of specific antibody (to the antigen of interest) in the immunoglobulin fraction of the serum. For this, consideration must be given to specificity of the reaction, the average intrinsic affinity of antibody molecules for this antigen, and, if the antigen is multideterminant or complex, the measurable strength or avidity of the antibody species studied.

The union of antigen and antibody is mediated chiefly by noncovalent binding phenomena and is roughly analogous to the binding of enzymes to their substrates. Thus the reaction is reversible and expressed generally by the following equation:

$$\text{Antibody} + \text{Antigen} \rightleftarrows \text{Antibody-Antigen} \quad (10.1)$$

The strength of union between an antibody and its antigen, or the antibody's affinity, is expressed as an equilibrium constant defined as the ratio of association over the ratio of disassociation. In reality, then, the affinity constant (K) is given as:

$$K = \frac{(\text{Antibody-antigen})}{(\text{Free antibody}) \quad (\text{Free antigen})} \quad (10.2)$$

By determining disassociation constant values for different ratios of antigen and antibody (usually performed by varying the antigen concentration while holding the antibody concentration constant), one can construct a binding curve. This binding curve is linearized by plotting of values of bound antigen concentration divided by free antigen concentration against total antigen available. The slope of this Scatchard plot line is the affinity constant for that particular reaction of antigen and antibody.

As a practical matter, most antigens of diagnostic interest contain multiple epitopes or antigenic determinants. For this reason, determination of equilibrium constants in a sample containing multiple antibody species reactive with multiple antigenic determinants is rarely performed.

In accomplishing this goal of measuring average antibody activity in a sample, the avidity of the antibody-antigen union becomes important. Another determinant is valency of the antibody species. IgG molecules have two binding sites and hence a valency of 2, whereas IgM has 10. The average binding value is determined by titration of the antibody (or serum) against a constant concentration of antigen. This is accomplished by regular dilution (twofold, tenfold, etc.) of antibody in a buffer solution before exposure to antigen: Two relative values are important. The first is the optimal dilution, which is defined as that dilution of reactants in which the average avidity of the antibody samples is the highest. The second value of importance in serology or immunochemistry is the last dilution of antibody or antigen to yield a detectable positive reaction. This value or titer is defined as the reciprocal of the last dilution of antibody yielding a positive reaction. For example, a titer of 256 means that the last twofold dilution that gave a positive reaction was 1:256 and was likely obtained through serial twofold dilutions according to the following: 1:2, 1:4, 1:8, 1:16, 1:32, 1:64, 1:128, 1:256, 1:512, 1:1024, etc. Although a titer is conventionally expressed in terms of dilution, it can also be expressed in terms of the amount of antibody bound (in nanograms or milligrams) per unit volume if a method for identifying bound antibody is available. Finally, it is important to note that antigen can also be titrated according to the same process and titers, expressed arbitrarily as units bound in a standard antibody solution or as actual protein values (e.g., milligrams per milliliter).

Careful study of in vitro serologic reactions has revealed that the interaction between antigens and antibodies occurs in two distinct time-related phases. Initial union of antigen with its antibody is referred to as the *primary binding phase* or reaction. It occurs rapidly, is largely independent of temperature (4°C through 37°C), is reversible, and is ordinarily invisible to the naked eye. The *secondary binding phase* that depends on the generation of a lattice or matrix of reacting antigen-antibody complexes and occurs slowly (1 to 24 hours), is generally enhanced by reaction at low temperatures (4° to 10°C), is irreversible, and will ultimately produce a resultant complex visible to the naked eye. By definition, then, primary reactions are more sensitive (in terms of detecting low levels of antibody) but require methods to separate bound from unbound reactants and also to render the reaction of interest detectable. In contrast, secondary reactions are less sensitive and by definition do not ordinarily require separation of reactant or elaborate detection techniques.

Early serologists depended on secondary phenomena to detect antigen-antibody reactions. These reactions have historical importance and are employed today in many clinical and diagnostic regulatory laboratories. They were used in two ways: qualitative and, with modification, quantitative. Qualitative reactions yield a "yes-or-no" answer; *yes*, the patient's serum contains antibody, or *no*, it does not. For this reason, qualitative assays have the greatest utility in diagnostic or screening tests. Quantitative assays answer the yes-no query and, in addition, provide data on the amount (titer) of antibody. This assay permits analysis of patterns of antibody responses and was preferred for investigative studies. Secondary assays, those producing a visible effect, are described first.

SECONDARY IMMUNOLOGIC ASSAYS

Within a 3-year period (1886-1889), the agglutination test, the precipitation test, and the complement fixation test were discovered by Max Gruber, Rudolph Kraus, and Jules Bordet, respectively. In all three cases, serum from vaccinated and/or convalescent animals was demonstrated to contain each species of antibody. For many years, antibodies were defined by the means used to detect them. It was believed that *agglutinins* (the name given to antibody measured by agglutination) did not function as precipitins, opsonins, or complement-fixing antibodies. Subsequently, this issue was clarified by a unitarian hypothesis stating that a single specific antibody is capable of performing all of the specific reactions described above, depending solely on how the antigen is "packaged." Thus antibodies agglutinate their antigen if the antigen is particulate. The same antibody will precipitate antigen if it is soluble. It is well recognized today that antibodies of the major classes of IgG and IgM are capable of all of the serologic functions illustrated in Figure 10-l. In light of current knowledge of immunoglobulins, the unitarian hypothesis has been modified. For example, IgA, IgE, and some minor subclasses of IgG of nearly all animal species fail to function as efficient agglutinins, precipitins, or complement-fixing antibodies.

AGGLUTINATION

IgG and IgM antibodies, specific for antigenic determinants on particulate antigens such as bacteria or erythrocytes, will—when mixed with these particles or with latex or polystyrene beads coated with soluble homologous antigen—produce visual agglutination or clumping. The cross-linking of antibody to the antigen-containing particles is counteracted by the presence of static electrical charges (negative or positive) on the particle. These static charges, known as the *zeta potential*, tend to repel the particles from one another. In that the strength of the repulsion is inversely proportional to the square of the distance between the particles, agglutinins need a strong binding affinity to cross-link particles. Therefore IgM antibodies, because of their larger size and higher valency, tend to be stronger agglutinins than are IgG antibodies.

As a serologic tool, the advantages of agglutination tests are severalfold: (1) the time interval between adding antibody to antigen and agglutination is usually less than 1 hour; (2) agglutination tests are less apt to be affected by conditions of excess antibody or excess antigen that may produce a false-negative reaction (prozone); and (3) agglutination tests are generally more sensitive than the conventional precipitation or complement fixation tests. Further, one can adapt agglutination tests to the detection of soluble antigens by attaching the antigens to inert carriers such as plastic beads or modified erythrocytes. Small amounts of proteinaceous antigen will irreversibly adhere to plastic or polystyrene surfaces. Commercially

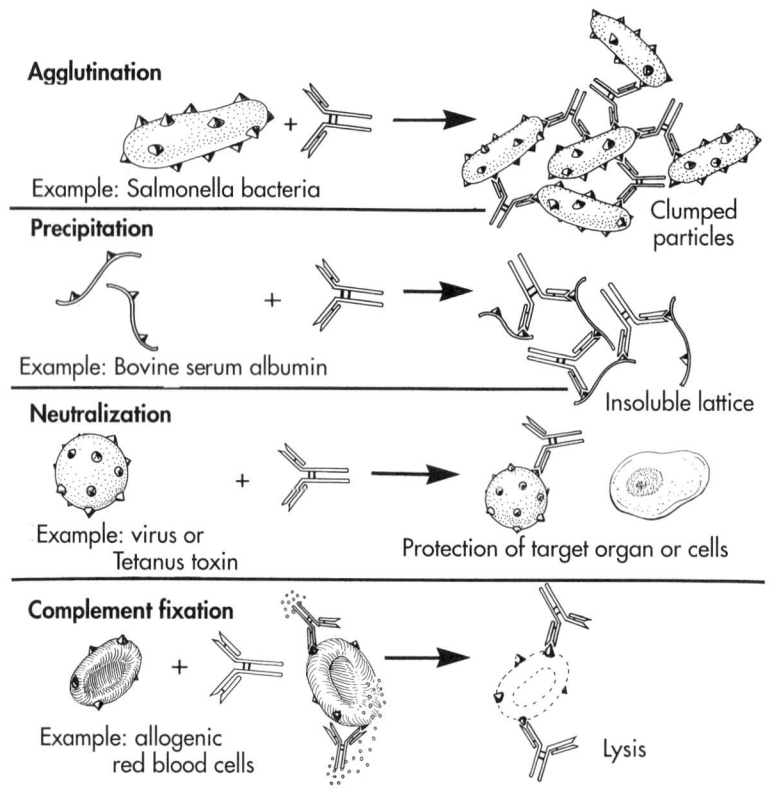

Figure 10-1 Antigen-antibody reactions. All basic serologic reactions between antibody and antigens depend on how the antigen is packaged. For example, particulate antigen agglutinates, whereas soluble antigens produce precipitation reactions.

available polystyrene beads are first incubated in a solution of antigen, washed during centrifugation to remove unbound antigen, incubated with an irrelevant protein (usually bovine serum albumin) to block residual sites on the beads, and then used. In another classic modification, irrelevant erythrocytes (usually ovine) are given long-term chloride treatment to make them "sticky" and then used as outlined above. A modification using buffered chromic chloride as the "tanning" agent is preferred because the resultant erythrocytes are stable for several months at 4°C.

QUALITATIVE AGGLUTINATION TESTS
Plate or card test

Qualitative plate or card agglutination tests involve the mixing of a known antigen with serum or whole blood, a short incubation period (five to ten minutes), and subsequent scoring. The technique is illustrated in Figure 10-2.

The identification of cattle with antibody to *Brucella abortus* by the plate or card test is a presumptive screening test that helps the veterinarian identify animals within a herd affected with brucellosis. A similar test is used to identify dogs infected with *Brucella canis*. Leptospirosis infections in cattle, dogs, pigs, and horses are likewise serodiagnosed by the presumptive plate or card agglutination test.

The matching of blood donor and recipient is quite easily achieved with the plate agglutination test. Washed red blood cells from the donor are incubated with serum from the recipient. The presence of incompatible antibody to donor cells in the recipient animal leads to rapid agglutination of donor cells. A qualitative agglutination test can detect the major blood group antigens in most animal species. This test is generally used only when the recipient animal has a history of previous transfusions. Animals that have had multiple transfusions may not produce antibody detectable by the plate test.

Milk-ring test

Brucella abortus infections in dairy herds can be presumptively identified with the milk-ring test. Antibody from infected cows can be detected by the addition of a suspension of hematoxylin-stained *B. abortus* organisms to milk. In the absence of antibody, the stained bacteria remain

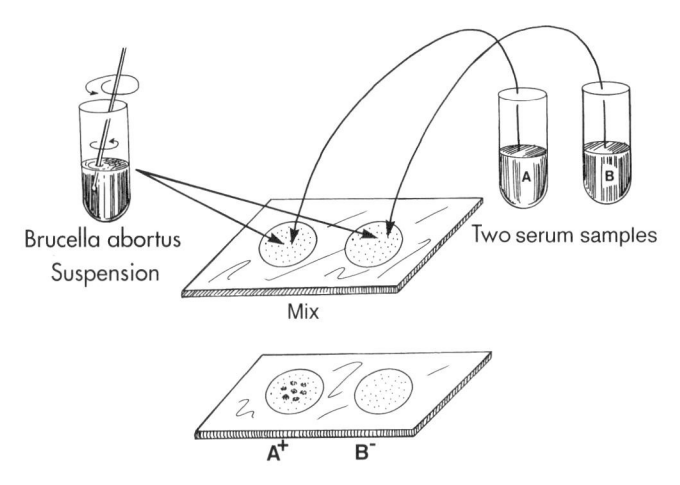

Figure 10-2 Qualitative plate agglutination test includes the simple mixing of serum with the appropriate antigen. This type of qualitative test is a basic tool in identifying *Brucella* antibody in ruminants. *A* is positive, *B* is negative. Though the test is simple, it does not permit the determination of antibody titers.

suspended in the milk portion. However, bacteria-antibody complexes (positive test) agglutinate on incubation and accumulate at the milk-cream interface, producing an easy-to-read blue ring.

Coombs' test

For bacteria, well as erythrocytes, antigen determinants are located on defined areas of the cell membrane surface. The agglutination of cells by IgG antibody often is prevented by the physical distance of antigenic determinants between cells. The IgG antibody to *Brucella* sp. frequently fails to cause effective agglutination, for the same reason. Likewise, IgG antibody to erythrocyte surface antigen (e.g., Rh antigen of human red blood cells) fails to agglutinate (Figure 10-3). Autoantibodies to erythrocyte determinants in many animal species (including cat and dog) behave similarly. In this case, erythrocytes coated with autoantibody do not spontaneously agglutinate, but they are fragile and tend to lyse in vivo, resulting in hemolytic anemia.

Bacteria or erythrocytes (sensitized, in serologic terminology) may contain specific nonagglutinating antibody on their cell surfaces. This antibody can be detected on treatment of suspect suspensions with a heterologous anti-IgG antibody. This antiglobulin—*Coombs' reagent*—reacts with the exposed Fc portion of the bound antibody and produces visible agglutination. There are two modifications of the Coombs test.

Direct Coombs' test

The direct Coombs test for autoimmune hemolytic anemia in all animal species is performed by treating patients' washed erythrocytes with the appropriate anti-IgG Coombs' reagent. Erythrocytes not sensitized with autoantibody fail to agglutinate in the presence of Coombs' reagent (see Figure 10-3), whereas sensitized erythrocytes agglutinate.

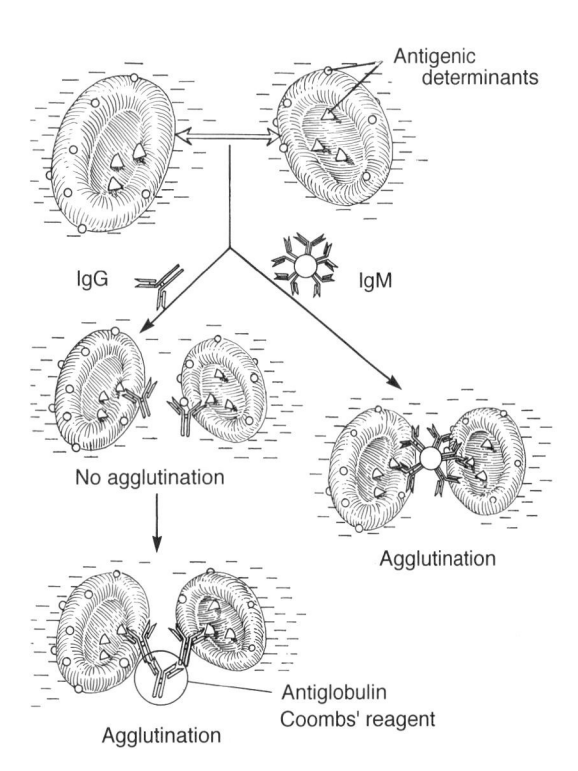

Figure 10-3 Direct Coombs' agglutination test detects antibodies (IgG) that fail to agglutinate. The direct Coombs' test uses an antiglobulin reagent that forms a bridge between particles and facilitates agglutination.

Indirect Coombs' test

The indirect Coombs test is performed by adding patient serum to normal erythrocytes, antigenically homologous to the cell type of the patient. After incubation of serum with red blood cells, the preparation is washed and treated with Coombs' reagent. Positive agglutination confirms the presence of autoantibodies in serum reactive with erythrocytes.

Coombs' reagent is a useful serologic tool. It is used as a link or bridge reagent for many serologic tests, which are described further below.

QUANTITATIVE AGGLUTINATION TESTS

In *Brucella* and *Salmonella* serology, positive qualitative tests are used as presumptive tests. A quantitative test is used as a confirmatory test. An important serologic tool in the diagnosis of disease is not only the identification of antibody to this pathogen, but determination of the change in antibody titer during the course of the disease. Rising titer generally implies current clinical involvement, whereas convalescence is associated with decreasing or constant titer with respect to time.

Tube agglutination test

The tube agglutination test is used to determine agglutinin titer. Serial twofold dilutions of serum are prepared in physiologic saline solution to which standardized antigen (i.e., *Brucella* or erythrocytes) is added. After incubation, the agglutination patterns are read without agitation (Figure 10-4). This type of test is used routinely in the serodiagnosis of leptospirosis in cattles, dogs, pigs, and horses, and of brucellosis in cattle and dogs.

2-Mercaptoethanol test

Brucellosis in cattle can be an acute or chronic disease. The evolution of antibody by immunoglobulin classes occurs during the course of the disease. IgM antibody appears first in infected animals and generally remains in serum as long as the animal is actively exposed to *Brucella* sp. antigens. During convalescence or after successful vaccination with *Brucella* bacterins, IgM antibody disappears from serum, leaving as the predominant *Brucella* agglutinin IgG antibody. To the clinician, it is of obvious importance to ascertain whether *Brucella* antibodies are of the IgM class (indicative of infection) or mainly of the IgG class (indicative of previous immunogenic exposure).

For detection of IgM agglutinins, two simultaneous tube agglutination tests are performed. A reducing agent such as 2-mercaptoethanol (2-ME) is added. At low concentrations, 2-ME reduces interchain disulfide bands of IgM, resulting in the destruction of its pentomeric structure. IgG is unaffected. Therefore, on comparison of agglutinating titers in 2-ME–treated and untreated tubes, the relative proportion of IgM agglutinins can be determined. This technique is simple and straightforward and is widely used in diagnostic serology for several diseases of clinical importance.

PRECIPITATION

Reaction of soluble antigen with antibodies in a serum sample results in the generation of soluble complexes. This occurs because the active antibodies possess two or more antigen-binding sites. Formation of this complex also depends on the antigen possessing multiple epitopes per molecule. Thus, precipitation cannot occur with haptens

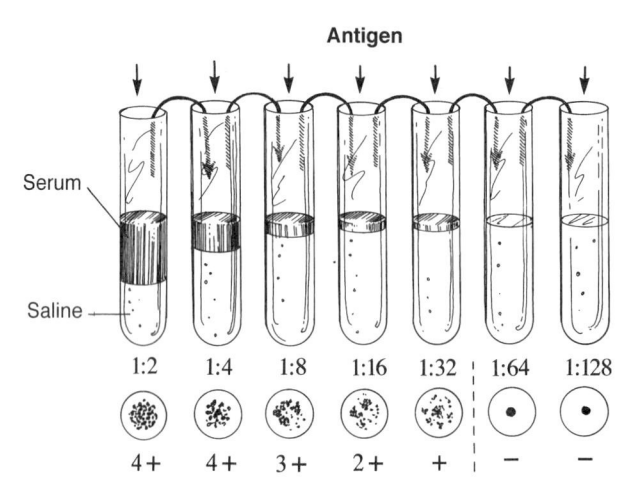

Figure 10-4 Quantitative agglutination test use serially-diluted antiserum and a standard dilution of antigen. The last dilution of serum that produces an agglutination pattern is the antibody titer end point.

or isolated free epitopes. Soluble complexes form almost immediately (Figure 10-5).

On subsequent incubation (hours), the cross-linking of primary complexes results in large secondary complexes (conglomerate-like lattices) that are observable as visual precipitate. Precipitation of the antigen-antibody secondary complexes is apparently due to the effective lack of interreaction of hydrophilic groups on the antigen-antibody molecules with hydronium ions.

Monovalent antigens, in contrast to multivalent antigens, fail to form visual precipitates in the presence of homologous antisera. Complexing of antibody and antigen occurs, yet insoluble complexes (precipitates) do not form. Other factors that prevent insoluble lattice formation are conditions of excess antibody or excess antigen (Figure 10-5). In the zone of excess antigen, too few antibody molecules are present to crosslink antigen into insoluble complexes. Complexes of this type consist of one antibody and two or more antigen molecules. In the presence of excess antibody, soluble complexes of two antibody molecules and one antigen molecule form.

The mixture of antigen and antibody in optimal proportions results in a zone of equivalence in which maximum precipitation forms. The zone of equivalence has in vivo and in vitro significance. The circulating soluble antigen-antibody complexes in great antigen excess, as a rule, are not trapped in extravascular tissue and do not have a part in immune-complex diseases. In in vitro precipitin tests, equivalence is necessary for precipitation to be seen. Therefore, in the presence of excess antigen, antibody, or both, a prozone effect may occur, producing a false-negative result (Figure 10-5).

QUALITATIVE PRECIPITIN TEXTS
Capillary tube precipitation test

Because of the difficulty in achieving the critical point of antibody-antigen equivalence necessary for maximum precipitation, the tube-precipitation test is rarely used. A modification of the tube test, called *capillary tube precipitation*, is commonly used in forensic medicine in the identification of animal species of origin of suspect meat (Figure 10-6). The test is also used in the Lancefield grouping of *Streptococcus*.

Using specifically prepared antisera to deer, cow, horse, or other animal species, forensic medicine specialists can identify, for example, venison or even ground venison mixed with ground beef. Saline solution extracts of suspect meat are layered over or mixed with known specific antideer serum. After a short incubation (approximately 1 hour), a visual precipitate forms, permitting positive identification of animal species meat or meat products. This sensitive technique can identify a ratio of up to 50:1 of ground beef and ground venison. This technique permits the positive identification of animal species antigen in extracts of dry blood or even in extracts of blood-sucking insects.

Gel precipitation (Ouchterlony) test

The problem of achieving antibody-antigen equivalence is overcome by immunoprecipitation in gels. Though various modifications of gel precipitation have been developed, the most commonly used method is Ouchterlony double immunodiffusion. The Ouchterlony technique is a double diffusion of soluble antigen and soluble antibody in saline-buffered agar gel (Figure 10-7). After diffusion, the antibody and antigen meet at a point of

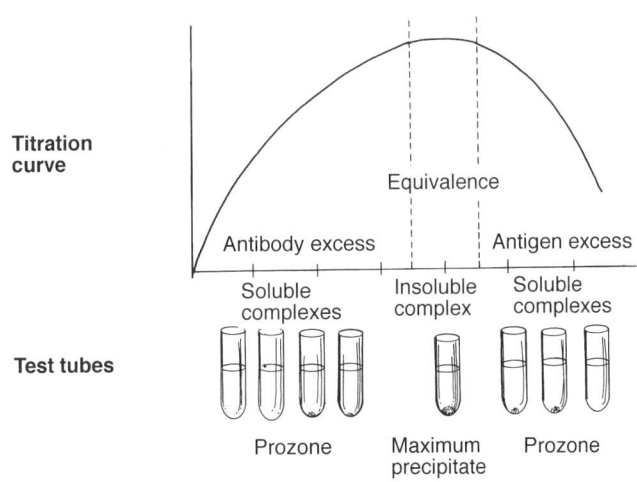

Figure 10-5 Quantitative precipitin curve. Maximum precipitation occurs where antigen-antibody concentration permits the formation of large, insoluble complexes (lattices). In the areas of either antibody or antigen excess, the amount of visible precipitate diminishes (prozone).

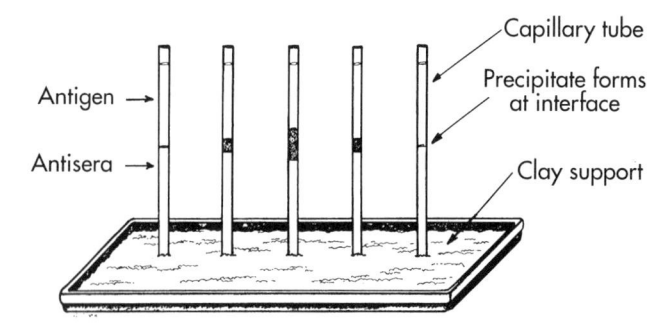

Figure 10-6 Capillary tube precipitation test. Soluble antigen is layered or mixed with increasing dilutions of antisera. Maximum precipitation occurs at the point of equivalence. This test is commonly used by forensic medicine specialists to identify meat adulterated with illegal meat substitutes.

equivalence where an observable insoluble precipitate line forms in the gel matrix. Moreover, each antibody-antigen system forms antigen reactions. For example, a mixture of three antigens may react with three different antibodies to form three different precipitin lines in the gel (Figure 10-7).

The major factors that influence the formation of a visual precipitate are several. Antigen and antibody must be soluble to diffuse into the agar matrix. The position of the precipitin line may vary, depending on antibody and antigen concentrations and rates of diffusion. Generally, antigen in weak concentration forms a line close to its own well. Likewise, a high concentration of antigen may only form equivalence with antibody close to the antibody well. Antibody and/or antigen concentrations below the point of equivalence do not form precipitin lines.

Because each antibody-antigen system forms a line of precipitation independent of other antigen-antibody systems, immunodiffusion in gel has been used as a powerful tool for antigenic analysis. For example, each protein from disrupted virus or bacteria or even soluble proteins in animal plasma theoretically forms a single precipitin line with appropriate homologous antisera. Moreover, the placement of antigen wells in proximal positions permits the analysis of common antigens (Figure 10-8). Two organisms that share common antigens produce a common line of identity in a immunoprecipitation test. Antigens that do not share common determinants may form lines that do not coalesce, *lines of nonidentity*. Under some circumstances, partial identity occurs, producing a "spur" effect. This is a result of the fact that soluble antigens generally contain several antigenic determinants. The spur formation indicates that two antigen molecules differ in some determinants but contain at least one common antigenic determinant (Figure 10-8).

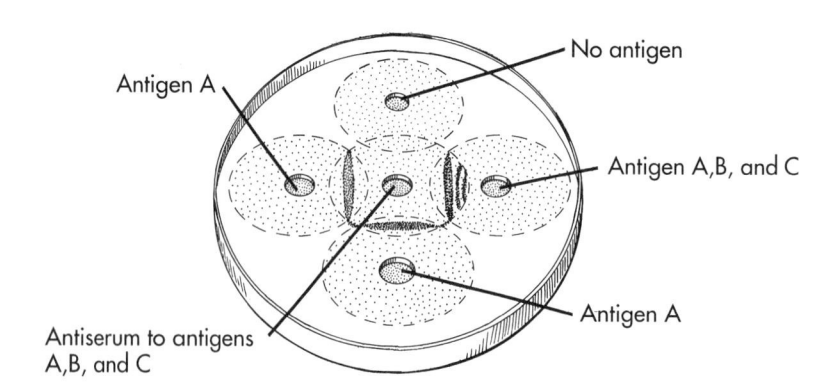

Figure 10-7 Ouchterlony two-dimension immunodiffusion in gel test. Antisera and antigen are placed in wells cut in a gel matrix. Both reactants diffuse into the gel; where they meet at the point of equivalence, a precipitin line occurs. Different antigen-antibody systems independently form their own lines of precipitation.

Coggins' test for equine infectious anemia

Ouchterlony immunodiffusion has been used in the diagnosis of several infectious diseases of veterinary importance. A major application is in the diagnosis of equine infectious anemia (EIA) in horses. Leroy Coggins, using the Ouchterlony immunodiffusion method, demonstrated that horses infected with EIA virus produce precipitin antibody to soluble EIA antigen. EIA antigen contains virus originally derived from EIA-infected horses.

In this test, the antigen is placed in the center well and standard EIA-positive sera are placed in peripheral wells, alternating with serum from suspect horses (Figure 10-9). It is important that the standardized sera are chosen such that they form a single precipitin line with the antigen. A positive test in suspect horse serum must form a line of identity with standard antisera. A line of nonidentity indicates a false positive test; absence of a precipitin line indicates a negative test (Figure 10-8).

The advantages of Coggins' test for EIA are several. Horses produce complement-fixing (IgG) and noncomplement-fixing (IgG_T) antibodies to EIA. Both of these isotypes function as precipitin antibodies. With the use of standardized anti-EIA serum, false positives can be identified. This is important because EIA antigen used today contains soluble antigens other than virus.

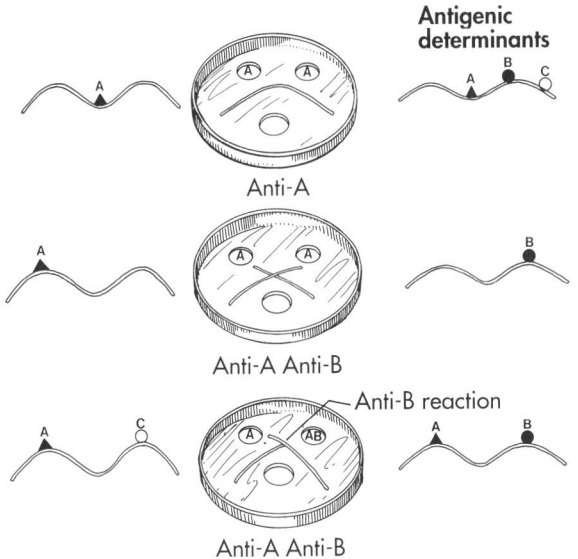

Figure 10-8 Antigenic analysis of two antigen mixtures. *Top*, Antigens that contain common antigenic determinants form a common line of *identity* in the immunodiffusion test. *Middle*, Antigens that do not contain common antigenic determinants produce precipitin lines that do not coalesce. These lines are referred to as lines of *nonidentity*. *Bottom*, Antigens generally contain multiple determinants. In situations where antigens contain both common and different antigenic determinants, precipitin lines of *partial identity* occur. The partial identity appears as a spur on one of the lines.

Figure 10-9 Coggins' test for equine infectious anemia (EIA). The center well contains a known standard EIA antigen. In the peripheral wells (*B*), known horse anti-EIA serum alternates with suspect horse sera (*C, D, E*). A line of identity between *B* and *C* shows that serum *C* contains EIA antibody; therefore, this is a positive Coggins' test. Lines of nonidentity between *B* and *E* are a false-positive test. No precipitin line with *D* is a negative test.

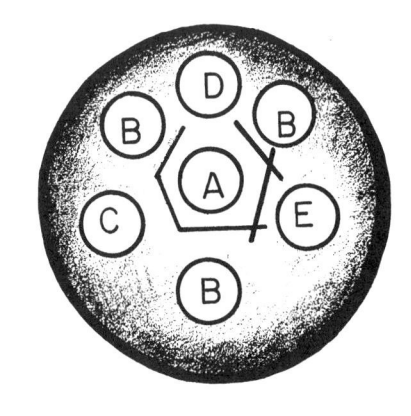

Immunoelectrophoresis

Immunoelectrophoresis is an extension of the Ouchterlony immunoprecipitation test. Immunoelectrophoresis first employs the advantages of separating antigen mixtures into individual components by means of conventional electrophoresis in gel (Figure 10-10). Each protein in the mixture contains a specific net electrical charge. Depending on its molecular size, configuration, and solubility, each protein migrates differently in an electrical field. Animal serum is separable into albumin, alpha globulins, beta globulins, and gamma globulins. Each of these fractions, except albumin, contains many different proteins. The subsequent diffusion of these components against appropriate antisera develops visual precipitin lines at points of equivalence, just as described earlier in, the discussion of the Ouchterlony immunodiffusion test.

Multiple precipitin arcs are discernible in each of the globulin fractions (e.g., upward of 16 to 20 separate antigens are discernible in animal serum). When serum is reacted with antiwhole serum, multiple bands are visible. When isotype-specific

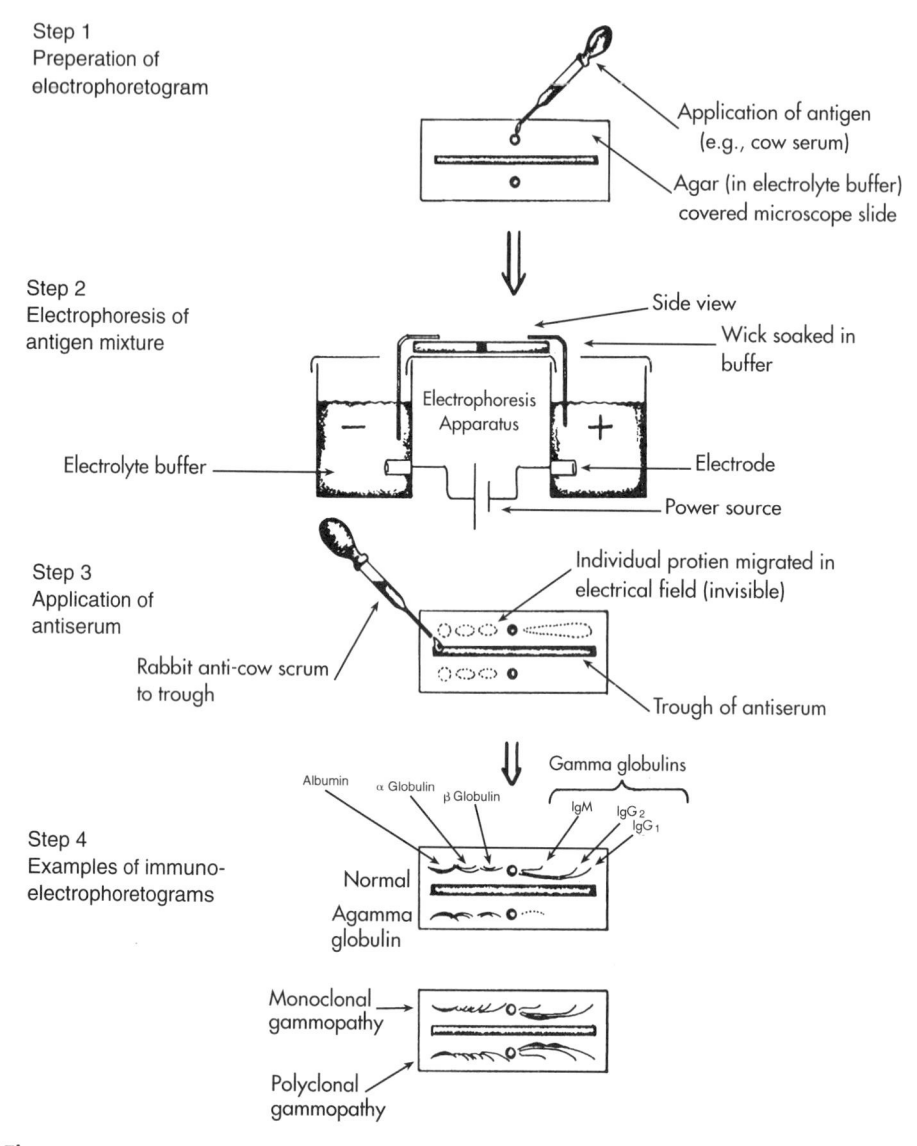

Figure 10-10 Immunoelectrophoresis couples the advantages of separating antigens electrophoretically in gel and forming lines of precipitation (precipitin arcs) by appropriate antisera. This method is commonly used in veterinary clinical immunology laboratories to identify gammopathies and to analyze the composition of complex proteinic mixtures.

antiserum is used, individual bands such as those for IgM and IgA are readily recognizable.

The clinical application of immunoelectrophoresis permits the analysis of various pathologic conditions of antibody-producing cells. For example, animals born without B cells and therefore lacking antibody-producing plasma cells, have a marked lack of gamma globulin proteins. Likewise, monoclonal and polyclonal gammopathies show up as areas of dense precipitation in certain portions of IgG or even IgM precipitin arcs (Figure 10-10).

QUANTITATIVE PRECIPITATION TESTS

Immunoelectrophoresis, like the Ouchterlony immunoprecipitation technique, is a powerful analytical tool for qualitative analysis of antigen mixtures. A limitation of both methods is the inability to quantitate antigens.

Radial immunodiffusion

The radial immunodiffusion method of Mancini employs the principles of immunodiffusion to quantitate antigens, notably immunoglobulins. For this, a standard antiserum: (e.g., rabbit anticow IgG) is mixed with molten agar. This mixture is poured into a carrier (microscope slide or dish) (Figure 10-11). Several wells are bored into the agar-antiserum gel.

To standardize the test, known quantities of cow IgG are placed in the wells. As the antigen diffuses into the gel, a ring of visual precipitation occurs where the antigen reaches equivalence with the antiserum in the gel matrix. The more concentrated the antigen, the larger the diameter. By measuring the diameters, one can draw a standard curve (Figure 10-11). With identical plates from which the standard curve was calculated, the testing of antigen of unknown concentration can easily be quantitated by measurement of the diameter of the precipitin ring and calculation of the concentration from the standard curve. Radial immunodiffusion kits for quantitative determination of immunoglobulin class levels in serum, secretions, joint fluids, and cerebrospinal fluid for all common domestic animal species are commercially available. For all, the sensitivity of the assays can be improved by means of staining of dried gels with a protein stain such as Coomassie blue.

Rocket immunoelectrophoresis

Techniques have been developed that combine quantitative gel diffusion with electrophoretic movement of proteins in the gel matrix. Countercurrent electrophoresis is a modification of agar gel diffusion, except that conditions (e.g., buffer pH) in the gel are manipulated so that antigen and IgG antibody migrate toward each other. Electric-field forced migration enhances the sensitivity of gel diffusion at least 10-fold.

For rocket immunoelectrophoresis (RIEP), antiserum is incorporated into the agar gel prepared in

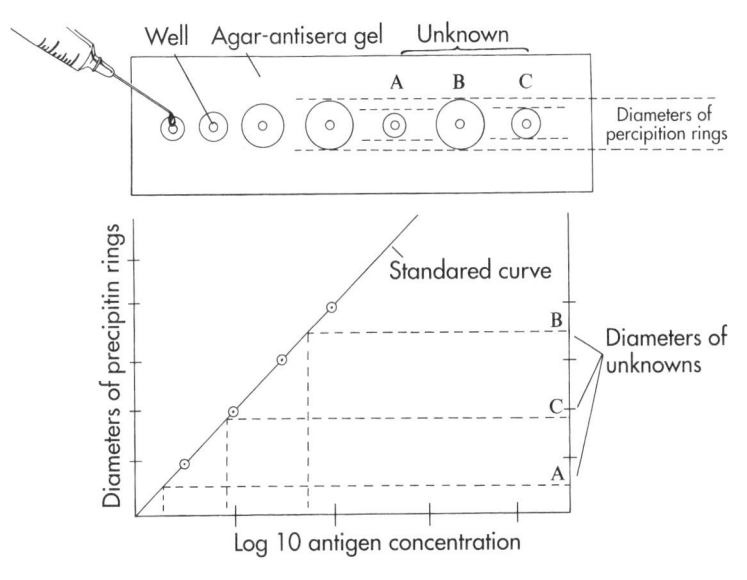

Figure 10-11 Radial immunodiffusion is commonly used in veterinary clinical pathology laboratories to quantitate serum Ig. With a standard curve, the diameters of the precipitin rings formed by test sera can be easily quantitated.

pH buffer, rendering the incorporated IgG immobile. Antigen solutions are placed in agar wells, and the plate is subjected to electrophoresis. The arcs of precipitation (rockets) formed in the gel are detected directly or after staining with Coomassie blue (Figure 10-12). Antigen concentration is proportional to peak height and is determined by the use of standards of known antigen concentration.

COMPLEMENT FIXATION TESTS

At the close of the last century, Pfeiffer and Bordet demonstrated that serum from an immune animal, when mixed with a thermolabile factor from guinea pig serum, was bacteriolytic. Bordet later showed that antibody in immune serum was capable of lysing bacteria, erythrocytes, or both in the presence of the thermolabile factor named *complement*. Neither complement nor antibody alone was lytic. The complement fixation (CF) test, as it is used today, is based on the principle demonstrated by Bordet that complement reacts with any antibody-antigen reaction. Complement (see Chapter 6) comprises at least nine serum components and is found in all animal sera. For the CF test, guinea pig serum is often used as the source of complement. This is because guinea pig complement is strongly lytic for antibody-coated (sensitized) sheep erythrocytes. With a few exceptions, antibody from any mammal, on reaction with antigen, activates (fixes) guinea pig complement.

Figure 10-13 illustrates the principle of the CF test. Under test conditions, only antibody-antigen complexes fix complement. Neither antibody nor antigen alone is capable of doing this. To determine whether the complement has been consumed in the test, sheep cells coated with antibody (sensitized SRBCs) are added to the antibody-antigen complement mixture. If the complement has been fixed by the test reaction, the SRBCs are not lysed.

Complement fixation test method

The complement fixation (CF) test is performed to determine the presence of complement fixation antibody in an animal serum, the serum sample is first heated in a 56°C water bath for 30 minutes to inactivate residual complement in the serum. After the inactivation step, 0.25 ml of serum is diluted in serial twofold dilutions in a buffer containing Ca^{++} and Mg^{++}. Added to each serum dilution is 0.25 ml of a known antigen and 0.50 ml of pretitrated guinea pig complement.

The complement titration is critical because the process requires enough complement to completely lyse the sensitized sheep erythrocytes in the indicator system yet be of low enough concentration to be completely fixed by the antibody-antigen reaction. Several methods are available to titrate complement. However, the most sensitive method, using the Von Krogh plot (Figure 10-14), determines the amount of complement in the guinea pig serum that lyses 50% of the SRBCs in the indicator system. This is expressed as CH_{50} units of complement. This plot facilitates the calculations required to determine what dilution of the complement stock contains one unit of complement, necessary for running the CF test.

After an incubation period of 1 hour at 37°C or overnight at 4°C, sensitized SRBCs are added to the antibody-antigen complement mixture. This is thoroughly mixed and incubated for 30 minutes; then the test is scored (Figure 10-15). If the serum contains antibody and reacts with the antigen, the

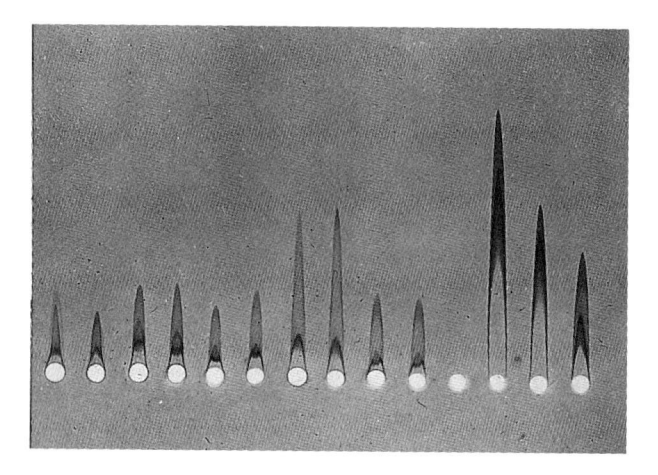

Figure 10-12 Rocket immunoelectrophoresis (RIEP) for the quantitation of serum albumin in the cerebrospinal fluids of dogs affected with viral encephalitis. The standard curve is on the right three wells. Stained with Coommassie blue.

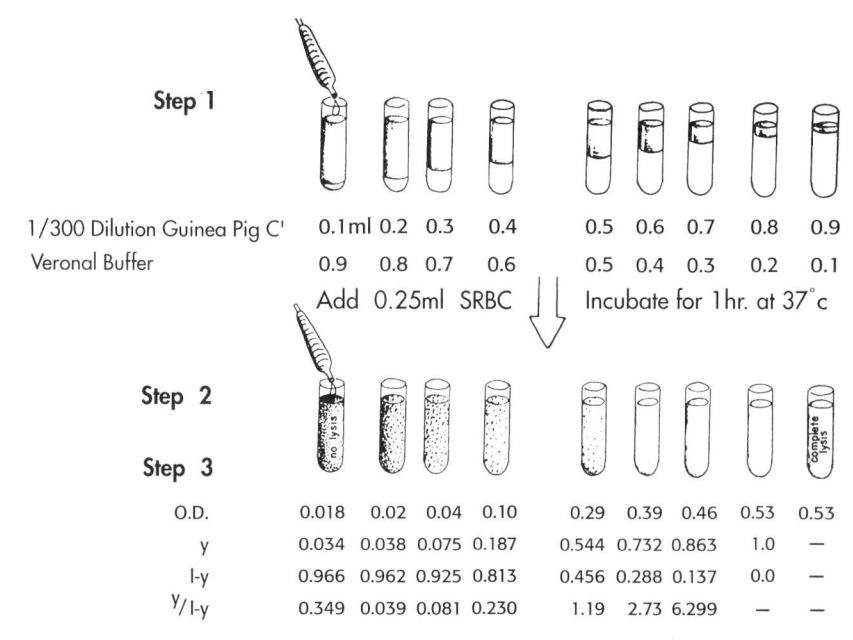

	Step 1									
1/300 Dilution Guinea Pig C'		0.1ml	0.2	0.3	0.4	0.5	0.6	0.7	0.8	0.9
Veronal Buffer		0.9	0.8	0.7	0.6	0.5	0.4	0.3	0.2	0.1

Add 0.25ml SRBC ⇓ Incubate for 1hr. at 37°c

	Step 2 / Step 3									
O.D.		0.018	0.02	0.04	0.10	0.29	0.39	0.46	0.53	0.53
y		0.034	0.038	0.075	0.187	0.544	0.732	0.863	1.0	—
l-y		0.966	0.962	0.925	0.813	0.456	0.288	0.137	0.0	—
y/l-y		0.349	0.039	0.081	0.230	1.19	2.73	6.299	—	—

Figure 10-13 Complement fixation test. Interreaction of IgM (and most subclasses of IgG) of all animal species with their appropriate antigens binds a complement receptor on the antibody that activates (fixes) complement. The fixation of complement can be determined by adding an indicator system (sensitized sheep red blood cells [SRBCs]) to the complement fixation test mixture. If complement is fixed by antibody-antigen reaction, the SRBCs do not lyse. However, if the initial antibody fails to react with antigen, the unfixed complement lyses the SRBCs.

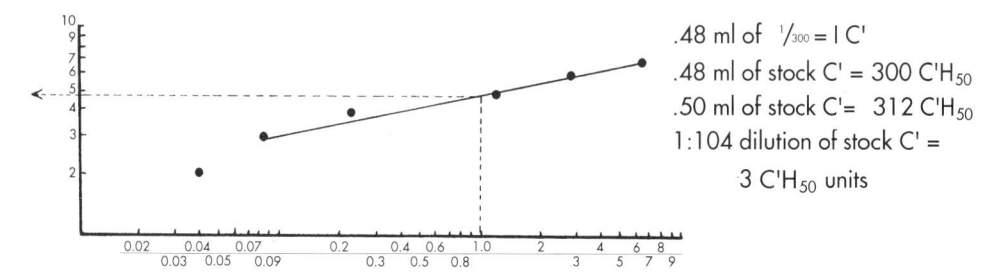

.48 ml of $1/300$ = 1 C'
.48 ml of stock C' = 300 C'H$_{50}$
.50 ml of stock C' = 312 C'H$_{50}$
1:104 dilution of stock C' =
   3 C'H$_{50}$ units

Figure 10-14 Complement titration. Varying amounts of stock guinea pig complement diluted 1:300 to 1:400 are incubated under the same conditions as the complement fixation (1 hour, 37°C). Added to each tube is a standard quantity (0.25 ml) of optimally-sensitized (SRBCs). The entire mixture is incubated an additional 30 minutes at 37°C. The optical density of the release of hemoglobin is used to calculate the percentage of lysis (y). To determine the amount of stock complement that lyses 50% of SRBCs, the value y/l-y is plotted against the quantity of complement used in the titration. One CH$_{50}$ unit, therefore, is that amount of complement that lyses 50% of the SRBCs under all controlled conditions of the titration. Three to five CH$_{50}$ units are generally used in most clinical complement fixation tests.

3 to 50 CH^{50} units of guinea pig complement are fixed. Therefore the SRBCs, when added to the test, are not lysed to release soluble hemoglobulin. The expression of antibody titer can be considered that dilution of serum that permits the approximately 50% lysis of SRBCs. The complement fixation assay can be used quantitatively. For this, the optical density of released hemoglobulin (540 mµ) in the test solution after centrifugation can be determined and related to antibody concentration.

Applications of the complement fixation text

The complement fixation test is applicable in the serodiagnosis of nearly all viral, bacterial, and mycotic diseases of domestic animals and human beings. The advantages are that it requires neither purified nor concentration reference antigen. In that all factors (complement, buffer, amount of antigen) can be standardized, the complement fixation test is very reproducible and has historically been used as a serologic test in diagnostic centers.

In the United States, the complement fixation test has been used in the serodiagnosis of leptospirosis, canine distemper, canine hepatitis, feline picornavirus, brucellosis, and Johne's disease. The appearance of complement fixation antibody in the serum occurs early in the clinical phase of the disease; generally, complement fixation antibody titer diminishes after convalescence. This is because IgM antibody is the most efficient activator of complement. Of course, without immunogenic stimulation IgM synthesis ceases. In the serodiagnosis of brucellosis, complement fixation antibody in cattle appears early after infection or vaccination, then decays faster than agglutination titer.

The disadvantages of the complement fixation test are several. The test is difficult to set up and requires expert technical ability for use on a routine basis. Antibodies from fowl, with the interesting exception of pigeons, are not compatible with guinea pig complement. Therefore conventional complement fixation testing is not suitable for serodiagnosis of avian diseases. Moreover, some

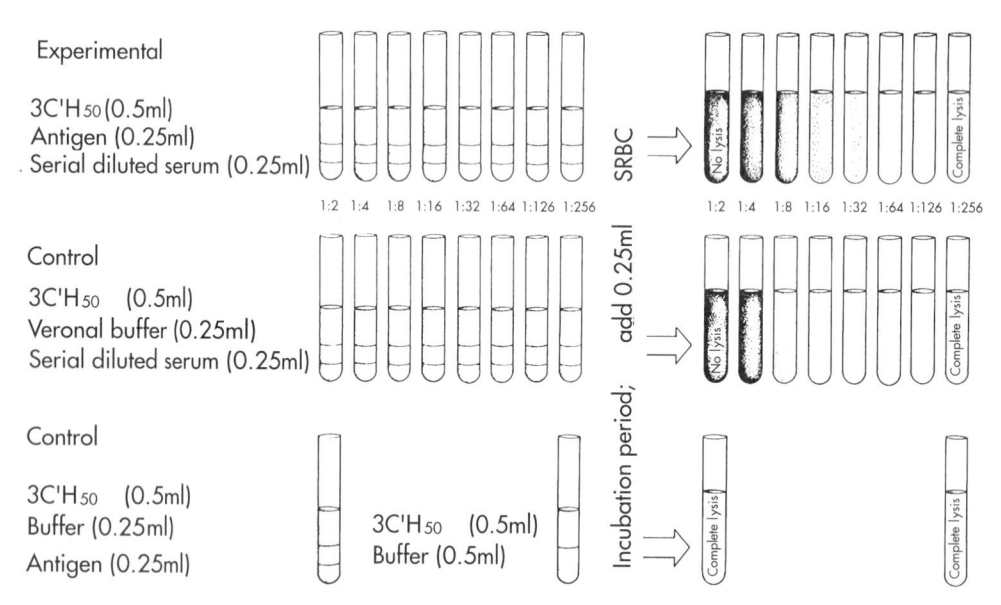

Figure 10-15 Complement fixation test. Serum from patient is diluted serially in replicate sets of serologic tubes. Into one set is added complement (3 units of CH$_{50}$) and antigen. The control tubes receive complement and buffer (instead of antigen). Additional controls include a tube with complement, buffer, and antigen, and a second tube with only complement and buffer. All tubes are incubated (usually 1 hour at 37°C), and the SRBCs are added to every tube. In the test, the last dilution that prevents the lysis of approximately 50% of the SRBCs may be considered as the complement fixation antibody titer. Controls determine whether serum alone or antigen alone fixed complement, and whether complement alone lyses to SRBCs. In the test illustrated above the complement fixation antibody titer is approximately 1:16, whereas the anticomplementary activity of serum was 1:2 to 1:4.

mammalian species produce subclasses of IgG that do not activate complement.

Horse IgG (T) and subclasses of IgG in the cat, dog, monkey, and cow limit the application of complement fixation test in serodiagnosis. For example, in EIA the appearance of IgG (T) contributes to false-negative test results for EIA. Similarly, the cat elicits a noncomplement-fixing response to feline leukemia, parainfluenza, leptospirosis, and pneumococci. Cats infected with feline picornavirus have been found to synthesize complementation fixation antibody (IgG and IgM) early in the clinical phase of virus infection, then switch to noncomplement-fixing IgG antibody that persists through late convalescence.

INDIRECT COMPLEMENT FIXATION INHIBITION TEST

Noncomplement-fixing antibody in all species can be identified and titered on the basis of the inhibition of reference complementation fixation test. For example, cats infected with feline leukemia virus (FeLV) produce an antibody that reacts with FeLV but does not activate guinea pig or cat complement. By incubating cat antibody with FeLV for 1 hour and then adding a rabbit anti-FeLV serum (CF antibody) and guinea pig complement, one can observe the inhibition of the CF test.

Similarly, noncomplement-fixing antibodies to arbovirus antigens in migratory bird sera (e.g., starling) have been identified. Thus, the complement fixation inhibition (CFI) test represents a powerful seroepidemiologic tool for those animal species to which the CF test does not apply. The level of technical expertise required to perform both tests is high. This fact, coupled with the time-consuming nature of the assay, restrict its use. Both assays have now been largely replaced with primary antibody-binding assays.

NEUTRALIZATION TEST

Neutralization assays have traditionally been used to measure the effects of specific antibodies on the biologic effects of toxins, bacteria, viruses, and enzymes. The basis of all the assays is the same: the neutralization of biologic events, for example, preventing a pathologic response in a suitable host or host cell.

Von Behring and Kitasato in 1890 effectively demonstrated the neutralization test in their studies with *Corynebacteria diphtheriae* exotoxin. They found that mixing immune guinea pig serum with toxin neutralized the toxin when the mixture was injected in susceptible nonimmune guinea pigs. The interaction of antibody with toxin did not destroy the toxin but prevented it from reaching the shock organ, which in the case of C. diphtheriae toxin was the adrenal glands.

Similar tests are used by epidemiologists to identify species of origin of clostridial toxins in food preparations. Suspect toxins are mixed with known specific types of clostridial antitoxins (antisera); after a suitable incubation period, the mixture is injected into mice. The protection of mice from the lethal effects of clostridial toxin is the basis of a positive identification of toxicogenic types of *Clostridia* sp.

The virus neutralization test (Figure 10-16) has the distinct advantage over other serologic tests for viruses in that it is the most specific. This is due to the fact that the antigenic determinant(s) on the virus surface is the only antigen involved in eliciting a virus neutralization response in animals. This surface antigen, from an evolutionary point of view, tends to show the greatest amount of variation. This is due in part to the immunologic pressures extended by the host. Internal viral antigens, as a general rule, are the most "conserved" antigens. In other words, internal antigens show less variation and tend to be similar in closely related viruses. Immunoprecipitation tests and complement fixation tests detect all viral antigens. Therefore it is not unexpected that all equine herpes (EH) viruses (types I, II, III and IV), for example, cross-react strongly in this test. The virus neutralization test, however, discriminates between them. Anti–EH-I serum, for example, does not neutralize EH-II or EH-III.

The virus neutralization test generally employs host cells grown in vitro under defined cultural conditions. The principle is to mix serum with virus and observe the degree of neutralization of viral cytopathic effects on the cell culture. The virus-induced cytopathic effects are observed as any of the following: cell killing; (e.g., by influenza virus in chick embryo cells), syncytial formation (production of multinucleated giant cells), and transformation into cancer cells (e.g., feline sarcoma and FeLV on feline embryo cells).

Because these types of cytopathic effects are discernible under the microscope, the virus neutralization antibody titer can be determined from the last dilution of serum that prevents formation of cytopathic effects (Figure 10-16). Other forms of virus neutralization tests may employ embryonated chicken eggs or laboratory animals such as mice. Virus neutralization tests are rarely used in routine diagnosis of animal diseases. However, virus neutralization tests are applicable to the epidemiologic identification of serotypes of equine influenza, EH viruses, transmissible gastroenteritis of hogs, and bovine rhinotracheitis virus.

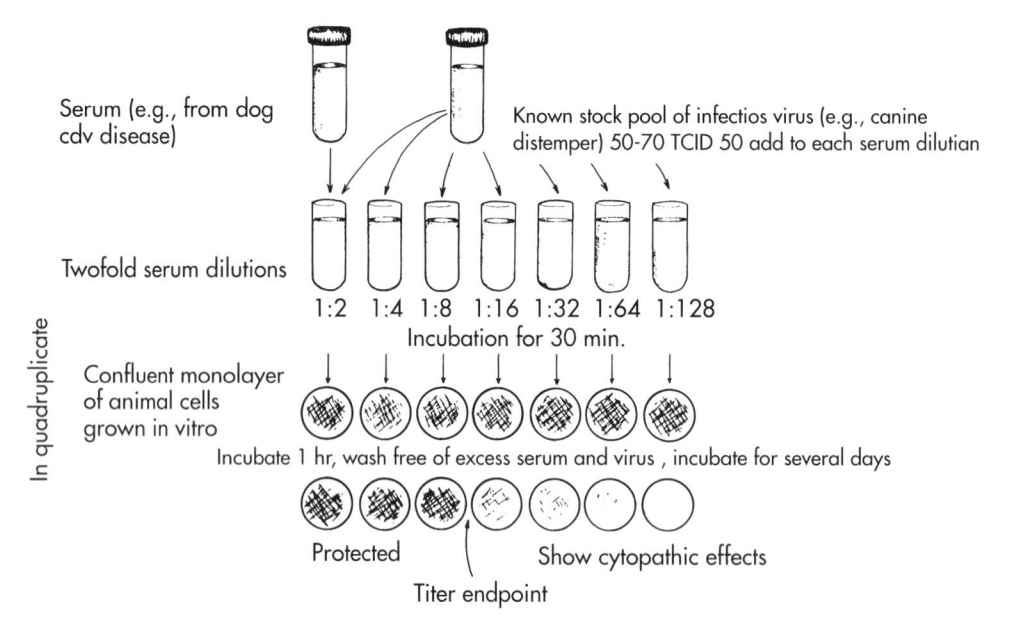

Figure 10-16 Virus neutralization test. In the test illustrated, varying dilutions of patient serum (such as a suspect dog with canine distemper virus [CDV]) are mixed with a stock dilution of CDV. The stock CDV used contains 50 to 70 tissue culture infectivity doses 50 ($TCID_{50}$). After an appropriate incubation period, the virus-serum mixture is added to cells that will support the growth of CDV. That dilution of serum that effectively prevents CDV growth (seen as cytopathic effects [CPE]) is considered as virus-neutralizing antibody titer.

PRIMARY SEROLOGIC ASSAYS

As described earlier, the first and primary interaction with antigen occurs rapidly and is largely independent of the concentration of the reactants. As a general rule, development of visible secondary phenomena depends on concentration or ratio of reactants; thus tests based on these phenomena are much less sensitive than primary antibody-binding assays. Thus the chief immunologic advantage of primary assays lies in their sensitivity. The chief practical importance of these assays lies in their easy adaption to automation or in-clinic performance capability.

Because the union of antigen and antibody is not visible, one or both of the reactants must be labeled or identified in some fashion. Furthermore, because the union is soluble and independent of the concentration of reactants, a method for separating and quantitating bound from unbound reactants in the solution must be available.

Labeling reagents

Table 10-1 lists the most commonly used approaches to labeling reagents of immunologic interest. One widely used method is the labeling of materials with radioactive isotopes. Antigens from viruses and bacteria are conveniently labeled in the internal method by the provision of ^{14}C, or ^{35}S-labeled amino acids into growth media. Inert antigens or isolated fractions of organisms are labeled externally with ^{121}I according to the chloramine T method. For this, the amino acid, tyrosine, must be exposed for iodination. Labeled reactants are measured by means of a variety of methods, including liquid scintillation and various autoradiographic techniques.

Isolated antibody preparations or antigens are commonly coupled to aniline dyes such as fluorescein isothiocyanate (FITC) or rhodamine isothiocyanate. These simple ringed compounds covalently bind lysine residues on proteins and emit energy when excited (475 v) by ultraviolet light and, fluorescence at 525 nm. For fluorescence microscopy (Figure 10-17), the resulting signal can be detected visually, thereby permitting precise anatomic localization of antibody binding site(s).

A general method of fluorescein conjugation suitable for use with most immunologic reactions is used. For this, antibody solution prepared by means of affinity chromatography, ammonium sulfate fractionation, or octanoic (caprylic) acid clarification is adjusted to 5 to 10 mg/ml and dialyzed in 0.05M bicarbonate buffer (pH 8.3). Reagent

Assays for Humoral Immunity, Including Serology   91

Table 10-1 Substances commonly used to label proteins

Category	Examples	Enzyme substrate	Detection as:
Radiolabels (isotopes)	^{131}I, ^{125}I, ^{35}S, ^{14}C	—	Counts per minute; autoradiography
Aniline dyes	FITC	—	Apple green (ultraviolet light)
	Rhodamine isothiocyanate	—	Red (ultraviolet light)
	Texas Red	—	Red (ultraviolet light)
Opaque	Ferritin colloidal gold	—	Electron opaque substance; electron microscopy
Enzymes	Horseradish peroxidase	3,-3, diamino-benzidine	Brown
		5-amino salicyclic acid	Purple-brown
		4-Chloro-1-naphthol	Blue
		3-Amino-9-ethylcorbazole	Red
	Alkaline phosphatase	5-Bromo-4-chloro-3-indolyphosphate	Blue
		p-Nitrophenyl phosphate	Yellow
	β-D-galaxtosidase	O-nitrophenyl β-D-galactopylamoside	Blue

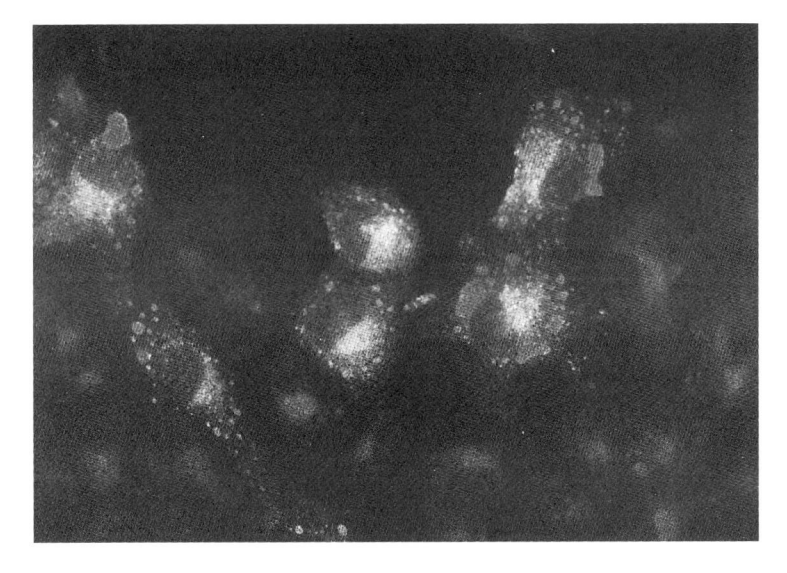

Figure 10-17 A direct immunofluorescence assay for the demonstration of canine-distemper virus in tissue culture cells.

grade FITC is dissolved in 10 volumes of bicarbonate buffer to a final concentration of 0.01 mg/ml. A dialysis bag filled with antibody solution is placed in the FITC solution and dialysis continued for 18 to 24 hours of 40°C. Unbound FITC can be removed from the labeled antibody by means of exhaustive dialysis or molecular sieve chromatography (Sephadex G-25). The FITC-labeled material is then titrated for binding, aliquoted, and frozen or lyophilized.

Ferritin is a high molecular weight (6.5 × 10^6 D) iron-rich storage protein isolated from equine spleen. It is covalently attached to proteins and used to localize antigens or binding sites on electron microscopy (EM). Ferritin molecules are electron dense and appear on EM as dark, black, fuzzy, spherical granules. Ferritin is coupled to protein by means of the gluteraldehyde crosslinking technique used for enzymes. Colloidal gold, coupled to antiglobulin or protein A, appears similar to ferritin but is smaller and is used when intracellular penetration of reagents is needed.

Enzymic labeling of immunologic reagents is widely used to construct labeled reagents with immunologic activity. Degradation of chromagenic substrates by the covalently attached enzyme yields soluble visible reaction products, which in turn permit accurate and sensitive detection of the enzyme. Suitable enzymes should be inexpensive, stable, and available in purified form and should utilize substrates that produce stable, easily measurable or detected breakdown products. Horseradish peroxidase, alkaline phosphatase, and β-D-galactosidase are commonly used. For most coupling reactions, the one-step glutaraldehyde technique developed by Avrameas is used. Gluteraldehyde crosslinks proteins by binding to the terminal amino group of lysine residues in proteins. For this, lyophilized enzyme is dissolved in antibody solution (2:1) and then a 1/20 volume of 1% (volume/volume) gluteraldehyde, and the mixture is held for 3 hours before addition of excess lysine to terminate the reaction. In most cases the resultant enzyme-antibody complex is a heterogeneous mixture of crosslinked proteins without appreciable free antibody or enzyme. Horseradish peroxidase (HRP) conjugations are the exception; much of the HRP is not crosslinked, presumably because of the relative lack of free lysine residues on the HRP molecule.

Separation strategies

Because equivalence is not a serious consideration for primary binding assays, soluble reaction mixtures frequently contain excess antigen, antibody, or both. Consequently, bound reactants must be separated from unbound reactants before quantitation. Table 10-2 outlines the major approaches to this problem. Of these, the last two, namely tissue section examination for immunocytochemistry and plate absorption will be detailed. Salt fractionation is largely of historical interest and is based on the principle of insolubility of gamma globulin in high-salt solutions. The chief use of polyethylene glycol (PEG) lies in its use to recover soluble immune complexes in serum from patients with immune complex disease. The PEG-precipitated material is then applied in plate absorption assays.

Immunofluorescence assays

The immunofluorescence (IF) assay is a primary binding test based on the principle that antibody, labeled with a fluorochrome dye such as FITC, can be identified visually after binding to its homologous antigen. The chief utility of IF lies in its ability to combine antigen detection capability with tissue or cellular morphology.

With chemically-fixed antigen (cells, tissues, bacteria, fungi), a positive IF reaction is seen as an apple-green fluorescence (Figure 10-18). The striking advantage of the IF antibody test over other serologic tests is that IF determines the exact site of antibody attachment in cells, a mixed population of bacteria or in tissues.

Two modifications of the IF test are commonly used. The simplest, the direct IF test, uses fluorochrome-conjugated antibody (see Figure 10-19). The advantage of this test is that it consists of a one-step procedure of incubating antibody to antigen, washing the excess antibody from the antigen preparation, and viewing in a fluorescent microscope. The direct test is suitable for identifying unknown antigen preparations such as *Clostridia* bacteria species in infected animals and rabies

Table 10-2 Approaches to separation of bound and unbound reactants in immunologic assays

Technique	Principle or mechanism of action	Predominant use
Ammonium sulfate fractionation	IgG is insoluble in 40% (volume/volume) ammonium sulfate; labeled antigen is not	Provides crude Ig preparation for variety of uses
Polyethylene glycol (PEG) preparation	Soluble complexes are less soluble than free reactants; PEG removes water of hydration and precipitates the complexes	Immune complex assays in conjunction with Clq
Solid phase absorption with protein A or carrier beads	Cowan strain I, *staphylococcus* aureus bacteria bind Fc-IgF; antigen covalently attached to dextran beads; for both, centrifugation removes bound reactants from solution	Radioimmune precipitation coupled with polyacrylamide gel electrophoresis (RIP-PAGE) for analysis of complex antibody-antigen reactions
Solid phase plate absorption	Soluble antigen or antibody absorbs plastic; excess is washed away	ELISA, RIA
Cell monolayer/tissue section absorption	Acetone-fixed cell monolayers, frozen tissue sections, or paraffin-embedded sections glued to glass slides; excess reactants are washed away	In situ immunocytochemistry

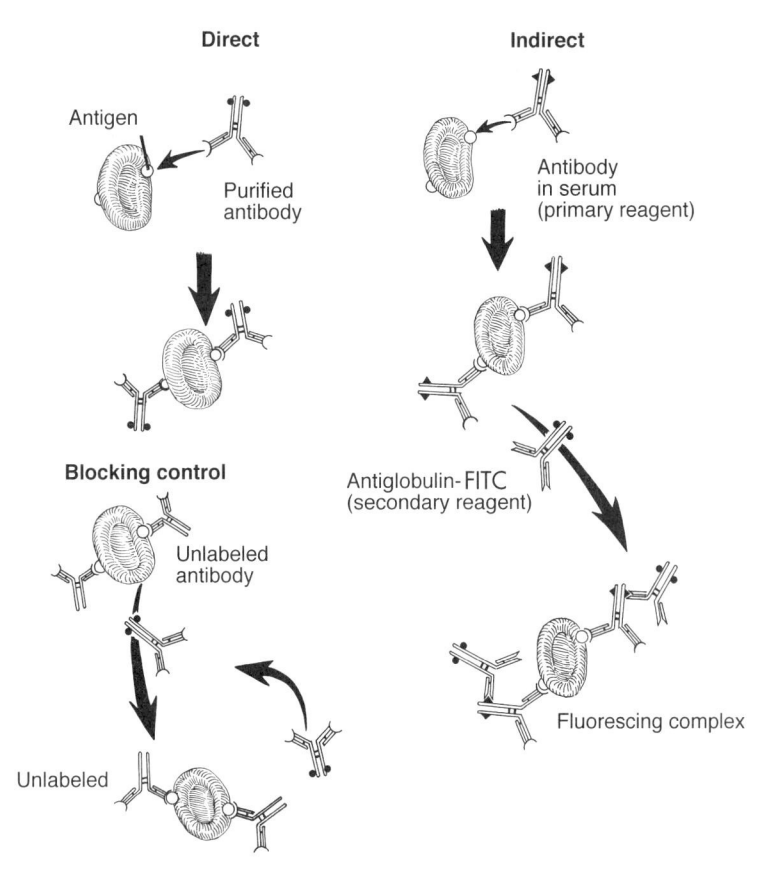

Figure 10-18 Fluorescent antibody tests. All fluorescent antibody (FA) tests are based on the ability to conjugate fluorochromes onto antibody without interfering with the antigen-binding sites. The direct IF test uses a reagent (purified antibody) that is conjugated with a fluorochrome such as isothiocyanate (ITC). The interreaction of this fluorochrome-labeled antibody with antigen can be seen directly with the aid of an ultraviolet microscope. To control the specificity of the direct FA test, the preincubation of unlabeled antibody blocks the attachment of labeled antibody. Globulin from nonimmune animals does not block this reaction. Indirect FA uses two reagents, an unlabeled primary serum that contains the antibody toward the appropriate antigen, and a fluorochrome-labeled secondary reagent (antiglobulin). The indirect FA is more sensitive than the direct FA in that multiple antiglobulin molecules may attach to a single antibody in the primary reagent. A striking advantage of the indirect FA test is that it does not require the purification and labeling of globulin from patient serum.

virus in animal brain tissues. The direct IF test is rarely used to identify antibody in animal serum.

The indirect IF technique employs animal serum (primary reagent) as the source of antigen-specific antibody and fluorochrome-conjugated antiglobulin (secondary reagent) (see Figure 10-20). As the staining reagent, the advantages of the indirect IF test follow.

1. A single secondary reagent can be used with many serum samples. This permits the screening of many animal sera for antibody.

2. The indirect test is up to 40 times more sensitive than the direct IF test. This is because many secondary antibodies react with a single primary antibody.

Controls must be performed with all IF tests to rule out the possibility of nonspecific attachment of antibody FITC to antigen. In the direct IF test, pretreatment of antigen with immune serum (nonconjugated antibody) blocks the subsequent attachment of FITC-conjugated antibody to antigen (Figure 10-18). Appropriate controls in indirect tests include the use of nonimmune primary reagent and incubation of the secondary along (no primary) with antigen. In either case, no fluorescence should be seen (Figure 10-18).

Direct and indirect IF techniques are largely restricted to frozen-section immunocytochemistry. That is, suspect tissue is frozen, cut on a cryostat, placed on slides, air-dried, and then treated or fixed with lipid solvents such as acetone or methanol. This special handling limits the adaptation of the technique to more routine cases.

Recently techniques have been developed that are suitable for use in aldehyde (formalin or glutaraldehyde)-fixed tissues. Thus tissue samples collected in formalin during necropsy or biopsy can be examined for antigens of biologic importance. A general procedure that can be used with IF or enzyme-labeled reagents is described below. Paraffin-embedded tissue sections, 4 to 6 μm thick, are mounted on glass slides coated with 5% (volume/volume) epoxy resin in xylene and deparaffinized. After extensive washing in saline solution, sections are treated with protease VII (or trypsin) and reduced with sodium borohydride. Sections are then stained for test antigen by means of an indirect IF procedure using primary goat antisera followed by rabbit antigoat IgG-FITC, or avidin-biotin-complex (ABC) peroxidase labeling techniques. With the latter techniques, the tissue section may be embedded in epoxy resin directly from the glass microslide, thereby permitting efficient and precise ultrastructural localization of labeled antigen. The advantages of these improved methods over previously employed procedures are, for IF, increased sensitivity combined with detailed morphologic preservation of tissue, and for peroxidase, efficient ultrastructural localization and analysis with retention of tissue architecture.

One example of a major use of IF is in the diagnosis of rabies. Rabies virus is found in animal brain tissue (Figure 10-19). Sections of brain tissue that may contain rabies virus are fixed in acetone. The fixation procedure increases the permeability of brain cells, thereby permitting the penetration of antirabies globulin. After incubation of the tissues with the fluorescein-conjugated rabies antibody, the slides are washed to remove unbound fluorescein antibody. Rabies antibody remains attached to rabies virus antigen. Virus-infected cells contain fluorescing Negri bodies (viral inclusions). Uninfected cells do not fluoresce.

One method of FeLV diagnosis is performed with an indirect IF test. Blood smears from suspect cats are fixed in methanol, incubated with specific rabbit anti-FeLV serum, and then stained with a fluorescein-conjugated goat antirabbit secondary reagent (Figure 10-20). After proper washing of the slide to remove unbound globulin, the slide is viewed under an ultraviolet microscope. A positive FeLV test detects fluorescing neutrophils and platelets. This test identifies FeLV infection even before the onset of clinical disease.

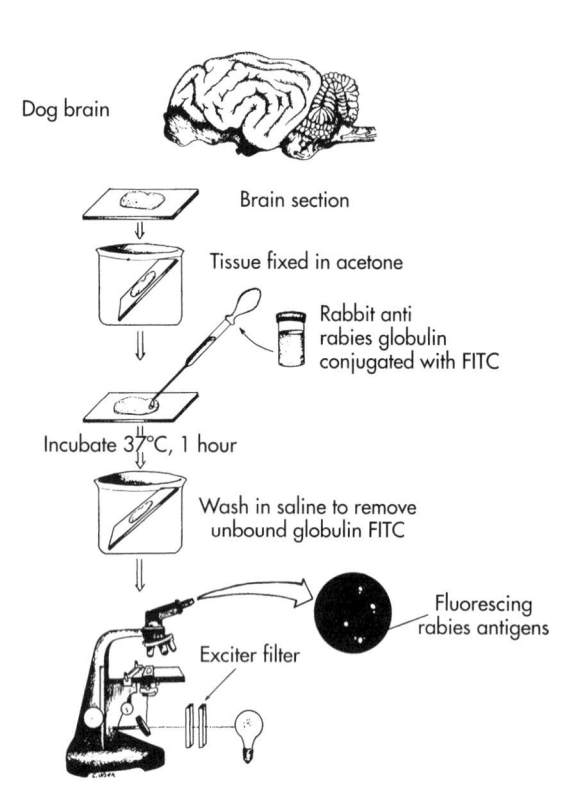

Figure 10-19 Direct FA test for rabies. Brain sections of animals suspected to have rabies are chemically fixed. Fixation denatures protein but preserves the morphologic features of the tissue and renders intact the antigenicity of the virus antigen. After the tissues are washed in buffered saline, an antirabies globulin conjugated with isothiocyanate (ITC) is added and Satt a allowed to incubate in a human chamber for 1 hour at 37°C. After the unbound globulin ITC is removed by washing in buffered saline, the specimen is examined in an ultraviolet microscope. In the case of rabies, the technician sees fluorescing Negri bodies within nonfluorescing brain cells. Negri bodies contain rabies antigen.

Solid phase plate assays

Both radioimmune assay (RIA)– and enzyme-linked immunosorbent assay (ELISA)–based serologic techniques are designed to take advantage of the fact that most protein antigens will adhere to polyvinyl, polycarbonate, and polypropylene surfaces. The plastic surfaces available as tubes, 96-well microtiter plates or solid sheets of plastic

Assays for Humoral Immunity, Including Serology   95

bound from unbound antigen or antibody is achieved (Figure 10-21).

Detection of antibody is achieved with linker or amplification reagents. Table 10-3 delineates commonly used materials. All are derived, in principle, from Coombs' antiglobulin reagent. Because the primary (i.e., patient serum) antibody is only present in small (nanogram) amounts, most of these linker reagents are designed to amplify the reaction by providing an "inverted pyramid" of bound reactants. Four general approaches to the amplification of the primary binding reaction are used. These are illustrated in order of increasing sensitivity (Figure 10-22). In the figure, the indicator system is an enzyme. If desired, isotopes can be used instead of the enzyme. Direct assays depend on the binding of the labeling reagents to the primary antibody. In the indirect variant, an antiglobulin is attached to the complex before addition of labeling reagents.

The sensitivities of RIA and ELISA are very high. Values of bound antibody in the nanogram range

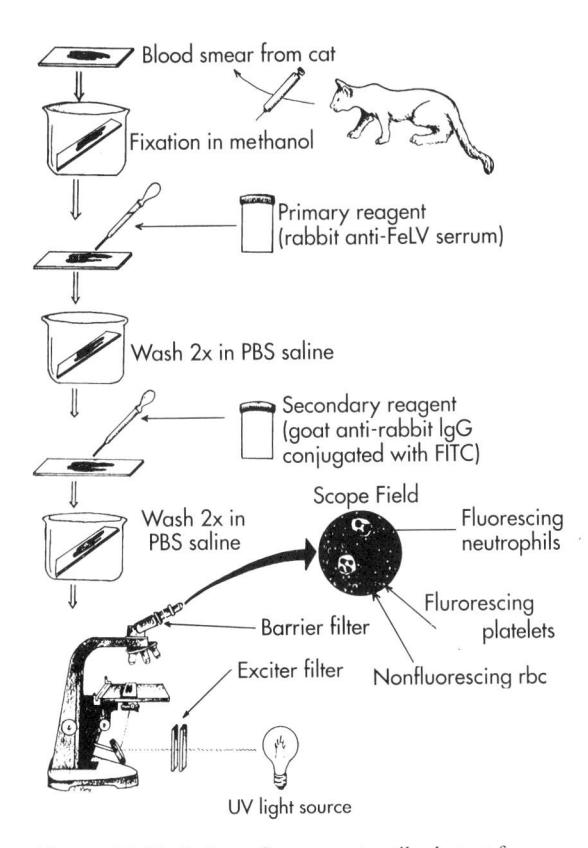

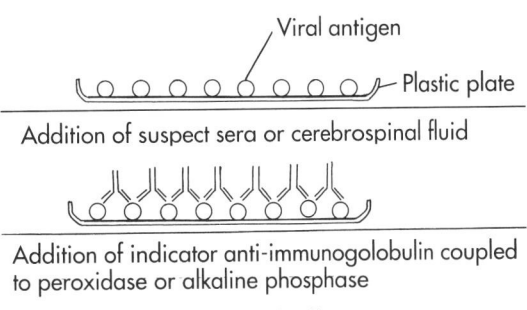

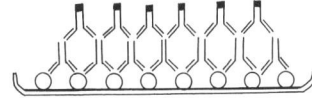

Figure 10-20 Indirect fluorescent antibody test for feline leukemia (FeLV). Blood smears from cats suspected of having FeLV disease are fixed in methanol, washed in buffered saline, and then treated with a primary reagent (rabbit anti-FeLV serum). After incubation and subsequent washing (to remove unbound globulin), the slide is then flooded with conjugated goat antirabbit IgG (secondary reagent). The slide is washed a second time to remove unbound conjugated globulin and is viewed under an ultraviolet microscope. In FeLV-positive cats, neutrophils and some platelets fluoresce.

film are suitable solid phase supports. Diluents with antigen contain an irrelevant protein, usually bovine serum albumin, and a detergent, Tween-20. Effective coating of the plates is complete within an hour or two. Because only a small amount of antigen binds to the plastic, antigen solutions can be decanted and used again—as many as four or five times. After washing, plates are incubated with a bovine serum albumin or other protein solution to ensure saturation of the plastic with protein, thereby avoiding nonspecific attachment of subsequent immunologic reagents. Once dried, the antigen-coated plates may be stored indefinitely. Thus, with simple washing of unbound reactants from the plastic, efficient separation of

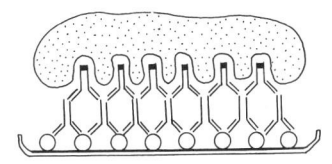

Figure 10-21 An ELISA-plate assay for demonstration of antibody to CDV. The plate, coated with CDV, has been incubated in sequence with canine serum containing anti-CDV antibody, rabbit anti-dog IgG conjugated to horseradish peroxidase and enzyme substrate (DAB).

Table 10-3 Commonly used linker or amplification reagents used in conjunction with immunoassays and immunocytochemistry

Type of reagent	Use of mechanism of binding
Antiglobulin	Anti-heavy chain for all "indirect" assays
Protein A (*S. aureus*)	Binds Fc regions of many IgG subclasses
Lectins	Binds glycoprotein residues
Peroxidase-antiperoxidase (PAP)	PAP complex binds IgG-Fc
Biotin	Binds avidin-labeled reagents
Dinitrophenol (DNP)	Binds to DNP-labeled antibodies

Complement components (Clq, C3)

or below, are routinely obtained. Manipulation of primary antibody by dilution will yield straight-line binding curves over a wide range of dilutions, thereby facilitating quantitative calculations. The requirement for small amounts of reagents has made automation a reality. Literally thousands of assays can now be performed by one laboratory technician. Finally, it is important to point out that all of the techniques outlined here can be reversed. That is, antibody attached to solid supports can be used to measure antigens of importance by this methodology (an example of this principle for a viral disease is given in Figure 10-23).

Choice of serologic assay

The almost infinite number of serologic assays appears confusing to both the student and the

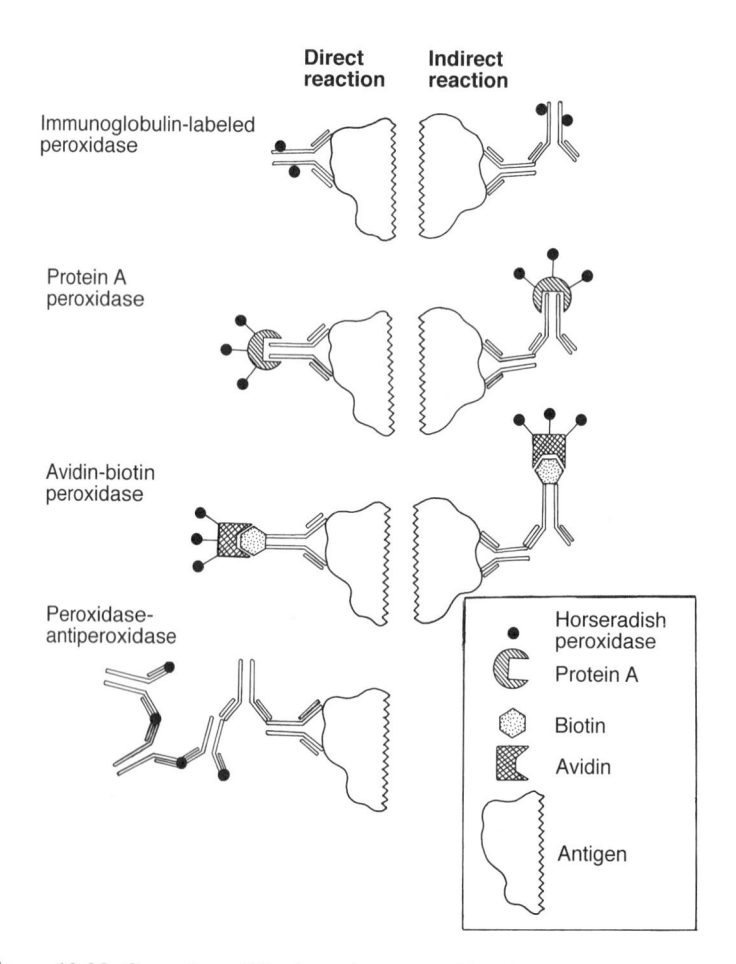

Figure 10-22 General amplification schemes used in primary binding immunoassays.

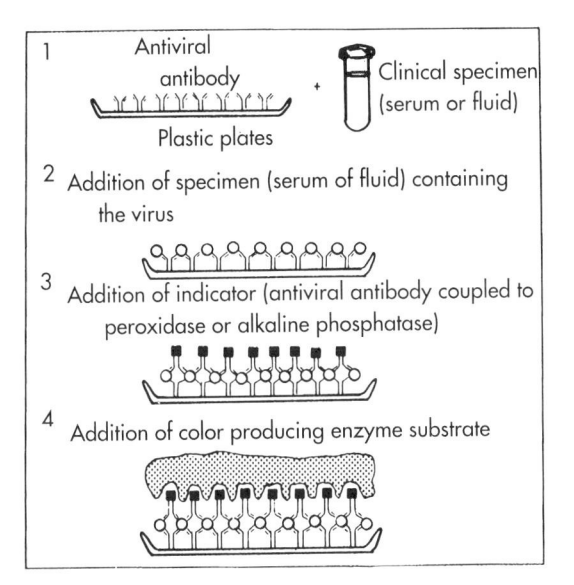

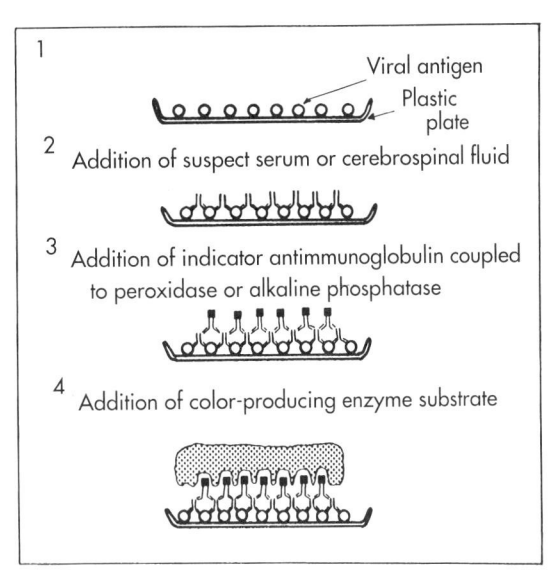

Figure 10-23 An ELISA for viral antigen (*left*) compared to an ELISA for viral antibody (right).

practicing veterinarian. For the latter, proper submission of the clinical sample to a reliable clinical pathology or diagnostic laboratory is important. Many serologic tests are now available in kit form. Today it is possible to determine pregnancy in a mare with a latex bead-based agglutination test for placental gonadotropin in urine. Commercially produced ELISA kits for FeLV and FIV can now be performed by animal technicians.

IF assays will likely be restricted to experimental or diagnostic settings. RIAs, though very sensitive, carry with them the need for specialized equipment and the dangers of dealing with radioactive materials. ELISA-based assays are equivalent in sensitivity to RIA, yet are safe and relatively easy to use. For this reason, ELISA has become the serologic method of choice for detecting antibodies or antigenic substances of biologic importance in both human and veterinary medicine.

SUGGESTED READINGS

Avramea S, Ternynck T, and Guesdone JL: Coupling of enzymes to antibodies and antigens. In Engvall E, Pesce AJ, editors: *Quantitative enzyme immunoassay*, 1978, Blackwell Scientific.

Axthelm MK, Krakowka S: Immunocytochemical methods for demonstrating canine distemper virus antigen in aldehyde-fixed paraffin-embedded tissue, *J Virol Methods* 13:215-229, 1986.

Beh KJ, Lascelles AL: The use of the antiglobulin test in the diagnosis of bovine brucellosis, *Res Vet Sci*, 14:239-244, 1973.

Carrier SP, Boulanger P, Bannester GL: Equine infectious anemia: sensitivity of the agar-gel immunodiffusion test, and the direct and the indirect complement-fixation tests for the detection of antibodies in equine serum, *Can J Comp Med*, 37:171-197, 1973.

Carpenter AB: Enzyme-linked immunoassays. In Rose NR, DeMacrio EC, Fahey JL, Friedman H, Penn GM, editors: *Manual of clinical laboratory immunology*, ed 4, Washington, DC: American Society of Microbiology, 1992, pp. 2-9.

Check IR, Piper M, Papadea C: Immunoglobulin quantitation. In Rose NR, DeMacrio EC, Fahey JL, Friedman H, Penn GM, editors: *Manual of clinical laboratory immunology*, ed 4, Washington, DC, American Society of Microbiology, 1992, pp 71-83.

Coggins L, Norcross NL: Immunodiffusion reaction in equine anemia, *Cornell Vet* 60:330-335, 1970.

Corbel MJ: Characterization of antibodies active in the Rose Bengal plate test, *Vet Rec* 90:484-485, 1972.

Corbell MJ, Lucas M, Cartwright SF: Immunoglobulin class in relation to neutralization of transmissible gastroenteritis virus, *Vet Rec* 90:658-659, 1972.

Corbel MJ, Wray C: The effect of natural infection with *Salmonella urbana* on the serological status of cattle in relation to tests for brucellosis, *Br Vet J* 131:324, 1975.

Engrall E, Perlmann P: Enzyme-linked immunosorbent assay (ELISA). Quantitative assay of IgG, *Immunochemistry 8*: 871-874, 1971.

Essex M, Klein G, Snyder SP, Harrold JB: Antibody to feline oncornavirus-associated cell membrane antigen in neonatal cats, *Int J Cancer* 8:384-390, 1971.

Hardy Jr WD, Hirshant Y, Hess P: Detection of the feline leukemia virus and other mammalian oncornaviruses by immunofluorescence. In Chieco-Bianchi RM, Chieco-Bianchi L, editors: *Unifying concepts of leukemia*, Basel, 1971, Karger, pp 778-799.

Holbrow EJ, Johnson GD: Immunofluorescence. In Weir DM, editor: *Handbook of experimental immunology*, Philadelphia, 1967, Davis pp 571-596.

Huck RA, Evans DH, Woods DG, King AA, and others: Border disease of sheep: comparison of the results of serological testing using complement fixation: immunodiffusion, neutralization and immunofluorescent techniques, *Br Vet J* 131:427, 1975.

Krakowka S, Fenner W, Miele J: Quantitative determination of serum origin cerebrospinal fluid proteins in the dog, *Am J Vet Res* 42:1975-1977, 1981.

Levine L: Micro-complement fixation. In Weir DM, editor: *Handbook of experimental immunology*, Philadelphia, 1967, Davis pp 707-719.

Morris JH, Stevens HE: Aggregation and the anti-complementary activity of an antigen used in the complement-fixation test for Johnes' disease, *Res Vet Sci* 21:117-118, 1976.

Musiani M, Zerbini M, LaPlaca M: Rapid diagnosis of viral infections by an alkaline phosphatase immunocytochemical methods, *J Immunol Methods* 88:255-258, 1986.

Neter E: Bacterial hemagglutination tests. In Frankel S, Reifman S, Sonnenwirth AC, editors: *Gradwohl's clinical laboratory methods and diagnosis*, vol 2, St. Louis, 1970, Mosby, pp 1554-1560.

Ouchterlony O: Immunodiffusion and immunoelectrophoresis. In Weir DM, editor: *Handbook of experimental immunology*, Philadelphia, 1967, Davis, pp 655-706.

Patterson JM, Degoe BL, Stone SS: Identification of immunoglobulins associated with complement fixation, agglutination, and low pH buffered antigen tests for brucellosis, *Am J Vet Res* 37:319-324, 1976.

Pfeiffer NE, McGuire TC, Bendel RB, Werkel JM: Quantitation of bovine immunoglobulins: comparison of single radial immunodiffusion, zinc sulfate toxicity, serum electrophoresis, and refractometer methods, *Am J Vet Res*, 38:693-698, 1977.

Poston RN: A buffered chronic chloride method of attaching antigens to red cells: use in hemagglutination, *J Immunol Methods* 5:91-96, 1974.

Potgieter SND: The influence of complement on the neutralization of infectious bovine rhinotracheitis virus by globulins derived from early and late bovine antisera, *Can J Com Med* 39:427-433, 1975.

Prokudina EN, Semenova NP, Zhdanor VM: Detection of viral antigens by solid phase radioimmunoassay on polyethylene film, *J Virol Methods* 13:27-33, 1986.

Rice CE: Studies of changes in serum proteins in cows and calves in a herd affected with Johnes's disease, *Res Vet Sci* 10:188-196, 1969.

Roitt I, Brostoff J, Male D: *Immunology*, ed 3, St Louis, 1993, Mosby.

Sonnenwirth AC: Miscellaneous serologic tests. In Frankel S, Reitman S, Sonnenwirth AC, editors: *Gradwohl's clinical laboratory methods and diagnosis*, vol 2, St. Louis, 1970, Mosby, pp 1561-1575.

Tannelli D, Diaz R, Bettini TM: Identification of *Brucella abortus* antibodies in cattle serum by single radial diffusion, *J Clin Microbiol* 3:203-205, 1976.

Valler A, Bartlett A, Bidwell DE: Enzyme immunoassays with special reference to ELISA techniques, *J Clin Pathol* 31: 507-520, 1978.

Wray C, Morris JH, Sojka WJ: A comparison of indirect haemagglutination tests and serum agglutination tests for the serological diagnosis of *Salmonella dublin* infection in cattle, *Br Vet J* 131:725, 1975.

11 Assays for T Lymphocyte Function

In vitro and in vivo assessment of lymphocyte functions and identification of lymphocytes and subpopulations of lymphocytes

IN VIVO IDENTIFICATION METHODS

Because lymphocytes are, for the most part, morphologically identical, their nature and role, if any, in the specific immune response remained unknown throughout the first half of this century. Conclusive demonstration of their function(s) was provided by irradiation, reconstitution, and ablation experiments pioneered by Medewar in the 1940s. The in vivo findings can be summarized by consideration of the effects of these manipulations on inbred strains of mice and chickens.

In mice, sublethal irradiation destroys lymphatic tissues and ablates the ability of these animals to respond to immunologic challenge. Reconstitution with bone marrow cells and thymus (but not thymus alone) restores immunologic capability. Removal of the thymus in the neonate eliminates cellular responses (e.g., skin graft rejection) without affecting antibody response to some, but not all, antigens. Reconstitution with syngeneic bone marrow is successful in restoring graft-rejecting ability, thus demonstrating the trophic influence of the thymus on the development of thymus-derived T-cell function. The avian species provides additional information on the compartmentalization and functions of lymphocytes. As with the mouse species, thymectomy of a developing embryo ablates T-cell function. However, unlike mammals, the bird species possesses a special organ, the bursa of Fabricius that, when removed in the embryo by surgery or testosterone injection, eliminates the humoral antibody (B lymphocyte) response.

Thus one method for in vivo identification of lymphocyte subpopulations involves ablation and subsequent examination of lymphoid tissues for any morphologic changes. Removal of the thymus results in depletion of paracortical lymphoid cells in lymph nodes and loss of cellularity around the periarteriolar regions in the spleen. When reconstituted with bone marrow, lymphatic tissue from irradiated, thymectomized mice shows well-developed germinal centers in the cortical regions of the lymph nodes. Lymphatic tissue from similarly treated mice, when reconstituted with thymus, shows well-developed paracortical areas.

Application of these techniques to the larger outbred domestic animal species is difficult, if not impossible, because of histocompatibility differences between individuals. In addition, thymic-dependent lymphocytes peripheralize in the developing fetus in utero, making postnatal thymectomy ineffective. In utero thymectomy experiments have been performed in dogs and sheep, and the data generated support observations made in chickens and mice. Thus because of these severe limitations of postnatal thymectomy considerable effort has been expended to develop methods for in vitro identification of lymphocytes.

APPROACH TO PURIFICATION OF MONONUCLEAR CELLS FROM PERIPHERAL BLOOD

In peripheral blood smears, lymphocytes are distressingly similar. The in vitro experiments described earlier suggested compartmentalization of lymphocyte functions and provided the stimulus to develop methods to identify these cell subpopulations in vitro. Most of the in vitro lymphocyte methodologies discussed are applied to peripheral blood, since this is a convenient source of lymphocytes for repeated analysis. However, single-cell suspensions from lymphoid tissues are often used experimentally. If short-term culture is anticipated, then careful attention to sterile technique is mandatory. In general, manipulations should be performed with a sterile, enriched tissue culture medium (RPMI-1640), supplemented with antibiotics, glutamine, and bicarbonate. Tissue culture phosphate-buffered saline (TC-PBS) devoid of calcium and magnesium ions is an excellent wash solution. At each step in the procedure, viability should be assessed by supravital staining with trypan blue combined with cell counts (viable cells per milliliter) to assist in calculating yield efficiencies.

Single-cell suspensions from lymphoid tissues are prepared by sterile mincing of the tissue followed by passing the pieces through stainless-steel mesh or sterile, gauze-covered, glass beakers to separate cells from connective tissue fragments. Before further processing, nonviable cells or cell aggregates should be removed by passage over a ficoll-gradient. Usually a 10 to 15 minute centrifugation is sufficient. If peripheral blood is used as the starting material, it is necessary to prevent coagulation. A variety of techniques are used. Blood samples may be drawn into a syringe containing preservative-free heparin (final dilution is 10 to 20 units/ml). However, heparin is somewhat toxic to cells, and the samples should be processed soon after collection. Similarly, the calcium chelator ethylenediaminetetraacetic acid (EDTA) is an excellent anticoagulant. Sodium citrate is also an effective anticoagulant (1 ml of 3.8% sodium citrate/10 ml blood). Finally, an unclotted sample may be drawn and placed in a glass beaker or Erlenmeyer flask containing glass beads and defibrinated for 10 to 15 minutes by gentle agitation. This last method has the advantage of removing platelets and many neutrophils, but markedly reduces total mononuclear cell yield per milliliter of blood.

Blood platelets complicate the efficient separation of cells because of their marked tendency to aggregate and, along with fibrin, produce sticky sites for nonspecific attachment of leukocytes. If the assays performed depend on adherence to plastic, glass, or target cells, platelet aggregates will interfere with this event. For this reason, it is frequently desirable to deplete peripheral blood of platelets before separation. As mentioned, platelets can be eliminated by defibrination. If cell yield is compromised by defibrination because of small sample size, platelet contamination may be reduced by a platelet separation procedure before mononuclear cell isolation. For this, EDTA-anticoagulated blood is subjected to a modified ficoll separation using a diluted Hypaque solution of specific gravity 1.014. The platelet-rich supernatant is removed and discarded. The cellular pellet is resuspended in TC-PBS and then processed further. It may be necessary to reduce or eliminate contamination of lymphocyte suspensions by monocytes; this is important for in vitro immunoglobulin (Ig) production assays, as monocytes clearly inhibit bursal-derived (B) cell differentiation. In this instance, monocytes are best removed before mononuclear isolation by the technique of carbonyl iron ingestion. For this, blood anticoagulated with EDTA is mixed with gas-sterilized iron filings (such as GAF carbonyl iron powder*) grade SF-Spec, GAF Corp. and incubated at 37°C for 60 minutes before further processing. Monocytes and neutrophils engulf these iron filings and subsequently migrate through Ficoll Hypaque to the bottom of the centrifuge tubes. It is important to point out that this technique is not 100% effective in removing these cell types. A general strategy for this isolation and separation of leukocyte populations is given in Figure 11-1.

ISOLATION OF MONONUCLEAR CELLS

Separation of lymphocytes from other blood elements is accomplished by taking advantage of density differences between these cells. A solution of sucrose polymer (ficoll) and diatrizoate (Hypaque) with a specific gravity of 1.0805 is effective. This solution can be made in the laboratory, but commercially available products for cellular separation are widely available and should be used, if feasible, to ensure day-to-day reproducibil-

---

*GAF Corporation, New York, New York.

Step 1 — Sterile heparinized blood is collected in a syringe

Step 2 — Dilute blood with phosphate-buffered saline

Step 3 — Underlaying with sterile Ficoll-Hypaque (sp. gravity 1.0805)

Step 4 — Centrifugation 400g × 40 min

Step 5 — Diluted Plasma / Lymphocytes / Ficoll-Hypaque / Erythrocytes and Neutrophils → Isolated lymphocytes

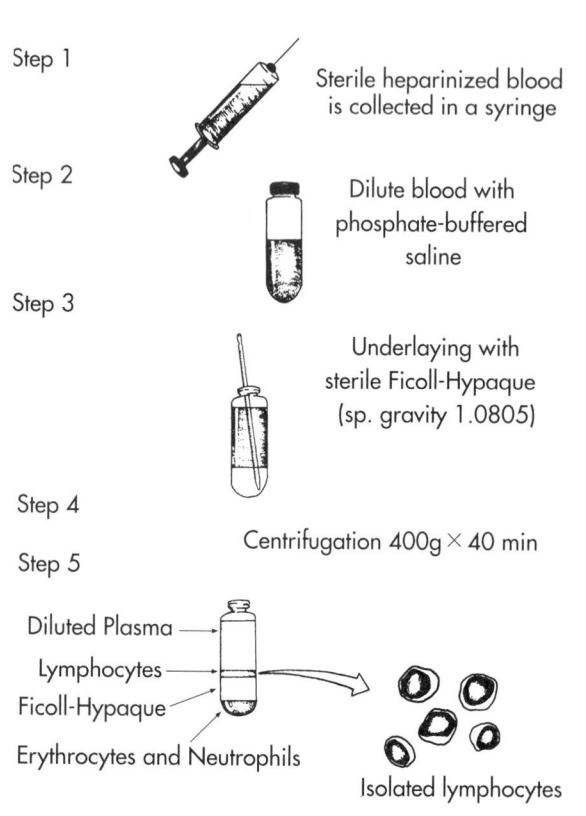

Figure 11-1 Isolation of lymphocytes from peripheral blood using Ficoll-Hypaque.

ity of results. Products such as Ficoll-Paque, Histopaque, and Lymphoprep all work well.

Heparinized or defibrinated peripheral blood is diluted in saline and placed in a centrifuge tube. Ficoll-Hypaque is layered under the blood sample with a syringe and needle, and the tube is centrifuged at 400 g for 30 to 40 minutes. As the blood moves through the separating solution, erythrocytes are agglutinated by Ficoll and, along with neutrophils, settle to the bottom of the tube. Lymphocytes and monocytes remain at the saline-ficoll interface (Figure 11-2). Depending on the species, 70% to 90% of the cells collected are lymphocytes. Cellular contaminants are monocytes (10% to 30%), neutrophils, and eosinophils, in that order. For routine manipulations, the latter two are disregarded. A crisp, well-defined mononuclear band is generally achieved in adults. However, the band is wide and diffuse when samples from young animals are processed. Frequently the band in young animals is heavily contaminated with erythrocytes. These should be removed before the culture because hemoglobin has a quenching effect on scintillation counting and is also somewhat toxic to cells. For erythrocyte removal the contaminated mononuclear band is collected and washed, and the cellular pellet is vigorously resuspended in 10 ml distilled water for 10 to 15 seconds before the addition of 2.9 ml of 3.5% (w/v) saline solution to reestablish isotonicity. Cells are then collected by centrifugation, resuspended in media, and then processed further. Lymphocytes collected in this manner can then be used for surface marker identification studies and tests for lymphocyte function.

In order to further define cell types involved in the various manifestations of the immune response, methods have been devised to separate B and T cells in vitro. Most of the techniques available take advantage of the different membrane characteristics of these cells. These differences have resulted in two general approaches to further purification. The first relies on distinguishing physical or behavioral characteristics of the cell populations of interest, and the second takes advantage of the immunologic marker systems such as Fc receptors, surface immunoglobulin and subpopulation-specific cell-membrane markers identified by monoclonal antibody panels.

SEPARATION OF MONONUCLEAR CELL POPULATION(S) BY PHYSICAL METHODS

Physical methods take advantage of specialized properties of cells such as adherence, relative density, and net surface electrical charge. Lymphocyte subpopulations differ in relative densities and can be separated by fractionation through sucrose or serum albumin gradients. This technique is difficult and exacting and is presently restricted to experimental situations. Likewise, differences in net surface charge have been detected in lymphocytes by submitting them to gentle separation in a semi-solid gel electrophoresis system.

In the presence of extracellular calcium ions, monocytes settle onto glass and plastic surfaces and subsequently attach to these surfaces quite firmly. This property of adherence is widely used to deplete a mixed population or, conversely, to enrich for monocytes. Two variant procedures are used. In the first, lymphocyte suspensions (5 to 10 × 10^6 cells) are dispersed into small (75 mm^2) plastic flasks with medium and incubated 1 to 2 hours at 37° C. Nonadherent cells (chiefly lymphocytes) are then decanted, and adherent cells are rinsed several times with TC-PBS. In the second variant, small syringes stoppered with a plug of spun glass or nylon wool are filled with Sephadex G-10 beads. After equilibration and warming at 37° C 1 hour in media, 1 to 2-ml cell suspensions (5 to 10 × 10^6 cells total) are applied

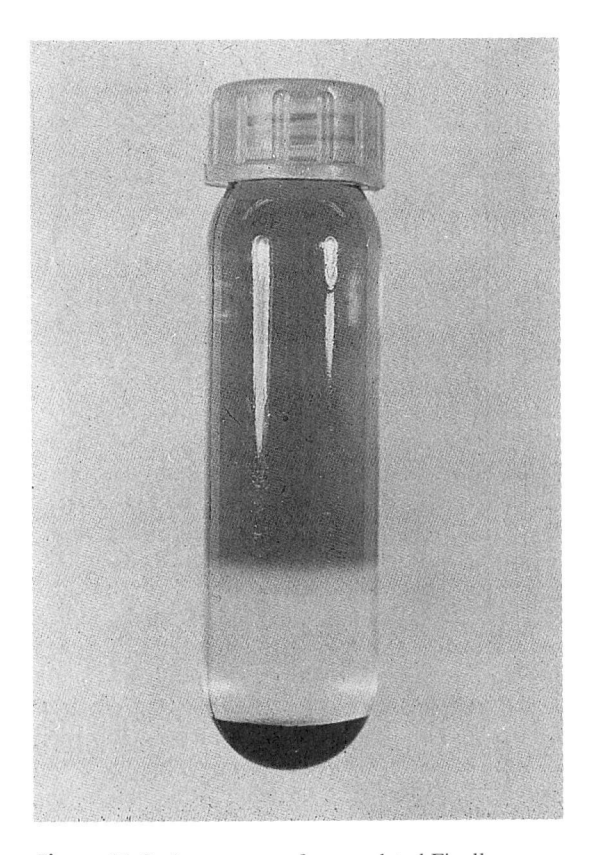

Figure 11-2 Appearance of a completed Ficoll-Hypaque centrifugation isolation of feline peripheral blood leukocytes. Mononuclear cells are harvested from the interface. (Courtesy GL Cockerell, DVM, PhD, Colorado State University.

to the column, stoppered, and then incubated 1 to 2 hours at 37°C. Nonadherent lymphocytes are washed through the columns with warmed media. Monocytes from either plastic or beads may be dislodged by rapid chilling at 4°C for 30 minutes followed by agitation, scraping (from plastic) or elution with medium containing 0.25% (volume/volume lidocaine). Adherence procedures do not produce pure populations of monocytes. Platelets, PMNs, and lymphocytes (chiefly B cells) will also adhere to plastic. We have noted substantial individual differences between dogs in the success of this technique for unknown reasons. Of course, species difference may also influence yield and purity.

Peripheral blood monocytes may be isolated from autologous plasma-diluted buffy coats by first aggregating the platelets with bovine thrombin, increasing the ionic strength of the suspension by addition of 2 to 3 volumes of 9% saline, and finally by Ficoll-Hypaque isolation (specific gravity 1.077, 700 g × 30 minutes.

SEPARATION OF MONONUCLEAR POPULATIONS BY IMMUNOLOGIC METHOD

More modern immunologic separation methods are based on expressed population-specific or shared cell-membrane markers on the surface of viable lymphoid cells. Cells of the immune system express receptors for complement components and also for the Fc region of IgG, as described in Chapter 3. Before the development of monoclonal antibody reagents, a convenient method for separation of cells involves rosette formation. In this method, isolated lymphocytes are rosetted with erythrocyte (E), erythrocyte-IgG antibody (EA), or erythrocyte-IgM-murine complement (EAC) complexes and then submitted to Ficoll-Hypaque gradient centrifugation. The rosetted cells are more dense than unrosetted cells and can be recovered in the pellet. Complete separation with this method is not achieved because not all T or B lymphocytes rosette with specific reagents. Thus their usefulness as a definitive method for isolation of homogeneous cell preparations is limited. Nonetheless, B cells particularly can be enriched with EAC rosette isolation and can be further purified by applying additional techniques to the EAC-positive population.

A more useful approach, now that well-defined polyclonal and monoclonal reagents are available, involves the application of specific antibody reagents to the isolation procedure. Although the development of the fluorescence-activated cell sorter (FACS) allows for sterile separation into any populations for which an antibody is available, this technique is not generally available. A more practical application for those without a FACS is the affinity isolation technique. For this, the IgG fraction of antisera is coupled to solid-phase support such as cyanogen bromide–activated Sepharose beads or are attached to plastic culture vessels (the panning technique). After washing and blocking unbound sites on the beads or plastic with an irrelevant protein such as bovine serum albumin, cell suspensions are applied to the support complexes. After incubation, unbound cells are removed by gentle washing and bound cells are eluted, ordinarily with a glycine-based buffer, 0.01 M, pH 2.2. The process is repeated with the unbound cells several times and the eluted cells are then pooled and analyzed for purity, viability, and yield (see Chapter 3). The success of the technique depends on the quality of the antisera used. Antiglobulin coated plates or beads will isolate B lymphocytes. Similarly, antisera to T-cell antigens such as CD3, CD4-helper, or CD8-suppressor/cytotoxic population(s) have been successfully used in this regard. A useful variation of this technique involves using magnetic beads coated with the appropriate antibody. The beads are incubated with the lymphocyte suspension and the appropriate cells bind to the antibody. A magnetic device is then used to retrieve the beads with bound cells. After washing, the cells are eluted from the beads. Fluorescence analysis (FACSCAN) then be used to evaluate the purity of the separated population.

Another general method for depletion of T or B lymphocytes from a mixed cell suspension involves use of cytotoxic (complement-dependent) antisera specific for unique cell surface antigens. The thy-1 system for T-cells in the murine species has been used in this type of procedure.

These methods are used experimentally to determine the specific cells involved in the generation of the immune response. These techniques have demonstrated the cooperative cellular interactions necessary in response to T-cell dependent and T-cell independent antigens, as well as the cellular origin of lymphokines. In addition, regulation of the responses through T-cell suppressor activity has been delineated in part by these methods.

Antigen-specific leukocytes may be isolated from a mixed cellular population by adherence techniques. If the antigen is known and is available in pure form, then the affinity-binding procedure using plastic or Sepharose beads is used. Cytotoxic T-cells and natural killer (NK) cells may be enriched by adherence to target-cell monolayers. For canine NK cells, the canine thyroid adenocarcinoma cell (CTAC) line is useful in this regard. For this, mononuclear cell suspensions are applied to confluent CTAC monolayers and incubated at 37°C for 2 to 3 hours. Nonadherent cells are removed, and adherent NK cells are identified by phase microscopy (see Figure 3-13). Binding is firm and a variety of cell marker assays may be applied to these cells. Elution from monolayers is achieved by washing monolayers in glycine buffer containing lidocaine.

Finally, the most definitive method for cellular separation uses the FACS (as mentioned earlier). After labeling cellular suspensions with fluorescein-bound antibody reagents, the FACS machine can be programmed to not only count negative and positive populations, but also to disperse them into separate culture vessels. Aside from the expense, technical problems are frequent. The quality of the starting immunologic reagent is the key variable in the success of this technique.

ASSAYS FOR LYMPHOCYTE FUNCTION(S) IN MIXED OR PURIFIED CELLULAR POPULATIONS

B lymphocytes

The extracellular product of B lymphocyte activation is, of course, immunoglobulin. Detection and quantitation of systemic or local antibody responses is known as serology; this subject is covered separately in Chapter 10. The recognition that B lymphocytes produce humoral antibodies led to the development of methods for detecting antibodies on lymphocyte surfaces. Of these, fluorescein-conjugated antiimmunoglobulin sera are in most widespread use. Lymphocytes are suspended in the antisera, and specific-membrane fluorescence is then detected under a microscope equipped for detecting fluorescence. Thymic-dependent lymphocytes lack surface immunoglobulin. Use of class-specific antisera allows quantitation of lymphocytes bearing IgG, IgM, IgA, and IgE on their surfaces. This method does not distinguish cytophilic antibody from that actively produced by the cell. Accordingly, a more accurate method of quantitating B cells requires brief trypsinization of the cells in vitro and testing for newly-produced surface immunoglobulin 24 hours later. In the mouse species data generated by this technique reveal that the major Ig determinant on the cell surface is IgD not IgG. In vitro trypsinization studies should be done before data on types of surface immunoglobulin appearing on peripheral blood B lymphocytes in domestic animal species can be relied on. Other cellular marker systems besides surface immunoglobulin will identify the B-cell population. These systems are outlined in Chapter 3.

B lymphocytes may be stimulated to differentiate into plasma cells using several different plant lectins. Of these pokeweed mitogen (PWM) is most widely used. Monocytes, probably through production of interferon and/or prostaglandins, down-regulate this event and so should be removed from the cellular suspensions by prior carbonyl iron ingestion. T lymphocytes potentiate the response by secretion of a lymphokine, B-cell growth factor (BCGF). The assay is performed in vitro. For dogs, cells (2×10^6/ml) plus PWM or media are cultured for 5 to 6 days at 37°C. Quantitation of the response is achieved by Ig-class–specific staining of cytospin preparations or smears with fluorescein-conjugated antiglobulin reagents (see Figure 3-10). Immunoglobulin released in culture fluids is detected and quantitated by an Ig-trap enzyme-linked immunosorbent assay (ELISA) (see Chapter 10). Other mitogens, notably bacterial lipopoly-saccharide will also induce B-cell differentiation. It is important to remember that these mitogens are polyclonal B-cell activators. This assay is useful in evaluating the effects of drugs, toxins, and immunoregulatory substances on the B-cell arm of the immune response.

In vivo evaluation of T-lymphocyte function

Perturbations of T-lymphocyte function in vivo are frequently reflected in the finding of lymphopenia. Besides this, three classic approaches for demonstration of cell-mediated immunity are: delayed-type hypersensitivity skin tests, allograft rejections, and graft-versus-host (gvh) reactions.

The intradermal skin test is widely used in veterinary medicine. Studies of tuberculosis in guinea pigs by Koch in the late 19th century established the skin test as a correlate of developing effective immunity to the tubercle bacillus. The skin test can be differentiated from skin responses induced by antibodies in the following manner. The maximum skin response occurs 24 to 72 hours after testing (delayed hypersensitivity), in contrast to several hours for antibody-mediated (immediate hypersensitivity) skin lesions. This activity is transferable to unsensitized hosts by cells and not by serum. Histologic examination of skin test sites reveals the presence of lymphocytes and macrophages instead of neutrophils and edema fluid characteristic to antibody-mediated lesions. Reconstitution experiments have demonstrated that this is a T-lymphocyte function and not a characteristic of B cells. Development of the response requires only a few specifically sensitized cells. Macrophages and additional lymphocytes are recruited to the area of antigen deposition by the release of soluble products by sensitized lymphocytes contacting the antigen, termed *lymphokines*.

A second classic manifestation of cell-mediated immunity is allograft rejection. If a skin graft from a histoincompatible donor is placed on a genetically unrelated recipient, the graft is rejected within 10 to 14 days of placement (Figure 11-3). The proximate cause of death of the graft is interference with its blood-vascular supply. Vascular changes of fibrinoid necrosis, thrombosis, and inflammation are mediated by lymphocytes sensitized to the foreign-tissue antigens. The reaction is T-cell dependent, as proven by ablation-reconstitution and passive cellular transfer experiments. Another attempt to graft tissue from the same donor to the recipient results in accelerated rejection 4 to 7 days after placement. In this case, T lymphocytes and specific antibodies participate in the accelerated rejection reaction. The graft rejection reaction is immunologically specific in that grafting of genetically unrelated tissue onto an animal rejecting the initial graft is rejected in the normal time period (10 to 14 days). Sensitization results in the generation of T-lymphocyte–mediated memory that lasts for long periods (years to life) after induction. In inbred mice, immunologic memory exceeds normal life span for this species; this memory response has been transferred by cells through several generations.

A third in vivo manifestation of cell-mediated immunity similar to graft rejection is the GVH reaction. In this system, immunologically immature or immunocompromised animals are given a graft of immunocompetent donor cells (bone marrow alone or bone marrow plus thymus). These grafted cells recognize recipient foreign antigens and produce an immune response to them. Thus in contrast to the above situation, the graft rejects the host. Animals with fulminant GVH develop a runting syndrome, characterized by decreased body weight, alopecia, chronic dermatitis, diarrhea, arthritis, and glomerulonephritis. The GVH reaction can be avoided in some cases by using fetal liver transplants as the source of immunocompetent cells or by depleting grafted populations of alloreactive cells by absorption or cytotoxic means.

In vitro assessment of T-lymphocyte function

Definitive dissection and characterization of the immune response in animals using only in vivo methods has many practical limitations. To circumvent this, methods for short-term propagation of lymphocytes and macrophages in tissue culture

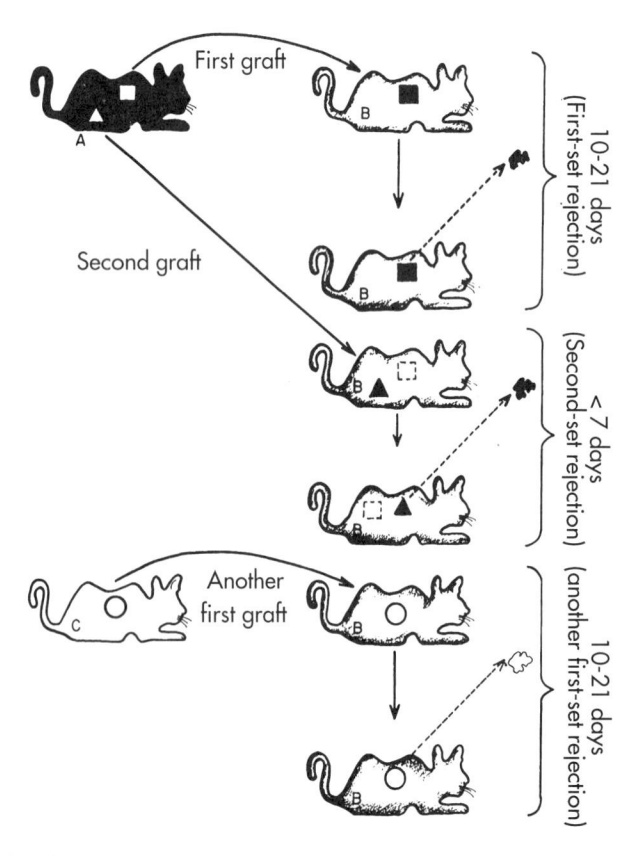

Figure 11-3 T-lymphocyte–mediated skin allograft rejection illustrating first-set rejecion, accelerated second-set rejection, and a third, antigenically-unrelated first-set rejection.

have been developed. Lymphocytes are isolated from peripheral blood as described earlier.

Tissue-culture medium used for lymphocytes is enriched with essential amino acids and other nutrients and buffered with sodium bicarbonate. Commercially-prepared media such as RPMI-1640 and L15 are in wide use. Inclusion of serum (2% to 20% volume/volume) is often necessary. As a general rule, lymphocytes grow better in homologous serum than in heterologous serum. Hemoglobin is somewhat toxic to cells and also interferes with scintillation counting; it should be eliminated by hypotonic shock lysis of erythrocytes and washing of lymphocytes before placement in culture. Lymphocytes suspended in media and incubated at 37° C, 5% to 10% CO_2 remains viable for 5 to 7 days (Figure 11-4).

While investigating the leukocyte and erythrocyte-agglutinating properties of plant lectins (high–molecular-weight polysaccharides), Nowell noted that incubation of lymphocytes with dilute quantities of these lectins stimulated growth and division (see Figure 3-8). Before this, the prevailing thought was that lymphocytes were end cells and, therefore, not mitotically active in vitro. This remarkable technical advance in lymphocyte culture methodology provided the stimulus for further in vitro studies of lymphocyte activity. Demonstration that the in vitro proliferative response correlated with intact cellular immunity lead to the widespread use of this method.

Initial studies quantitated the blastogenic response by counting stimulated cells versus unstimulated cells on stained smear. Blasts have a large nucleus, a pronounced nucleolus, and abundant cytoplasm (see Figure 3-8). Recognition that the essential feature of blastogenesis is DNA synthesis led to the use of radioactive DNA precursors (usually tritiated ^{3}H-thymidine) to quantitate this response. Early studies used a photographic emulsion technique. With development of the slides, incorporated ^{3}H-thymidine was determined by counting the number of cells in a smear with silver grains over the nucleus.

Currently, blastogenesis is quantitated using microcultures (1.5×10^5 cells/well) and an automated cell-harvesting machine. Cells or trichloroacetic acid-extracted DNA is deposited on a carrier (usually fiberglass paper strips). These strips are then transferred to vials containing scintillation fluid "cocktail," and the amount of incorporated ^{3}H-thymidine is quantitated in a liquid scintillation counter. Disintegrating ^{3}H-thymidine in the cocktail causes the generation of photons of light, which are detected by the machine and translated to disintegrations or counts per minute (cpm). There are several different methods used to express the data generated by ^{3}H-thymidine incorporation. A common calculation is the stimulation index where counts per minute (cpm), mitogen treated is divided by cpm, media control. The net or Δ (delta) cpm is calculated by cpm, mitogen minus cpm, media.

Plant lectins or phytomitogens, specifically bind and cross-link carbohydrate residues on cellular surfaces. Those in widespread use include

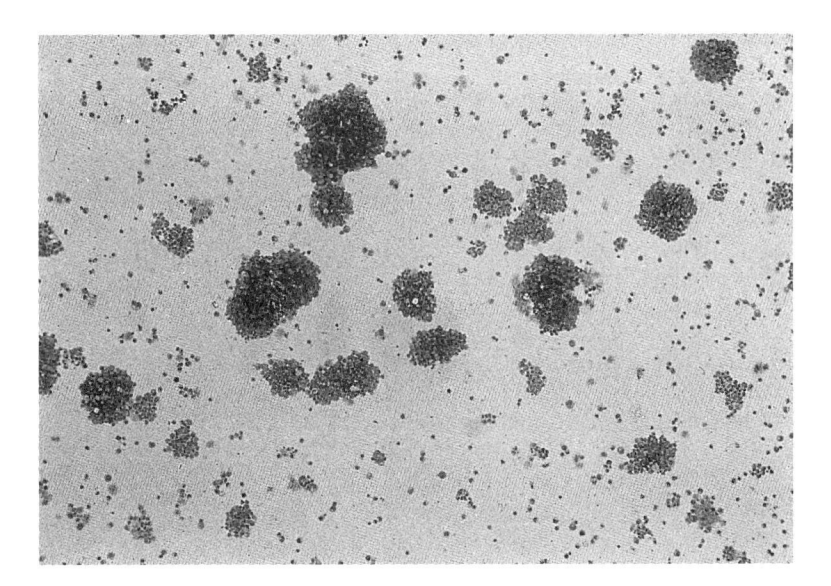

Figure 11-4 Phytohemagglutinin-P–stimulated canine lymphocyte culture demonstrates the agglutinating properties of the mitogen and its colony-forming ability.

Table 11-1 Binding specificities of some commonly used plant lectins in veterinary medicine

Lectin	Plant/animal source	Binding specificity	Lymphocyte mitogenic activity for: T cells	B cells
Concanavalin A	Jack bean	α-D-Mannose	+++	
Phytohemagglutinin	Phaseolus vulgaris	N-acetyl D-galactosamine	++	+
Lentil lectin	Lens culinaris	α-D-mannose	++	+
Helix pomatia	Vineyard snail	N-acetyl D-galactosamine	++	+
Limulus polyphemus	Horseshoe crab	Sialic acid		
Ricinus communis	Castor bean	D-galactose		
Pokeweed mitogen	Phytolacca americana	Unknown	+	+++

phytohemagglutinin (PHA), PHA-P or PHA-M, concanavalin A (Con A), PWM, lentil lectin, and SPA. The glycosyl-binding specificities of some commonly used mitogens in veterinary medicine are given in Table 11-1. In contrast to antigens, these mitogens are nonspecific stimulators of lymphocytes. That is, they stimulate 60% to 90% of the cells in culture into blastogenesis. For optimal stimulation, some degree of contamination with phagocytic cells is essential. Thus, although only lymphocytes undergo the blastogenic response, this response is macrophage-dependent. Mitogens are useful in distinguishing T and B lymphocytes in culture. In general, PHA and Con A stimulate T cells, whereas PWM is a B-cell mitogen. The distinction is not absolute, however, because some T lymphocytes respond to PWM, and some B cells are stimulated by PHA. Another class of mitogens unrelated to those plant extracts is bacterial endotoxins or lipopolysaccharides (LPS). Lipopolysaccharides are mitogenic for B cells in some species.

Several technical aspects in development of this assay for routine clinical or laboratory use are worth mentioning. Consideration should be given to dose of mitogen per culture, number of cells cultured, and time in culture. A typical schematic dose-response curve for use of PHA-P with canine lymphocytes is given in Figure 11-5. The lymphocyte blast transformation (LBT) test should be standardized for these variables in each laboratory. In spite of the widespread use of this procedure, it is important to emphasize the fact that adoption of this technique to clinical situations is difficult. Tremendous variability in stimulating efficiency (as determined by ^{3}H-thymidine incorporation) is the rule. Sources of this variation are attributed to individual idiosyncracies, subtle variations in day-to-day laboratory technique, varying ratios of cell types in the responding population, and circadian or diurnal fluctuations in the individual under study. Variations may be minimized by aliquoting mitogen and serum supplements and discarding the extra after one use and by running a panel normal control animals (3 to 4) for each assay.

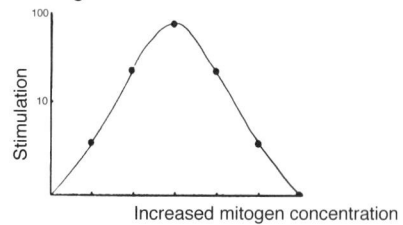

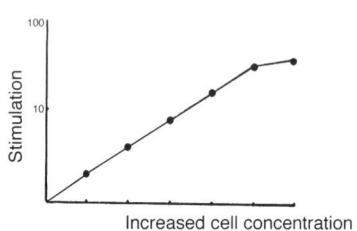

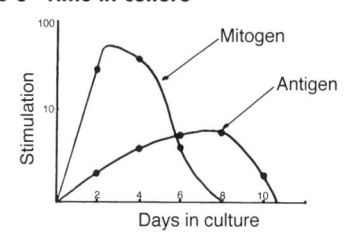

Figure 11-5 Variables in mitogen- or antigen-induced lymphocyte blastogenesis in vitro. Variables include mitogen concentration, cell concentration, and time in culture.

In spite of these limitations, the assay is widely used as an in vitro correlate of cell-mediated immunity. The "anergy of infection" associated with conditions such as canine distemper, measles virus infection, infectious bovine rhinotracheitis, feline leukemia, and generalized demodectic mange can be measured. The method can be used to evaluate the immunologic status of animals affected by neoplasias and congenital immunodeficiencies.

In addition, this assay is used to monitor the effects of drugs such as cyclophosphamide or cortisone on lymphoid tissues. The biologic effects of antilymphocyte serum, immune complexes, and immunoregulatory substances are readily assayed by LBT. Also, mitogen-stimulated cells are used to propagate lymphotrophic viruses such as canine distemper and as a method for isolation of bovine leukemia virus (BLV) from leukemic cells.

A third important use of this system is for the generation of lymphocyte products (lymphokines) for in vitro and in vivo study. Mitogen-stimulated cells are efficient producers of such factors as lymphotoxin, macrophage-inhibiting or macrophage-aggregating factors, interleukin-2 IL-2, gamma interferon (IFN-γ), and other interleukins (IL-3, IL-4, IL-5, IL-6, IL-10, etc.). Production of interleukins is currently thought to be important in the kind of immune response that is generated in an infection. For example, when one sub-population (helper T, type I cells) produces IFN-γ and IL-2, cell-mediated immunity and enhanced protection is facilitated in certain infectious diseases. When an alternate population of T cells (helper T, type II cells) produces IL-4 and IL-10, cell-mediated immunity is depressed and an immediate type of hypersensitivity response is facilitated. Differentiation of these two kinds of CD4 T lymphocytes is currently based only on the their cytokine profile. Species differences appear to occur in the delineation of these subpopulations.

Antigen-specific reactions of lymphocytes in vitro

Antigen-specific activity of isolated lymphocytes is readily monitored using methods similar to those of mitogen stimulation. The blastogenic response of immune lymphocytes to antigens is similar to phytomitogen-induced stimulation. The antigen-specific nature and the magnitude of the response is of importance. Because antigen-specific cells are in the minority (< 0.1%) in culture, the time necessary to detect a proliferative response is longer, and the magnitude of stimulation, as measured by incorporated ^{3}H-thymidine, is much lower (Figure 11-5). Both T and B cells participate in antigen-induced stimulation. As with mitogens, several different cell types are necessary for maximum development of the response in vitro. Antigens such as keyhole-limpet hemocyanin induced by immunization as well as environmentally-encountered immunogens such as tuberculin, streptokinase-streptodornase, and viral antigens are effective. The discriminatory ability of lymphocytes to recognize antigenic determinants approaches that observed with humoral antibodies. Antigen-specific transformation also stimulates lymphokine production and release, although to a lesser degree than do mitogens.

Mixed lymphocyte reactions

A widely used in vitro correlation of histocompatibility differences comparable to the graft rejection reaction is the mixed leukocyte culture (MLC) test. In the two-way test, lymphocytes from donors and recipients are cultured together in vitro, then labeled with ^{3}H-thymidine for incorporation into newly-synthesized DNA. For the one-way test, donor cells are irradiated or treated with mitotic inhibitors such as mitomycin C, and then used as target cells. The magnitude of stimulation of recipient lymphocytes is a different indication of the genetic or histocompatibility differences between individuals. The assay is used to screen large numbers of donors to arrive at the best tissue match for grafting and transplantation purposes. In addition to this practical use, supernatant fluids from mixed leukocyte cultures contain lymphokines; this culture system can be used to generate them for further study.

Interleukin 2

Interleukin 2 or T-cell–growth factor is a hormonelike lymphokine released by activated T cells. In an immunologic context, its chief function is to promote proliferation of activated T lymphocytes. Thus, it amplifies T-cell–mediated immune responses in vitro and in vivo. Production of IL-2 in vitro is usually demonstrated by assaying supernatant fluids of T-cell populations stimulated to blastogenes by the T-cell mitogens Con A or PHA-P. Bioassay for IL-2 is achieved by measuring ^{3}H-thymidine incorporation into IL-2-dependent murine T-cell lines. If these are not available, then the assay can be performed on freshly isolated mononuclear cells cultured for 24 to 48 hours with a suboptimal mitogenic concentration of Con A or PHA. In this instance, an increase in ^{3}H-thymidine incorporation (versus IL-2 media controls) is measured and attributed to the presence of IL-2. Recombinant IL-2 products of human and murine origin are commercially available. Both recombinant or produced IL-2 preparations are used to establish permanent T-cell lines for subsequent immunologic analysis.

Monocyte function: in vitro correlates

Approximately 10% to 20% of isolated mononuclear leukocytes are monocytes. In addition to this antigen-presenting function, monocytes serve as sources of immunoregulatory substances (prostaglandins, interferons, and IL-1) and also as phagocytic and cytotoxic effector cells. Evaluation of dysfunction of phagocytic functions by these cells is discussed in Chapter 9.

Monocytes/macrophages are the primary source of IL-1 or T-cell–activating factor. In an immunologic context, IL-1 activates uncommitted or resting T cells. IL-1 is a pleuripotential monokine with pyrogenic (fever inducing) and fibroblastic activity. Activated macrophages produce large quantities of the substance. Production of IL-1 is stimulated by exposing cultured monocytes to bacterial endotoxin (Escherichia coli, LPS). Peak production is achieved if the prostaglandin synthetase system is inhibited by inclusion of indomethacin in the culture media. Bioassay of IL-1 is assessed by dose-dependent enhancement of ^{3}H-thymidine incorporation by lectin-stimulated thymocytes. IL-l responsive murine thymocyte cell lines are also used for the bioassay.

Monocytes also possess the capability of cytotoxic lysis of certain target cells. Macrophages are cytotoxic to many different tumor cells. The nature of the specificity for tumor cells is unknown, but no doubt it is a reflection of specific tumor cell-monocyte receptor interactions. Unlike T-cell–dependent cytotoxicity, however, the monocyte cytotoxic event takes 4 to 5 days of in vitro coculture to effect a positive result. The general approach for performance of cytotoxicity assays is outlined below.

Target cell cytotoxicity assays

T cells, NK cells, and cells possessing an Fc receptor for IgG (killer [K] cells) are all capable of destroying appropriate target cells in vitro. This method is described in a separate section because the techniques used are largely similar, and the actual effector mechanism of target cell destruction seems to be similar, regardless of the effector cell type under study.

Before the advent of radiolabeled release techniques, morphologic and tissue culture survival methods, although cumbersome, were in wide experimental use. Reduction in target cell survival was commonly measured as an index of cytotoxic activity, despite the fact that the number of surviving cells is not directly proportional to cytotoxicity activity.

More precise quantitation of cytotoxic activity is achieved by use of radiolabeled target cells. For this, suitable targets (tumor cells, histoincompatible lymphocytes, viral-infected cells or NK-susceptible cells such as K562 or CTAC, etc.) are prepared as single-cell suspensions and then incubated with 400 to 600 microcurie (μCi) of sodium ^{51}chromate (^{51}Cr). Cells internalize the ^{51}Cr rapidly and then slowly release it into the supernatant over the next 24 to 48 hours. Leakage of ^{51}Cr can be retarded somewhat by cold-stabilizing the cells before coculture with effectors. For this, labeled cells are washed 2 to 3 times in cold media (0° to 4°C) and cellular pellets held in an ice bath for 1 hour before use. Target cell ratios (100:1 to 1:1) are commonly used. Cytotoxicity is facilitated by close cellular contact between effectors and targets. This is achieved by gentle centrifugation (100 to 200 × g) of the mixtures into U-bottom microculture plates. A portion of released ^{51}Cr will be internalized by viable effector cells, thereby reducing the total of released ^{51}Cr detected in the supernatants. This variable can be assessed by inclusion of a control panel using effector (spacer) cells incapable of cytotoxicity such as CT-45S lymphoblastoid cells or unlabeled target cells. Cytotoxic capabilities are quantitated by determining the amount of free ^{51}chromium in cell-free supernatants after a suitable incubation period. Data are expressed as net cpm, that is, (cpm effector minus cpm spacer) minus (cpm media minus cpm spacer media). Another way to express the data are percentage terms of total ^{51}chromium available for release. The latter number is generated by osmotic lysis of labeled target cells.

Cytotoxic T-cell assay

Lymphocytes from immunized animals are cytotoxic for cells bearing homologous antigenic determinants in vitro. This cytolytic phenomenon is antigen-specific, requires direct contact between living lymphocytes and target cells, and is independent of antibody or the complement system. The cytolytic event is rapid and is a property of lymphocytes of T-cell origin. Lymphocytes themselves are not killed during the course of the reaction. The microcytotoxicity assay has been used to detect cellular immunity in animals to histocompatibility antigens, viral infections, chemical and viral-induced tumors, and, in humans, a number of different neoplasms.

The interaction of a cytotoxic lymphocyte (CTL) and a target cell involves a series of reactions that have only recently been elucidated. Formation of a conjugate occurs after the interaction and this is followed rapidly by a Calcium-dependent step that requires the use of ATP and results in membrane damage to the target cell. After this interaction, the CTL is free to find another target cell, while the original targets undergo a process of lysis. The lytic event occurs between 15 minutes and 3 hours after the "lethal hit." The reaction is characterized by a progressive increase in target-cell membrane permeability, with release of low–molecular-weight components like ATP initially and eventually leaking of high–molecular-weight substances. Ultrastructurally, actual cell membrane bridges have been found between target cells and adherent lymphocytes, suggesting the direct transfer of cytocidal substances from the lymphocyte to the target. The recognition events that occur in conjugate formation involve the TCR-CD3 and the CD8 cell surface molecules on the CTL. The integrin receptor, leukocyte function-associated antigen (LFA-1), also binds to the membrane of the target cell. Apparently, after TCR binding, the LFA-l increases in avidity for its ligand on the target cell; this is a short-lived increase and a return to lower avidity occurs within minutes, allowing the CTL to dissociate. The "lethal hit" by the CTL actually involves the release of material contained in storage granules of the CTL. Granule contents that are released include perforin, a family of six esterases containing high–molecular-weight proteoglycans, and cytotoxic cytokines (tumor necrosis factor [TNF] beta). The perforin system is similar to the C9 component of the complement system (see Chapter 6). Cylindric pores are created in the cell membrane after polymerization of the perforin subunits. The end result is lysis of the target cell.

Natural killer cell assay

The test for NK activity is performed essentially as described for cytotoxic T cells. Crucial to the success of this assay is a source of NK-susceptible target cells, hopefully of homologous species origin. The CTAC cell line appears to be the target cell line of choice for dogs. NK activity in cattle, swine, and horses has been measured using a murine origin K562 cell line.

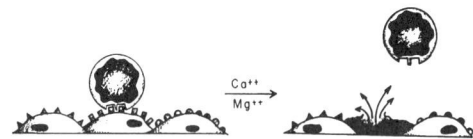

Antibody-directed cellular cytotoxicity

Immunoglobulins can trigger a number of different cellular attack mechanisms. The effect is mediated by the exposed Fc portion of IgG and is complement-independent. Specificity is established by IgG attached to the target cell, yet cytotoxicity is accomplished by cells possessing the Fc receptors, including neutrophils, macrophages, B lymphocytes, and lymphocytes known as K cells. K cells are nonphagocytic lymphocytes of uncertain B- or T-cell origin that do not adhere to glass. It is important to recognize that the cytotoxic effector cells are not immune. That is, cells from animals without previous exposure to the immunogen are effective in target cell killing, providing that the IgG used reacts with a surface antigen on the target cell. Methodology for assaying and quantitating ADCC activity is similar to that used for lymphocyte-mediated cytotoxicity. These various types of cytotoxic cellular interactions are schematically outlined in Figure 11-6.

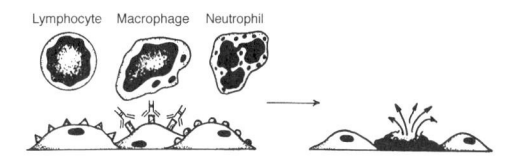

Figure 11-6 Three mechanisms of lymphocyte-mediated cellular cytotoxicity. *1*, Lymphotoxin is nonselective. *2*, Specificity for T-lymphocyte–mediated cytotoxicity is achieved by cellular receptors for target cell antigens. *3*, Specificity for antibody-directed cellular cytotoxicity is provided by specific antibody, but cell killing is accomplished by lymphocytes, macrophages, or neutrophils.

SUGGESTED READINGS

Bowles CA, White GS, Lucas D: Rosette formation by canine peripheral blood lymphocytes, *J Immunol* 114:399-402, 1975.

Campus M, Rossi CR, Lawman MJP: Natural cell-mediated cytotoxicity of bovine mononuclear cells against virus-infected cells, *Infect Immun* 34:1054-1059, 1982.

Cockerell GL, Hoover EA, Krakowka, S, and others: Lymphocyte mitogen reactivity and enumeration of circulating B and T cells during feline leukemia virus infection in the cat, *J Natl Cancer Inst* 57:1095-1099, 1976.

Coligan JE, Kruisbeek AM, Margulies DH, and others: In vitro assays for T cell function. In Coligan JE, Kruisbeek AM, Margulies DH and others, editors: *Current protocols in immunology*, vol 1, New York, 1991, John Wiley.

Dean JH, Silva JS, McCoy JL, and others: Functional activities of rosette separated peripheral blood lymphocytes, *J Immunol* 115:1449-1455, 1975.

Eady RP, Hough DW, Kilshaw PJ, and others: Recovery of immunoglobulin removed from lymphocytic surfaces by proteolysis, *Immunology* 26:549-561, 1974.

Eby WC, Chong CA, Dray S, and others: Enumerating immunoglobulin-secreting cells among peripheral human lymphocytes: a hemolytic plaque assay for a B-cell function, *J Immunol* 115:1700-1703, 1975.

Fletcher MA, Klimas N, Morgan R, and others: Lymphocyte proliferation. In NR, Rose DeMacario EC, Fahey JL, and others, editors: Manual of Clinical Laboratory Immunology, ed 4, Washington D.C., 1992, American Society for Microbiology.

Gershwin LJ, Lance P, Rokito AJ: Comparison of analysis of bovine surface immunoglobulin bearing and peanut agglutinin binding lymphocytes by flow cytometry and fluorescence microscopy, *Vet Immunol Immunopathol* 5:185-196, 1983-1984.

Grewal AS, Rouse BT: Characterization of bovine leukocytes involved in ADCC, *Int Arch Allergy Appl Immunol* 60:169-177, 1979.

Hoover EA, Krakowkap S, Cockerell GL, and others: Thymectomy in pre-weanling kittens: technique and immunologic consequences, *Am J Vet Res* 38:99-103, 1978.

Jondal M, Hohn G, Wigzell H: Surface markers on human T and B lymphocytes. I. A large population of lymphocytes forming nonimmune rosettes with sheep red blood cells, *J Exp Med* 136:207-215, 1972.

Krakowka S, Cockerell G, Koestner A: Effects of canine distemper virus on lymphoid function in vitro and in vivo, *J Infect Immun* 1069-1078, 1975.

Krakowka S, Guyot DJ: Rosette-formation assays in the dog: lack of specificity of E-rosettes for T lymphocytes. *Infect Immun* 17:73-77, 1977.

Krakowka S, Wallace AL, Ringler SS, and others: Evaluation of B lymphocyte levels and functions in gnotobiotic dogs, *Am J Vet Res* 39:1181-1183, 1978.

Krakowka S: Mechanisms of E-rosette formation by mitogen-stimulated canine lymphocytes, *Immunology* 39:255-261, 1980.

Krakowka S: Mechanisms of in vitro immunosuppression in canine distemper virus infection, *J Clin Lab Immunol* 8:187-196, 1982.

Krakowka S, Wallace AL: In vitro properties of diffuse cytoplasmic esterase-positive canine mononuclear leukocytes, *Vet Immunol Immunopathol* 5:1-13, 1983.

Krakowka S: Natural killer (NK) cell activity in adult gnotobiotic dogs, *Am J Vet Res* 44:635-648, 1983.

Mossman TR, Coffman RL: Different patterns of lymphokine secretion lead to different functional properties, *Annu Rev Immunol* 7:145-173, 1989.

Nara PL, Krakowka S, Power TE: The effects of prednisolone on the development of immune responses to canine distemper virus in beagle puppies, *Am J Vet Res* 40:1742-1747, 1979.

O'Toole C: Standardization of microcytotoxicity assay for cell-mediated immunity, *Natl Cancer Inst Monogr* 37:19-24, 1966.

Parks DR, Herzenberg LA: Flow cytometry and fluorescence activated cell sorting. In Paul W, editor: *Fundamental Immunology*, ed 2, New York, 1989, Raven Press.

Ringler SS, Krakowka S: Cell surface markers of the canine natural killer (NK) cell, *Vet. Immunol Immunopathol* 9:1-12, 1985.

Romagnani S: Human T_{H1} and T_{H2} subsets: doubt no more, *Immunol Today* 12:256-257, 1991.

Shimizu M, Pan IC, Hess WR: T and B lymphocytes in porcine blood, *Am J Vet Res* 37:309-317, 1976.

Shimizu M, Shimizu Y: Demonstration of cytotoxic lymphocytes to virus-infected target cells in pigs inoculated with TGE virus, *Am J Vet Res* 40:208-213, 1979.

Steele RW, Hensen SA, Vincent MM, and others: A ^{51}CR microassay technique for cell-mediated immunity to viruses, *J Immunol*,110:1502-1510, 1973.

Whiteside TL, Rinaldo CR, Herverman RBA: Cytolytic cell functions. In Rose NR, DeMacario EC, Fahey JL, and other editors: *Manual of clinical laboratory immunology*, ed 4, Washington DC, 1992.

Young JD, Liu C: Multiple mechanisms of lymphocyte mediated killing, *Immunol Today* 9:140-144, 1988.

PART THREE

Immunopathology

12 Inherited Immunodeficiencies, Myelomas, and Lymphomas

Normal immune function relies on the presence and proper function of each component of the immune system. The lack of one or more cells or molecules of the immune system often causes life-threatening disease. Neoplasia of the immune system can result in an overgrowth of particular cells and sometimes the subsequent overproduction of immune effector molecules.

PRIMARY IMMUNODEFICIENCY DISEASES IN VETERINARY MEDICINE

Immunodeficiency disease syndromes are rare disorders of the immune system that have a demonstrated or presumed genetic basis. The defects can be relative or absolute in nature and theoretically can involve a stem cell defect, an isolated thymus-derived (T) or bursal-derived (B)-cell problem, or any combination thereof. It is important to distinguish between defects in lymphocytes themselves and defects, that occur at the sight of maturation of these cells, such as abnormal thymic epithelium. In humans a number of different inherited deficiencies have been described and it is possible, with the appropriate reagents and tests, to classify the defect in a definitive manner. Although there is no doubt that the full range of possible defects occurs in animals, they often go unrecognized as a result of the lack of research tools available to screen large numbers of prospective candidates for immunodeficiency. In spite of the intense interest in inherited disorders of immunity for use as clinical experiments of nature, conditions are rare and are essentially nonexistent in clinical veterinary practice. Of far more biologic and economic importance are immune deficits in the neonate associated with failure of passive transport (FPT) of maternal protective immunoglobulin (see Chapter 17) and deficits associated with a number of different infections and parasitic diseases (see Chapter 16). These disorders, defined as secondary immunodeficiencies, are described in detail in subsequent chapters.

Equine immunodeficiency diseases

Combined immunodeficiency disease of Arabian horses

Perhaps the best-characterized immunodeficiency disease is the combined immunodeficiency syndrome (CID) of Arabian foals. The disease was recognized as the underlying problem in the apparent increased susceptibility of neonatal Arabians to fatal adenovirus infection. Breeding trials have demonstrated that the defect is inherited as an autosomal recessive trait. Carrier animals are indistinguishable from normal adults.

Foals are born with lymphopenia (<1000/mm^3) and demonstrate no detectable immunoglobulin (Ig) synthesis. Maternal antibody provides passive protection for several months; however, as the levels of maternal Ig decline, severe and eventually fatal infections occur. The antibody-synthesizing defect has been observed in foal sera by the absence of natural antibodies to rabbit erythrocytes and by an absence of IgM. Defective cellular immunity is documented by the failure of peripheral blood or lymph node lymphocytes to respond to T-cell mitogens and by the lack of intradermal response to phytohemagglutinin.

Lesions at necropsy are helpful in making the diagnosis. In addition to lesions associated with the cause of death (e.g., adenovirus or *Pneumocystis carinii pneumonia*), lesions in the lymphoreticular system must be compatible with CID. Lymph nodes lack both lymphoid follicles and germinal centers, and the paracortical (T-cell) areas are severely depleted. Follicles and periarteriolar sheaths are absent from the spleen. The thymus is extremely hypoplastic and has been replaced by fatty tissue. The epithelial components, including Hassall's corpuscles, are present, and the thymic superstructure is intact.

The underlying genetic defect has not been identified. Investigators suggest that because thymic epithelial tissues are present, the thymic hypoplasia and resultant CID are caused by the failure of bone marrow–derived lymphocytes to populate the thymus. Thus the defect is at the stem cell level.

The diagnostic triad necessary to identify an Arabian foal with CID (and hence the sire and dam as carriers) is lymphopenia (<1000 lymphocytes/mm^3) absence of IgM in serum, and histologic demonstration of lymphoid hypoplasia. Recently, a young Appaloosa filly was diagnosed with CID based on these criteria. It is not known if the filly had Arabian sire ancestry or if this represents a CID mutation of Appaloosas. This case report emphasizes the need for careful clinicopathologic examination of all foals with lymphopenia and recurrent infections.

Currently, the only reliable method available for detecting the carrier trait in normal heterozygote mares and stallions is exhaustive breeding trials with known carrier animals, combined with progeny testing. A carrier test would be of great importance in eliminating this trait from the breed.

In humans approximately one half of the children with CID lack the enzymatic pathway to degrade adenosine, one of the purines. Adenosine deaminase activity in tissues, erythrocytes, lymphocytes, and platelets was measured in foals with CID as a possible biochemical marker for the defect. No differences were found between healthy foals and foals with CID or between carrier adults and adults that were not carriers. A defect in purine metabolism has been detected in cell cultures established from foals with CID. However, abnormalities in specific metabolic pathway(s) remain undefined. Immunotherapy has been attempted in foals with CID. One foal was given sibling bone marrow, and another was given fetal thymus. Although evidence was obtained for graft survival in both cases, both foals died; the foal given fetal thymus developed a graft-versus-host (GVH) reaction.

Equine primary agammaglobulinemia

Primary agammaglobulinemia has been described in a 1-year-old thoroughbred stallion. The clinical history included repeated bouts of bacterial pneumonia and arthritis. The horse died at 17 months of age. Immunologic data collected suggested that the case was very similar to X-linked agammaglobulinemia of human beings.

The B-cell defect was characterized: (1) absence of serum IgM, IgA, and IgG(T), with low levels of serum IgG; (2) absence of antibody following antigenic challenge and absence of natural antibodies to rabbit erythrocytes; (3) absence of plasma cells, follicles, and germinal centers in an antigen-stimulated lymph node; and (4) absence of surface immunoglobulins on lymphocytes.

Thymic-dependent immunologic function was intact in that isolated lymphocytes responded both to mitogens and sensitizing antigens by cellular proliferation and new DNA synthesis. Macrophage inhibition factor (MIF)-like activity was demonstrated in supernatants from antigen-stimulated lymphocyte cultures. The horse also responded to intradermal challenge with the mitogens phytohemagglutinin (PHA) and concanavalin A (ConA). Serum complement level, as measured by both total hemolytic complement method and radial immunodiffusion for C3 was normal.

This case differed from the CID case presented earlier in that the breed was thoroughbred, not Arabian, the survival was to 17 months of age versus 4 to 5 months of age in foals with CID, and T-cell functions were present. The mode of inheritance is unknown, but the evidence suggests that it is sex-linked, similar to Bruton's agammaglobulinemia in humans.

Equine transient hypogammaglobulinemia

A disorder similar to agammaglobulinemia in a foal-designated transient hypogammaglobulinemia has also been described. The defect was characterized by low serum Ig levels between 54 and 96 days of age, a time during which normal foals produce adequate levels of immunoglobulin.

After 96 days of age, Ig production increased, and the foal responded normally to antigenic challenge at 106 days of age. The foal was destroyed at 185 days of age as a result of runting and failure to thrive acquired during the transient defective stage of development.

Selective IgM deficiency of horses

Five instances of selective IgM deficiency associated with respiratory disease in 4 to 8 month-old foals have been described. The diagnosis was made at the time of onset of clinical disease. Although the conditions superficially resembled Wiskott-Aldrich syndrome in humans, all foals demonstrated delayed-type hypersensitivity reactions and lacked thrombocytopenia and eczema. IgM deficiency is distinguished from CID by demonstrating normal total lymphocyte levels and T-lymphocyte responses to mitogen.

Bovine immunodeficiency diseases

A45 lethal trait

A lethal autosomal recessive genetic defect (A45) occurs in Black Pied Danish cattle. Calves are born healthy but develop progressive wasting and widespread cutaneous manifestations of exanthema, alopecia, and parakeratosis by 1 month of age. They do not respond to skin tests designed to measure cellular immunity and die within the first 4 to 6 months of life. Serum Ig levels are within the normal range, and affected calves respond with a normal antibody response to immunization. These calves have been experimentally infected with the liver fluke *Fasciola hepatica*. Compared to normal controls, immunodeficient calves failed to respond to the fluke; no peripheral blood eosinophilia was detected, and the calves failed to respond to skin tests with fluke antigen for both cutaneous allergy (IgE-mediated) and delayed-type hypersensitivity.

Necropsy findings in affected calves reveal hypoplastic thymi, systemic depletion of T-cell–dependent regions in all lymphoid tissue, and evidence of secondary bacterial infection, although the calves are not lymphopenic. A remarkable clinical feature of this disease is the response to treatment with daily oral doses of zinc. Calves so treated reportedly undergo complete remission of the immunologic defect and cutaneous lesions in 2 to 3 weeks.

Bovine leukocyte adhesin deficiency

A family of cell-surface molecules that are responsible for cell-cell interaction have recently been identified. The beta$_2$ integrin family includes glycoprotein molecules that are responsible for the adherence of leukocytes to endothelial cells and their emigration through blood vessels, in response to the chemotactic stimuli associated with bacterial invasion. These integrins are classified as CD11/CD18 (alpha and beta subunits). An abnormality in the beta subunit (CD18) has been identified in holstein calves. This abnormality is an amino acid substitution in a 26-amino acid sequence of the CD18 molecule; this particular sequence shares homology with human and murine CD18 and is the site at which several mutations in the human gene occur. Animals with this defect exhibit a persistent neutrophilia with a lack of pus formation in areas of infection, despite overwhelming bacterial infection. Peridontitis, stomatitis, and diarrhea are commonly seen in affected calves. The inheritance of this defect is autosomal recessive, and a polymerase chain reaction assay has been developed to identify affected carrier animals. The syndrome is remarkably similar to the leukocyte-adhesin deficiency described in human infants and appears to be similar to the syndrome reported in the Irish setter breed of dogs.

Other reports of bovine immunodeficiency

One survey study using immunoelectrophoresis detected a relative deficiency of IgG in 15% of the mature cattle tested. No clinical disease was associated with the defect, and differentiation between primary and secondary immunodeficiency was not made. In addition, cows with selective deficiency of IgG$_2$ subclass have been described. These IgG$_2$-deficient cattle were more susceptible to gangrenous mastitis and recurrent pyogenic bacterial infections.

Agammaglobulinemia has been reported in a 3-month-old calf that subsequently died, but evaluation of cellular immunity was not performed. A 1-year-old Angus bull with persistent virus-induced papillomatosis was reported as a case of selective immunodeficiency of cellular immunity. Serum Ig levels were normal, and the animal responded to antigenic challenge with antibody production. Deficient cellular immunity was established by lack of a positive tuberculin skin test following immunization, a humoral suppressive factor that inhibited homologous lymphocyte stimulation in vitro, the presence of lymphoid follicles in thymic tissues. Unfortunately, this study did not distinguish between a primary immunodeficiency disorder and the more common (and in this case more likely) occurrence of immunosuppression secondary to persistent Papillomavirus infection.

Ovine immunodeficiency disease

Transient IgG$_2$ deficiency has been reported in young lambs. IgG$_2$ production was not detected until the lambs reached 3 to 4 weeks of age. Since no clinical disorder was observed, this may represent normal maturation of the immune response with age.

Canine immunodeficiency disease

Deficiency of the third component of complement

The third component of complement (C3) is the pivotal serum protein in both the alternate and classical pathways of the complement cascade and links both the coagulation and kinin systems to the complement proteins and cells of the inflammatory response (see Chapter 6). During the course of breeding trials in a colony of Brittany spaniels with hereditary, canine, spinal muscular atrophy, a number of individuals were found to be lacking detectable levels of C3. The trait is inherited in an autosomal recessive fashion and is separate from the spinal atrophy gene(s). Heterozygotes possess C3 levels that are one-half normal, and serum from C3-deficient dogs lacks any C3 inhibitor activity. C3-deficient serum is largely devoid of hemolytic, opsonic, and chemotactic activities. In spite of this, some C3-like functional activity (6% to 10% of that considered normal) is present, raising the possibility that a C3-like protein, antigenically distinct from native C3, exists in these dogs, or that another unidentified serum protein has some C3 activity.

Clinical manifestations of C3 deficiency fall into two general categories. By far the most important of these is heightened susceptibility to recurrent bacterial infections and sepsis. These occur under defined laboratory husbandry conditions, unlike complement deficiencies (C-5 mice, C-4 and C-2 guinea pigs, and C-6 rabbits) in other laboratory animal species. Aggressive antimicrobial and supportive therapy at the first sign (elevated rectal temperature) usually will help dogs through these septic crises.

The second general category of disease associated with C3 deficiency is progressive renal impairment. Histologic examination of moribund dogs or percutaneous renal biopsies has revealed that renal disease exhibits both interstitial (fibrosis and lymphoplasmacytic infiltrates) and glomerular (membranous to membranoproliferative with fibrosis) components. A portion of the dogs eventually develop systemic amyloidosis with prominent renal glomerular involvement. The nonamyloid glomerular lesion has a presumed, immune-complex etiology. Glomerular mesangial deposits of IgG, IgM, and occasionally, IgA are present in asymptomatic dogs. The lesion progresses to diffuse membranous or globular deposits of immunoglobulin in the glomerulus. Although not proven, these data suggest that an important function of C3 in maintenance of health is not only opsonization of immune complexes for eventual disposal, but also resolubilizing in situ deposits for eventual destruction.

Canine severe combined immunodeficiency syndrome

Severe combined immunodeficiency syndrome (SCID) is an X-linked recessive trait in beagle-basset crossbreeds that has recently been detected. The defect appears to reside in the T-cell arm of the immune response. Affected dogs have histologic lesions of thymic hypoplasia, T-cell depletion and lymphopenia, and isolated cells are unresponsive to canine T-cell mitogens Con A and PHA. The B-cell compartment is likely to be normal because B–lymphocytes are activated to IgM synthesis in vitro by pokeweed mitogen (PWM). Because the trait is X-linked recessive, all of the females in affected litters are phenotypically normal, and one half of them carry the trait. For males, one half are genotypically and phenotypically normal whereas one half are genotypically and phenotypically abnormal. All affected males studied to date develop life-threatening bacterial and viral disease as maternal, passively-acquired immunity wanes; eventually they die of infection at an early age (8 to 16 weeks).

Canine immunodeficient dwarfism

Immunodeficient dwarfism is a syndrome described in an inbred colony of weimaraner dogs that is characterized by growth hormone deficiency, congenital absence of thymic cortex, and a deficient in vitro response of canine lymphocytes to T-cell mitogens. Although the mode of inheritance has not yet been defined, it is likely to be an autosomal recessive trait. Affected pups develop a wasting syndrome that is (characterized by unthriftiness, emaciation, lethargy, and persistent often fatal infections). Therapy with a thymus extract, thymosin fraction, results in clinical improvement and increased thymus cellularity, but lymphocyte responses to mitogens are not improved.

Canine selective IgA deficiency

Selective IgA deficiency is the most common, inherited, immunologic disorder in humans. For humans the pattern of inheritance varies, but both autosomal dominant and recessive modes have been identified. Although a large proportion of IgA-deficient humans are clinically asymptomatic, a number of syndromes encompassing recurrent respiratory, dermatologic, and gastrointestinal disorders have been noted. In most instances cellular bases for the defect are not known, but they are thought to be either a primary deficit of B cells destined to develop into IgA lineage progeny or a T-cell defect in helper function in the Ig-class switch from an IgM-basal response to IgA responses.

Primary IgA deficiency has been described in three separate breeds of dogs. In German shepherds, the deficiency is relative (i.e., low but detectable) and is often clinically asymptomatic. However, increased susceptibility to enteric infection has been described. An autosomal, recessive, IgA deficiency was discovered in a large breeding colony of beagles, with recurrent dermatitis and pulmonary infections. In these dogs, all other parameters of immunity are within the normal range. Some of these IgA-deficient beagles exhibit immune-mediated atopic disease and increased incidence of lupus-like autoantibody formation with attendant clinical syndromes of hemolytic anemia and glomerulonephritis. IgA deficiency was identified in two colonies of Shar Pei dogs. Several affected dogs had recurrent respiratory disease and chronic, atopic, cutaneous disease, partially responsive to passive therapy with hypoallergenic diet. Serum IgA levels in affected dogs were very low (<5 mg/dl), parents with no symptoms also had low IgA levels.

Undefined canine immunodeficiency syndromes

A litter of six dachshunds fatally affected with *P. carnii* pneumonia has been reported. Because infection with this protozoan is only observed in immunodeficiency or following immunosuppression, the authors suggested that an underlying immunodeficiency disorder existed in these dogs. However, functional or morphologic data were not presented. Hypogammaglobulinemia and generalized lymphoid depletion was found in a 16-week-old dog with canine distemper. Because both of these features occur in normal dogs persistently infected with this virus, the authors' claim that this case represents an instance of genetic immunodeficiency seems tenuous at best.

Canine cyclic neutropenia

Cyclic neutropenia is an autosomal, recessive, hereditary disorder associated with hypopigmentation in the grey collie, color-variant dog. These dogs exhibit recurrent episodes of absolute neutropenia, most likely as a result of a defect within the regulatory mechanisms that control hematopoietic cell differentiation in bone marrow. Dogs are very susceptible to bacterial infections during the neutropenic phase of the cycle. Erythrocyte differentiation and platelet production is also affected by this cyclic phenomenon. The disease may be cured by transplantation of bone marrow from unaffected littermates.

Canine leukocyte adhesin deficiency

An inherited deficiency in the CD11b/CD18 beta$_2$ adhesin protein has been described in the Irish setter. A lack of both alpha and beta chains of the integrin (CDllb and CD18) renders the dogs' neutrophils totally unable to adhere to endothelial cells and to respond to chemotactic stimuli. This syndrome is much like that described in humans (leukocyte adhesin deficiency) and that described in cattle (bovine leukocyte adhesin deficiency). Severe recurrent bacterial infections are characterized by a lack of pus formation in the presence of extremely high levels of neutrophils in peripheral blood. The mode of inheritance is thought to be autosomal recessive.

Canine granulocytopathy syndrome

In 1975, an Irish setter dog with recurrent bacterial infections was found to exhibit a defect in neutrophil bacteriocidal function. The defect was found to reside within the neutrophil because these cells efficiently phagocytosed various bacteria. The defect is an inherited, autosomal, recessive trait and is associated with reduced glucose oxidation by the hexose monophosphate shunt pathway. Thus the phagocyte fails to exhibit the respiratory burst phenomenon. Lysosome formation is normal unlike most other neutrophil defects such as the Chédiak-Higashi syndrome. This syndrome may be caused by a defect in the integrin molecule, as described earlier for the Irish setters with canine leukocyte adhesin deficiency.

Neutrophil function defect

A neutrophil function defect has been identified in weimaraner dogs. It is characterized by recurrent bacterial sepsis and diffuse granulomatous inflammation. The mode of inheritance is unknown, but males seem to be disproportionally affected. Like the neutrophil defect described in Irish setters, neutrophils from these dogs fail to undergo a respiratory burst following phagocytosis. In addition, serum IgG levels are approximately one-half normal values, and acute-phase serum reactants appear to be absent.

Miscellaneous primary immunodeficiency disorders

A Siberian tiger cub with thymic hypoplasia, lymphopenia, and lymphoid depletion of both T-cell and B-cells–dependent areas were found. The cause of death was neutrophilic meningoencephalitis. Although no functional studies were performed the lesions at necropsy were comparable to those of CID in Arabian foals.

Plasma Ig levels, a relative deficiency of IgG, have been noted in a strain of chickens with hereditary muscular dystrophy. Serum IgA and IgM levels were normal. The cause of this deficiency was not determined.

Few primary immuno-deficiency diseases are recognized in swine and cats. The Chédiak-Higashi syndrome, a condition in which abnormal lysosomes and granulocyte primary granules occur, is seen in Persian cats and in several other species. Abnormalities in coat pigment and fundic pigmentation accompany this syndrome. It is likely that the full spectrum of disorders occurs in cats but the diagnosis is not made because of the well-documented and clinically similar effects of feline leukemia virus (FeLV) and feline immunodeficiency virus (FIV) infection in this species.

Finally, it is important to point out that a large number of hereditary defects in various levels of immune response occur in inbred strains of mice. Delineation of these defects is beyond the scope and nature of this book.

Neoplastic diseases of the lymphoreticular system

Neoplastic transformation and subsequent proliferation of cells of the immune system are relatively common cancers of domestic animals. Approximately 6% to 10% of all solid malignant tumors are of this type. In many species there is a strong etiologic association between viral infections (retroviruses and herpesviruses) and subsequent development of neoplasms. The classification, delineation, and identification by immunologic and cytochemical means is an ongoing clinical research effort. Thus far, unanimity in nomenclature is elusive in veterinary medicine because of the many species involved, associations with viral infection, and paucity of defined immunocytochemical markers. As a general concept, lymphoreticular neoplasms in animals, regardless of histologic appearance, are considered clinically malignant. The vast majority of these tumors are aleukemic until the terminal stages of disease. This means that routine hemogram analysis is unlikely to be of diagnostic help during the occult stages of the disease process. The disease exhibits a bimodal age distribution. Generally these tumors arising in the young are more likely the result of viral infection than of neoplasms associated with old age. Figure 12-1 delineates a provisional general classification of lymphoreticular and myeloid neoplasms. Clinical and pathologic features of tumors of the myeloid system, excluding those of monocytoid origin, will not be described.

PLASMA CELL MYELOMAS
Neoplasms of terminal B-lymphocyte differentiation

Plasma cell myelomas (multiple myelomas or plasmacytomas) are uncommon tumors of the bone marrow in domestic animals. They are neoplastic cells of B-lymphocyte lineage and occur most frequently in marrow tissue actively engaged in hematopoiesis. The cells are highly differentiated morphologically and biochemically. The cytoplasm of these cells contains an abundance of rough endoplasmic reticulum that is associated with secretory protein synthesis equivalent to their non-neoplastic counterparts.

The extracellular product of these neoplastic cells is called myeloma protein, a form of immunoglobulin. It was formerly thought that these Ig molecules were devoid of antibody activity; however, a number of these proteins isolated from plasmacytoma-bearing patients have been shown to bind both synthetic determinants (e.g. dinitrophenol and bacterial cell-wall antigens).

The clinical features of hyperproteinemia and proteinuria that are found in association with many myelomas are a consequence of abnormal protein production. Careful analysis of other normal serum Ig classes has revealed an absolute decrease in circulating levels, most likely the result of poorly understood, homeostatic, control mechanisms for IgG production. Myeloma-bearing animals have a markedly depressed ability to mount a humoral immune response to thymic-dependent or thymic-independent antigens. T-lymphocyte functions are normal. In this respect, the tumor-mediated immunodepression observed with myelomas is noteworthy because most other solid tumors are associated with T-cell deficits.

Myeloma proteins are of great experimental importance because they are a convenient source of

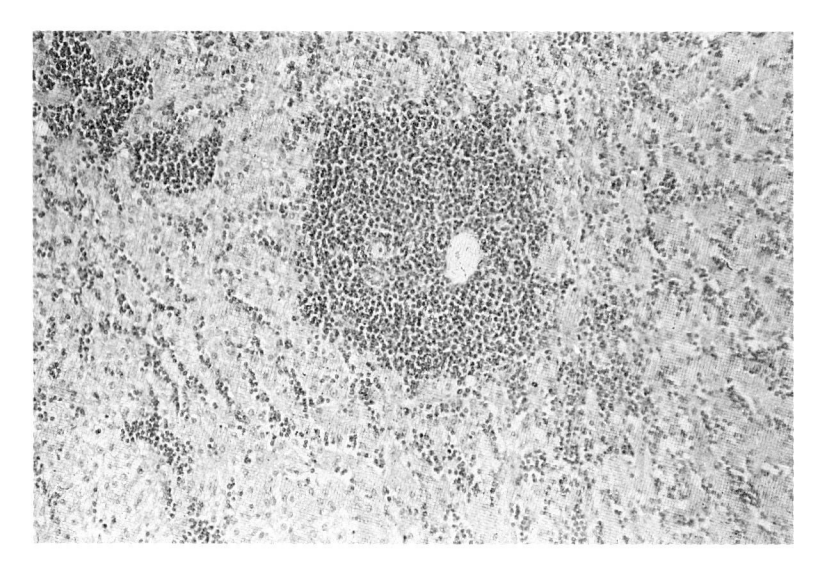

Figure 12-1 A canine T-cell leukemia illustrating the invasion of the hepatic sinusoids with neoplastic cells. This slide was stained with hematoxylin and eosin.

abundant amounts of homogeneous subclass-specific Ig protein, not only for detailed analysis of the biochemical and structural features of immunoglobulin, but also for study of intracellular events controlling Ig synthesis and release. Occasionally, monoclonal gammopathies (hypergammaglobulinemia of restricted electrophoretic mobility) are seen in the serum of patients with a variety of non-neoplastic diseases including unrelated cancer, chronic (obstructive) liver disease, rheumatoid arthritis, and certain viral diseases like equine infectious anemia (EIA), etc. The significance of these gammopathies lies in the need to differentiate them from true B-cell origin neoplasms.

Murine plasma cell tumors

A brief consideration of plasma cell neoplasms in mice as an experimental model or the study of these tumors is warranted. Spontaneous plasmacytomas in mice are rare. One strain, the BALB/c, is uniquely susceptible to the experimental induction of plasmacytomas using noncarcinogenic materials. Intraperitoneal injection of plastic, mineral oils, mineral oil adjuvants, or proteins such as casein will induce plasmacytomas. These agents are peritoneal irritants that produce a granulomatous reaction on gut and body walls. Neoplastic plasmacytes arise from these reactive tissues and can be identified as tumors 4 to 5 months after injection. Tumors can be transferred to histocompatible recipients or preserved in liquid nitrogen tanks using cryopreservation methods. Analyses of Ig products reveal Ig proteins of IgG, IgM, and IgA classes. Subclass specificities as well as dimers of kappa and lambda light chains (Bence Jones proteins) have also been identified.

Today the major use of murine myeloma cell lines is in the generation of monoclonal antibodies for clinical and experimental use. A full discussion of the theory, general method of production, and uses, including advantages and disadvantages of monoclonals, is found in Chapter 4. In brief, a number of metabolically-deficient myeloma cell lines, usually hypoxanthine-aminopterin-thymidine (HAT)-dependent, are available for use. These cells are fused with splenic B lymphocytes from mice immunized with the antigen in question. On a probability basis, a small number of B cells will fuse with myeloma cells and provide them with antigenic specificity and the missing HAT-enzyme pathway(s). Unfused splenic lymphocytes die within several weeks; unfused HAT-seropositive myeloma cells are killed by growth in HAT-deficient cell medium. Clonal selection for monoclonals of the desired specificity is performed by a variety of antigen-based antibody detection assays (usually radioimmune or enzyme-linked immunosorbent assay [ELISA]). When properly performed, a panel of myeloma Ig-secreting cell lines are established with specificity (V-region gene products) provided by the original immune splenic B cells and with immortality provided by the myeloma cell line.

Canine plasma cell myelomas

In veterinary medicine, canine myelomas are the most completely studied tumors of this nature. The tumors occur in middle- to older-aged dogs and most frequently involve hematopoietically active bones. Clinical signs are variable, but lameness, pain, and pathologic fractures usually are observed. Clinical signs that are less common include anemia, hemorrhagic tendency, depression, and weight loss, or, rarely, signs of renal failure. Classic cases of myeloma are associated with multiple osteolytic lesions that are visible on a radiograph without a rim of osteosclerosis in long bones or bones of the vertebral column. Tentative diagnosis can be made by identification of the abnormal paraprotein in serum or urine, and definitive diagnosis can be achieved by biopsy (Figure 12-2).

A hyperproteinemia (up to 12 mg/ml) with reduced ratio of albumin to globulin is usually observed. Cellulose or starch gel electrophoresis should demonstrate a dense homogeneous band of protein with restricted electrophoretic mobility that distinguishes myeloma from the diffuse hypergammaglobulinemic response observed occasionally in chronic infectious diseases or hepatocellular dysfunction. The paraprotein is further identified by agar gel or immunoelectrophoresis as belonging to IgG, IgM, or IgA classes.

Occasionally a paraprotein cross-reactive with only light-chain determinants is observed. These proteins usually occur as dimers in serum and urine and are termed Bence Jones proteins. Light-chain disease may be associated with serum protein levels within the normal range, these small-molecular-weight proteins are readily filtered by the renal glomerulus. Bence Jones proteinuria can be tentatively identified by heating an acidified urine sample to 50° to 60°C and observing it for protein precipitates. A more reliable method is to perform an electrophoretic or immunoelectrophoretic analysis of a urine sample.

Canine myelomas secreting Ig classes G, M, and A have been identified. Most frequent are those of the IgA series. Occasionally, more indolent varieties of this tumor, designated as gammopathies, have been encountered. Gammopathies, like their more malignant counterparts, are products of monoclonal B-cell proliferation. However, unlike the former, they do not produce osteolytic

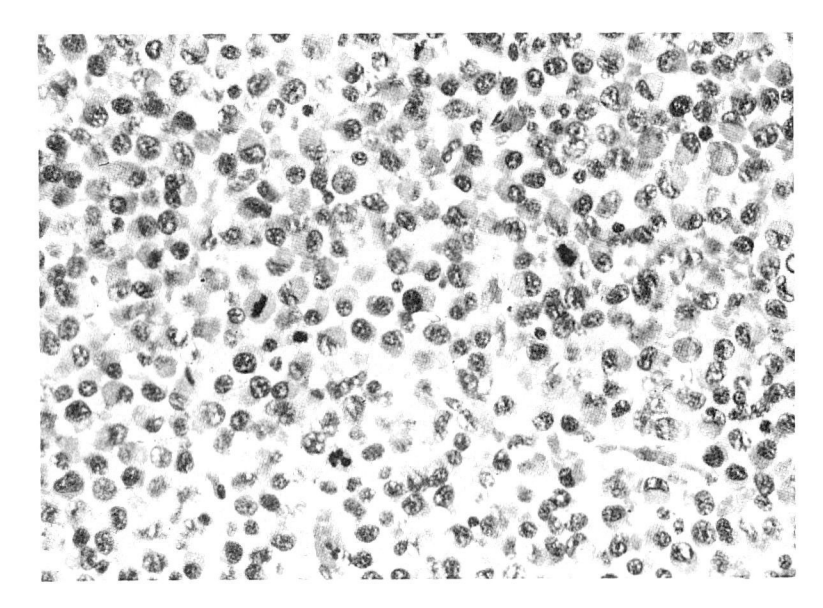

Figure 12-2 A photomicrograph of a canine-origin plasma cell myeloma. Stained with hematoxylin and eosin.

lesions, Bence Jones proteinuria, or increasing serum Ig levels over time. Thus the clinical course is usually benign. In addition to intact Ig-secreting myelomas, heavy-chain only and light-chain only dyscrasias are known to occur. For the latter, Bence Jones proteinemia and proteinuria of lambda specificity have been described.

Cryoglobulins are serum proteins or protein complexes that reversibly precipitate at low temperatures (4°C) but redissolve when heated to room or body temperature. Cryoglobulins of both the IgM and polymeric IgA types have been described in dogs. Although a cold precipitable myeloma may be asymptomatic, affected animals have exhibited clinical neurologic signs and serum hyperviscosity syndrome (anemia, thrombocytopenia, and bleeding diathesis) presumably related to the unusual biophysical characteristics of this protein.

Plasma cell myelomas in other species

Reports of plasma cell myelomas in other species include the cat, horse, and several other species. Identification of the tumor by its Ig product has revealed an IgG_T myeloma in a horse, as well as IgG and IgA myelomas in cats. Multiple myelomas in the pig and calf have been reported but are rare.

LYMPHOMAS

Malignant lymphomas (lymphosarcomas or lymphomas) are among the most common neoplastic diseases of animals. Lymphosarcomas arise in lymphoid tissues such as lymph nodes, spleen, and thymus and frequently metastasize to the gastrointestinal tract or to nonlymphoid organs such as the liver, heart, or kidneys. Lymphadenopathy (Figure 12-3) and splenomegaly are cardinal clinical findings. In contrast to humans, circulation of neoplastic cells (true leukemia) is not a constant feature of lymphoma in animals. Affected lymphoid tissues are enlarged, soft, and pale, and distinction between cortex and medulla is lost. Necrosis is also a feature. Histologically, the neoplastic cells consist of large, densely-packed, invasive cords of lymphoblastic cells with frequent mitotic figures. Typically the cells do not respect normal tissue boundaries, and invasion of

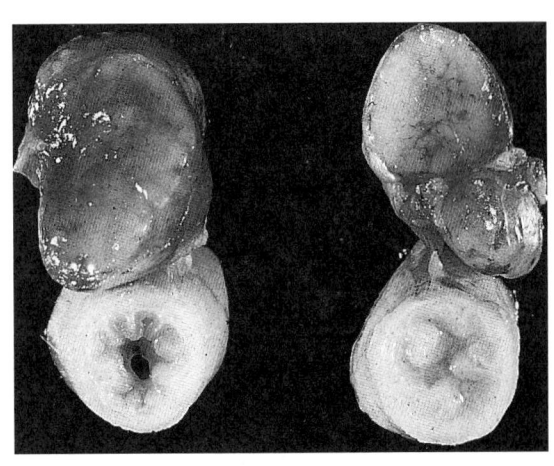

Figure 12-3 Lymphosarcoma in the mesentery lymph node of a cat, resulting from feline leukemia virus.

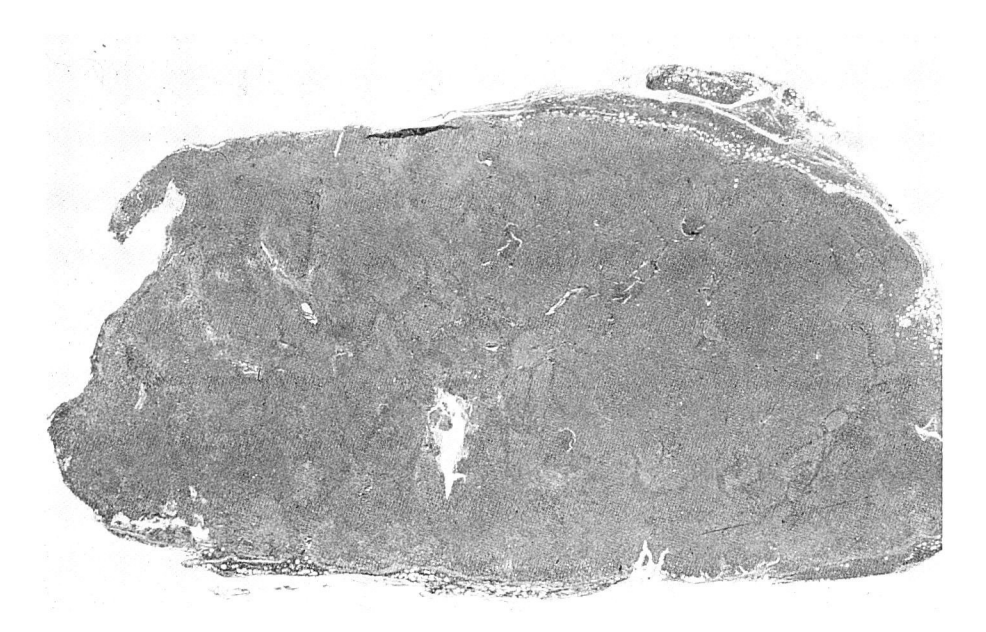

Figure 12-4 Lymphosarcoma resulting from feline leukemia virus that illustrates the destruction of normal lymph node structure by invading neoplastic cells. This slide was stained with hematoxylin and eosin.

the capsule and surrounding tissue can be found (Figure 12-4).

Lymphomas have been induced by radiation injury and many different types of chemicals. However, the putative cause for lymphosarcomas in chickens, mice, cats, and cattle are C-type oncornaviruses or retroviruses (see Figure 3-2). These ecotropic viral agents are transmitted vertically or horizontally and grow in a wide variety of nonlymphoid tissues. Viral replication proceeds through a viral enzyme, reverse transcriptase, which is a distinguishing biologic feature of this group of viruses.

Herpesviruses constitute the other type of viral-induced lymphomas. A number of different herpesviruses isolated from subhuman primates induce lymphosarcomas when inoculated into unnatural hosts. Marek's disease, a herpesvirus of chickens, produces neoplastic-like lesions in chickens susceptible to Marek's disease. Continuous lymphoblastoid cell lines infected with Marek's disease have been established in vitro.

In humans, Epstein-Barr herpesvirus (EBV) infection is strongly associated with infectious mononucleosis (a benign lymphoproliferative disorder) and Burkitt's lymphoma, (chiefly found in Africa). In addition, nasopharyngeal carcinoma, and cervical carcinoma, are thought to be induced by EBV. Of course, the AIDS-related human retrovirus (HTLV-II) is now thought to be responsible for an unusual form of adult T-cell leukemia in Japan.

Viral infection is different from virus-induced malignant transformation because transformation requires alteration of host genetic information. For retroviruses, DNA, proviral copies are inserted into host cellular DNA and they can be detected by molecular nucleic acid hybridization. Similarly, in herpesvirus induced lymphoma, it is possible to find viral DNA segments in host DNA.

No discussion of etiology of lymphosarcoma in veterinary medicine would be complete without a mention of the effects of infection of bovine lymphocytes by *Theileria parva*. *T. Parva* is a hemotropic protozoal parasite responsible for East Coast fever. The *T. parva* merozoites infect bovine lymphocytes and transform them into immortalized lymphoblastoid cells. Infected cells replicate indefinitely unless cured of the parasitism by naphthoquinones treatment. Transformed cells represent a minority T-cell population that binds both peanut and soybean agglutinins. It is thought that only these cell types possess cellular receptors for the infectious organisms.

In addition to immunologic markers such as surface immunoglobulin and monoclonal reagents to T-cells, use of enzyme or cytochemical staining methods are used as an aid to differentiate neoplasms of lymphoid origin from those of myeloid origin. Of these cytochemistry, (ANAE) is useful in identifying neoplasms of T-cell origin, and the cytoplasmic peroxidase stain (positive in myeloid or granulocytic series) is useful in distinguishing neoplasms of this cell type (Table 12-1).

Table 12-1 Expression of cell-surface markers on canine lymphosarcoma cells

Case Number	Surface Ig EAC	Surface Ig G	Cytoplasmic Ig M	Cytoplasmic Ig G	M	T-cell markers Thy-1	T-cell markers EA	T-cell markers ANAE
1	−	−	−	−	−	−	−	+
2	+	+	+	+	−	−	−	−
3	+	+	−	+	−	−	−	+
4	−	+	−	−	−	−	−	N
5	−	+	−	−	−	−	−	N
6	−	−	−	−	−	+	+	N

ND, not done.

Lymphomas in domestic animals

Lymphomas induced by feline leukemia virus
Lymphosarcoma (LSA) associated with feline leukemia virus (FeLV) is the most common neoplastic disease of cats. It is predominantly a disease of young cats, without breed or sex distribution.

Tumors can be transmitted by cell-free filtrates and are the result of infection and subsequent malignant transformation by FeLV virus. Experimentally, fatal disease progresses from primary infection (chiefly in cells of the bone marrow) to a phase characterized by thymic atrophy and systemic virus-mediated immunodepression. Under natural conditions, the virus is shed from infected carrier cats into all excretions and secretions. Infectious saliva is thought to be the chief means of horizontal transmission. It is thought that most cats infected naturally experience a self-limiting subclinical infection. The virus does persist in these cats in a latent or unexpressed form and can be activated by prednisolone treatment in vivo or in vitro. Thus infected cats, even though asymptomatic, are at risk for eventual development of FeLV-related disease and many, under certain conditions, transmit the infection to other cats in the environment.

Neoplastic disease is an infrequent and late manifestation of naturally occurring FeLV disease. The majority of cats infected with FeLV are affected with an immunologic wasting syndrome termed FAIDS (feline acquired immunodeficiency syndrome). This immunosuppressive state is mediated by direct viral infection of lymphocytes and also by a noninfectious viral polypeptide (p15E). This systemic immunodepressive phase increases susceptibility of cats to non–FeLV-related diseases such as feline infectious peritonitis (FIP) a nonspecific wasting syndrome, or fatal nonregenerative anemia. Thus death may supervene before the tumor is evident.

FeLV-induced neoplasms are of T-cell origin and are frequently manifested as a thymic mass (Figure 12-5). Previous classification schemes using histologic scoring methods suggested that neoplasms are of both T- and B-cell types. Lymphomas of B-cell distribution but of T-cell origin have been produced in thymectomized kittens and have been shown to possess surface markers for T cells and not B cells. Lymphomas tend to develop in deep lymphoid tissues associated with the gut, spleen, and mediastinum. There is a predilection for the thymus. Peripheral nodes are largely spared. Most feline lymphosarcomas are aleukemic.

The capacity of cats to develop LSA depends in part on the age of the animal at the time of inoculation, the route, the quality and nature of the immune response to viral antigens, and a virus-coded antigen expressed on the surface of transformed lymphocytes termed *feline oncornavirus-associated cell membrane antigen* (FOCMA).

Cats make antibodies to both viral envelope antigens (detected by virus neutralization) and to FOCMA. A vigorous antibody response to FOCMA following oncogenic challenge is associated with protection. FOCMA antibody can be measured by a membrane immunofluorescence test or a modification of it, complement-dependent cytotoxicity. The target cell that is used varies, but the FeLV-transformed FL-74 cell is most commonly used.

Serologic diagnosis and prognosis in an FeLV-infected or FeLV-exposed cat is performed by using an immunofluorescence test for group-specific viral antigen in neutrophils on a methanol-fixed blood smear (see Figure 10-20). Newer diagnostic kits use an ELISA-based system for identification of viral antigen in affected sera. These tests tell the veterinarian only if the cat is viremic and has been exposed to FeLV. Cats that remain test positive eventually die of lymphoma or FeLV-related disease. FOCMA antibody levels in serum are much more useful for prognostic purposes. A rising FOCMA titer is associated with protection regardless of the state of viremia at the time of testing. The role of cell-mediated immunity in protection against FeLV-induced disease has not been fully evaluated.

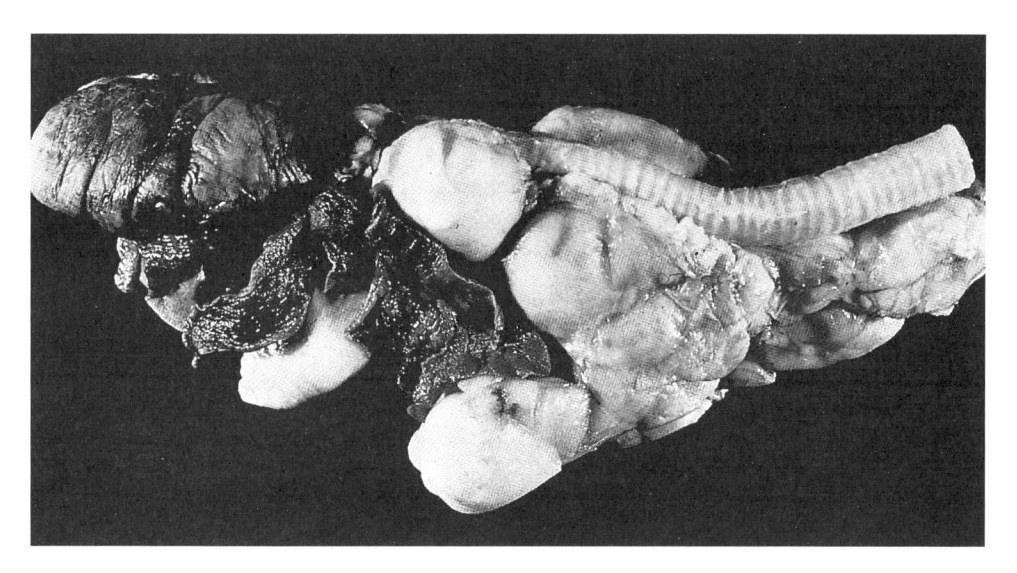

Figure 12-5 Thymic lymphosarcoma, a T-cell neoplasm, resulting from feline leukemia virus.

An effective vaccine (Leukocell, manufactured by Norden Laboratories, Inc.) is available for use in FeLV-susceptible cats (see Chapter 17). Vaccination not only protects cats from the adverse effects of FeLV infection but also prevents establishment of the latent or carrier state in challenged individuals.

Bovine lymphomas

Oncornavirus-induced lymphoma in cattle is a disease of great economic importance in some areas of the United States and Europe. Field studies indicate two different patterns of involvement. The disease may appear as an enzootic infection in certain herds or regions, or it may be sporadic. In the United States the incidence of lymphoma in western-range cattle is very low when compared to closed dairy herds in the midwest or east. Infection with bovine leukemia virus (BLV), a retrovirus similar to FeLV, results in an asymptomatic carrier state, a benign form known as persistent lymphocytosis, or a fatal lymphoid neoplasia known as enzootic bovine leukosis. Like FeLV, the BLV proviral genome is integrated into host cell DNA. Unlike the feline virus, BLV-infected cattle do not develop a non-neoplastic wasting syndrome. Lymphoid neoplasms occur in fetuses, calves, and adults, with the average age being 4 to 8 years. Tumors are widely disseminated and involve both peripheral and deep nodes. Frequently, neoplastic cells invade nerves which result in paralysis, the abomasum, which causes bloat, and the right heart myocardium, which causes progressive congestive heart failure. Unlike cats, approximately 30% to 40% of cows with lymphoma have the leukemic form.

Using cellular membrane markers, neoplastic lymphocytes from adult cows possess surface immunoglobulins and, thus, are B cells. The form of the disease found in calves which is characterized clinically by thymic involvement, is of T-cell origin. Transmission experiments indicate that both vertical and horizontal modes are important.

BLV is a retrovirus. The virus can be readily isolated from lymphocytes by short-term culture with the mitogen PHA. Stimulation results in increased viral production, which can be detected by electron-microscopic or immunologic methods. Apparently, BLV lacks the interspecies antigen common to other members of the mammalian oncornavirus group.

A number of different serologic tests have been devised to detect viral infection in cattle. Antibodies to BLV have been measured using gel diffusion, complement-fixation, and indirect immunofluorescence. The antigen used is ether-treated virus. For complement fixation a modified, direct test is used. In this test, unheated normal bovine serum is added to guinea pig complement. Virus can be identified by electron microscopy on mitogen-stimulated leukocytes or by gel diffusion. Several subtle immunologic abnormalities have been reported in leukocytic BLV-infected cattle. Leukocytosis is the result of an absolute increase in the number of surface Ig-positive B lymphocytes. In vitro culture of these cells without mitogen are characterized by elevated spontaneous uptake of ^{3}H-thymidine. Isolated B cells are hyporesponsive to PWM-induced IgM synthesis in vitro; this is also reflected by the finding of depressed serum IgM levels in vivo. However, asymptomatic infected cattle are clinically indistinguishable from uninfected cattle in all parameters of milk, reproductive, and beef performance.

Sheep are susceptible to infection with BLV. BLV produces lymphosarcomas when inoculated into fetal or neonatal sheep. Lesions and course of the disease are similar to those observed in cattle. A leukosis outbreak in Sweden has been traced to an inoculation of sheep with blood of a calf infected with bovine *Babesia* from a BLV-positive herd. Young adults inoculated with BLV rapidly seroconvert following infection but do not differ from controls when a number of different immunologic assays were applied to them.

Porcine lymphosarcoma

Lymphosarcoma in young slaughter pigs is a common neoplasm. A genetic predisposition has been noted; however, transmission experiments failed. Endogenous (nononcogenic) porcine retroviruses have been found in continuous porcine cell lines. The leukemogenic potential of these viruses is unknown.

Canine lymphoma

Lymphosarcoma in dogs is a disease of middle age. Clinical signs, gross legions, and histopathologic findings are consistent with lymphosarcoma in other species. Initial clinical signs of lymphoma are nonspecific and consist of weight loss, peripheral lymphadenopathy, anemia, and gastrointestinal dysfunction. There are a few scattered reports of isolation of a canine retrovirus similar to FeLB or BLV. These agents are poorly characterized and their oncogenic potential is unknown. Classification of canine lymphomas using immunologic and cytochemical marker systems have been attempted. Data from one small series of dogs studied in our laboratory (S.K.) are outlined in Table 12-1. A proportion of cases lack definitive markers for either B or T cells and thus are classified as null cells. However, the vast majority of lymphoid neoplasms expressing cellular markers appear to be of B-cell origin. Only one true T-cell leukemia was identified (Table 12-1).

A number of researchers initiated investigations on immunophenotyping canine lymphoid neoplasms, correlations with the working formulation classification scheme for lymphoma in widespread use in humans and response to chemotherapy or chemotherapy combined with autologous bone-marrow transplantation. Using a combination of cytochemical and immunocytochemistry procedures (surface or cytoplasmic immunoglobulin for B cells and monoclonals; DT2, DLy-1, F3-20-70 for T cells), approximately 80% of canine lymphomas are identified as of B-cell origin, 7% to 15% are of T-cell origin (Fig. 12-6), and the remainder are of undetermined (null) cell origin. The vast majority of B-cell neoplasms stain positively for IgG.

The working formulation for classification of lymphoid neoplasms is based on morphologic appearance of neoplastic cells obtained from biopsy before clinical intervention. Three grades of malignancy (low, intermediate, and high) are recognized. In humans, low-grade malignancies are least responsive to chemotherapy yet have the longest mean survival time. High-grade malignan-

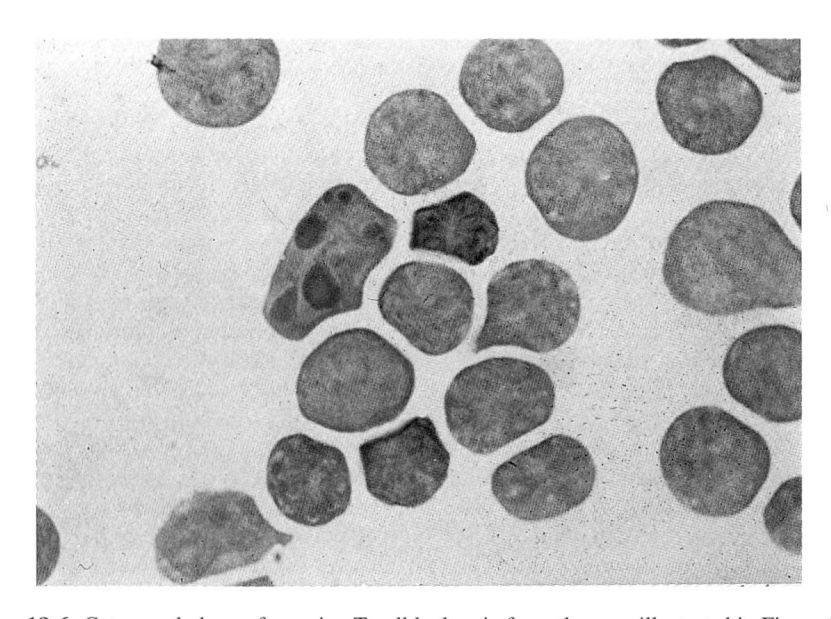

Figure 12-6 Cytomorphology of a canine T-cell leukemia from the case illustrated in Figure 12-1.

cies are most responsive to chemicals yet patients experience rapid relapses. In humans, malignancy grades are approximately equal (i.e., one third) for each group. In contrast, high-grade malignancies (>50%) characterize the canine condition.

For dogs the average survival time after diagnosis is less than 3 months. Chemotherapy marginally extends survival to 5 to 6 months. Lymphoma-bearing dogs are used to evaluate modes of experimental chemotherapy with or without bone marrow or peripheral blood stem-cell transplantation suitable for use in humans. Using a combination of chemotherapy, total body irradiation, and autologous bone marrow (5×10^8 cells/kg) transplantation, 25% long-term (>2 years) survival rates have been achieved. There is no doubt that continuous refinement of this approach will eventually yield a therapeutic regimen suitable for adaption to small-animal practice.

Avian leukosis

Lymphosarcoma (visceral lymphomatosis or lymphatic leukosis) is the most common neoplasm of chickens. It is caused by a vertically transmitted retrovirus. Four viral subgroups (A through D) have been identified based on host-cell range, viral interference studies, and the presence of virus-neutralizing antibodies in serum. In addition to lymphomas, oncornaviruses have been identified as causative agents in osteoporosis, erythroblastosis, myelocytomatosis, hemangiomas, and nephroblastomas.

Selective breeding trials have resulted in strains of chickens that are highly resistant to visceral lymphomatosis. Hens are more susceptible than roosters; testosterone treatment of hens decreases the incidence of lymphomas, probably by its effects on lymphopoiesis in the bursa.

Lymphomas are of B-cell origin because bursectomy prevents lymphoma induction. Surviving and vaccinated birds develop effective immunity to the virus and a FOCMA-like antigen expressed on neoplastic lymphocytes. Recently a cell-mediated immune assay to this cell-surface antigen has been developed.

Murine leukemia virus infection

A number of different neoplastic, immunoproliferative, and autoimmune diseases in mice are caused by oncornaviruses. Detailed discussion of these diseases is beyond the scope of this book.

Simian retrovirus viral lymphoma

Captive macaque monkeys develop an acquired immunodeficiency syndrome analogous to human AIDS. It is characterized by outbreaks of unusual opportunistic infections, leukoencephalitis, retroperitoneal fibrosis, and lymphomas. Affected monkeys have hematologic changes similar to those observed in AIDS patients, including reduced helper T-cell numbers. Lymphomas develop in a portion of the animals, and the neoplasm can be transmitted with cell-free filtrates, strongly suggesting a viral origin. Subsequent work resulted in the isolation of a retrovirus (termed simian T-lymphotropic virus-III) that is remarkably similar to human HTLV-III, the human AIDS virus.

Herpesvirus-induced lymphomas

Herpesvirus saimiri and *Herpesvirus ateles* are natural asymptomatic infections of squirrel monkeys and spider monkeys, respectively. The infection is lifelong and is transmitted horizontally. Experimental infection of marmosets and owl monkeys induces malignant lymphomas with a frequency of over 90%. The course of the disease is rapid and is characterized by a true leukemia and concomitant diffuse infiltration of many tissues. In vivo viral infection is abortive because mature virions are not produced. However, viral genetic material can be demonstrated in host cellular DNA, and viral antigens can be found on malignant lymphocytes by culturing these cells in vitro. The cells are of T-cell origin.

Marek's disease is a member of the herpesvirus group that causes lymphoid tumors in chickens. Infection is spread by contact transmission. The actual production site of infectious virus following viremia is not lymphoid tissue but rather feather follicle epithelium. Lymphoblasts of T-cell origin do not contain virus when examined by electron microscopy, nor can viral antigens be identified by immunofluorescence. Viral genetic information is contained in these cells, as demonstrated by recovery of the virus using cocultivation techniques and by demonstration of cell-associated infectivity.

There is a systemic effect of infection on the bird's immunologic system. Impairment of both antibody production and graft rejection times is seen in birds infected with Marek's disease. Passive antibody offers some protection.

A major advance in tumor research was achieved by demonstrating the efficacy of vaccination of chickens susceptible to Marek's disease with a closely-related herpesvirus of turkeys. Infection was not prevented but neoplasia was prevented. This discovery marked the first conclusive demonstration of specific immunity in abrogating cancer. Analysis of both the turkey herpesvirus and, later, an attenuated Marek's disease has revealed that both vaccine viruses have lost one antigen present on virulent Marek's disease virions. The mechanisms of resistance to neoplasia following vaccina-

Neoplasms of monocytic origin

Canine cutaneous histiocytoma

Cutaneous histiocytomas are common, benign, cutaneous neoplasms of young dogs (Figure 12-7). Histologically, the masses consist of nests and islands of pleomorphic mononuclear leukocytes (histiocytes). Mitotic figures are numerous. Histiocytoma cells stain positively for alpha-$_1$-antitrypsin protein, and this is a helpful diagnostic aid in differentiating them from other cutaneous "round-cell" tumors of dogs, notably transmissible venereal sarcoma (TVS). The TVS cells are reported to stain positively for vimentin. However, histiocytomas do not metastasize and rarely recur following surgical removal. After a variable period of growth, these neoplasms regress. Regression is associated with infiltration of the tumor by lymphocytes and neutrophils.

Malignant histiocytosis

Malignant histiocytosis is a rare, systemic, neoplastic proliferation of atypical monocytes (histiocytes). The disorder has only recently been identified in dogs. The salient cytologic features of this neoplasm are tissue infiltration by large mononuclear cells with abundant foamy cytoplasm and eccentric nuclear placement. Occasional multinucleate forms are seen. Recently a continuous cell line was established from a canine case of histiocytosis. In vitro, the cells were actively phagocytic for IgG-coated erythrocytes and latex beads, yet they lacked receptors for complement and were negative for surface immunoglobulin (B-cell marker) and terminal deoxynucleotidal-transferase, a T-cell marker enzyme.

A histiocytic proliferative disease syndrome has been identified in Swiss Bernese mountain dogs. Two clinical forms of the disease are recognized. The clinically benign form, designated as systemic histiocytosis, occurs in young (4-year-old) dogs and is characterized by histiocytic infiltration of nodular and diffuse patterns in the skin and adnexa. However, other tissues contain neoplastic cells. These cells resemble activated histiocytes and stain positively for acid phosphatase and nonspecific esterase. Several dogs in this series responded successfully to treatment with bovine tymosin fraction 5.

The second form of histiocytosis is malignant and strongly resembles malignant histiocytosis, which was described earlier. Malignant histiocytosis of the Bernese dogs almost exclusively affects older males and follows a rapidly-progressive clinical course. Although cutaneous lesions are present, the bulk of the neoplasm is found in lungs, hilar lymph nodes, and lymphoreticular tissues, including the liver. Neurologic manifestations are common. Neoplastic cells closely resemble activated histiocytes and stain positively for cytoplasmic lysozyme, a cytochemical marker for monocytes/macrophages.

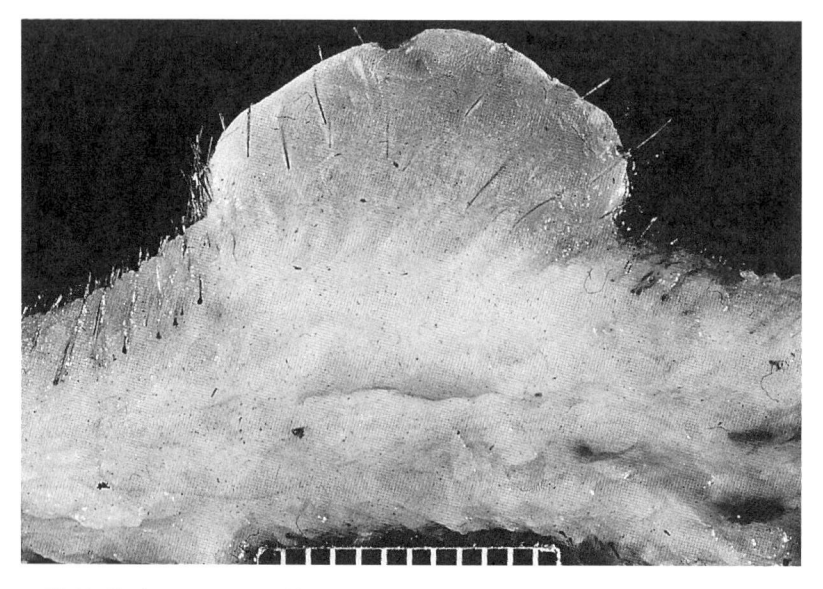

Figure 12-7 Canine cutaneous histiocytoma, a benign proliferation of monocyte-origin cells.

SUGGESTED READINGS

Applebaum FR, Deeg HJ, Stork, and others: Cure of malignant lymphoma in dogs with peripheral blood stem cell transplantation, *Transplantation* 42:19-22, 1986.

Ardans AA, Trommershausen-Smith A, Osburn BL, and others: Immunotherapy on two foals with combined immunodeficiency, resulting in graft versus host reaction, *J Am Vet Med Assoc* 170(2):167-175, 1977.

Banks KL, McGuire TC, Jerrels TR: Absence of B lymphocytes in a horse with primary agammaglobulinemia, *Clin Immunol Immunopathol* 5:282-290, 1976.

Blum JR, Cork LC, Morris JM, and others: The clinical manifestations of a genetically determined deficiency of the third component of complement in the dog, *Clin Immunol Immunopathol* 34:304-325, 1985.

Bostock DE, Owen LN: Porcine and ovine lymphosarcoma: a review, *J Natl Cancer Inst* 50:933-939, 1973.

Braund KG, Everett RM, Bartels JE, and others: Neurologic complications of IgA multiple myeloma associated with cryoglobulinemia in a dog, *J Am Vet Med Assoc* 174:1321-1325, 1979.

Bue CM, Davis WC, Magnuson NS, and others: Correction of equine severe combined immunodeficiency by bone marrow transplantation, *Transplantation* 42:14-19, 1986.

Cockerell GL, Parodi AL, Levy D: Immunocompetence of sheep experimentally infected with bovine leukemia virus, *Vet immunol Immunopathol* 13:189-202, 1986.

Couto CG, Krakowka S, Johnson, and others: In vitro immunologic features of weimaraner dogs with neutrophil abnormalities and recurrent infections, *Vet Immunol Immunopathol* 23:103-112, 1989.

DeMartinini JC: Hypoplasia and lymphopenia in a Siberian tiger, *J Am Vet Med Assoc* 165(9):824-826, 1974.

Dewhirst MW, Stump GL, Harvitz AI: Idiopathic monoclonal (Iga) gammapathy in a dog, *J Am Vet Med Assoc* 170:1313-1316, 1977.

Duncan JR, Corbeil LB, Davies DH, and others: Persistent papillomatosis associated with immunodeficiency, *Cornell Vet* 65(2):205-211, 1975.

Essex M: Neoplasms of cats caused by oncornaviruses, *Pathobiology Annual* 5:169-195, 1975.

Essex M, Cotter SM, Carpenter JL: Feline virus-induced tumors and the immune response: recent developments, *Am J Vet Res* 36:809-812, 1973.

Falk LA, Wolfe LG, Deinhardt F: Herpesvirus Saimiri: experimental infection of squirrel monkeys (Saimiri Sciurellus), *J Natl Cancer Ist* 51:165-170, 1973.

Felsberg PJ, Glickman LT, Jezyk PF: Selective IgA deficiency in the dog, *Clin Immunol Immunopathol* 36:297-305, 1987.

Ferrer FJ: Antigenic comparison of Bovine Type C virus with murine and feline leukemia viruses, *Cancer Res* 32:1871-1877, 1972.

Flastad T, Anderson S, Nielson K: The course of experimental *Fasciola hepatica* infection in calves with a deficient cellular immunity, *Res Vet Sci* 13:468-475, 1977.

Grindem CB, Perman V, Stevens JB: Morphological classification and clinical and pathological characteristics of spontaneous leukemia in 10 cats, *Am Anim Hosp Assoc* 21:227-236, 1985.

Grindem CB, Stevens JB, Perman V: Cytochemical reactions in cells from leukemic dogs, *Vet Pathol* 23:103-109, 1986.

Hurvitz AI, Kehoe JM, Capra JD: Characterization of three homogeneous canine immunoglobulins, *J Immunol* 107:648-654, 1971.

Hurvitz AI, Kehoe JM, Capra JD, and others: Bence Jones proteinemia in a dog, *J Am Vet Med Assoc* 159:1112-1116, 1971.

Hurvitz AI, MacEwen G, Middaugh CR, and others: Monoclonal cryoglobulinemia with macroglobulinemia in a dog, *J Am Vet Med Assoc* 170:511-513, 1977.

Jacobs RM, Couto CG, Wellman ML: Biclonal gammapathy in a dog with myeloma and cutaneous lymphoma, *Vet Pathol* 23:2311-231, 1986.

Jones JB, Yang TJ, Dale JB, and others: Canine cyclic hematopoiesis: marrow transplantation between littermates, *Br J Haematol* 30:215-223, 1975.

Jubb KVF, Kennedy PC: *Pathology of domestic animals*, ed. 2, New York, 1970, Academic Press.

Kehoe KM, Hurvitz AI, Capra JD: Characterization of three feline paraproteins, *J Immunol* 109:511-516, 1972.

Kehrli ME, Schmalstieg FC, Anderson DC, and others: Molecular definition of the bovine granulocytopathy syndrome: identification of deficiency of the Mac-1 (CD11b/CD18) glycoprotein, *Am J Vet Res* 51:1826-1836, 1990.

King NW: Simian models of acquired immunodeficiency syndrome (AIDS): a review, *Vet Pathol* 23:345-353, 1986.

Klein G: Herpesviruses and oncogenesis, *Proc Natl Acad Sci U S A* 69:1036-1064, 1972.

Laufs R, Melendez LV: Latent infection of monkeys with oncogenic herpesviruses, *Med Microbiol Immunol (Berl)* 158:299-308, 1973.

Lingeman CH: Plasma cell neoplasms of man and animals, *Natl Cancer Inst Monogr* 32:303-311, 1969.

Mackey LM: Feline leukaemia virus and its clinical effects, *Vet Rec* 96:5-11, 1975.

Magnuson NS, Perryman LE: Metabolic defects in severe combined immunodeficiency in man and animals, *Comp Biochem Physiol* 83:701-710, 1986.

Mansa B: Hypo-7S-globulinemia in mature cattle, *Acta Pathol Microbiol Scand* 63:153-158, 1965.

McGuire TC, Banks KL, Davis WC: Alterations of the thymus and other lymphoid tissue in young horses with combined immunodeficiency, *Am J Pathol* 84(1):39-50, 1976.

McGuire TC, Banks KL, Evans DR, and others: Agammaglobulinemia in a horse with evidence of functional T lymphocytes, *Am J Jet Res* 37(1):41-46, 1976.

McGuire TC, Pillara B, Moore JJ, and others: Valuation of adenosine diaminase and other purine salvage pathway enzymes in horses with combined immunodeficiency, *Infect Immun* 13(2):995-997, 1976.

McGuire TC, Poppie MJ: Hypogammaglobulinemia and thymic hypoplasia in horses: a primary combined immunodeficiency disorder, *Infect Immun* 8(2):272-277, 1973.

McGuire TC, Poppie MH, Banks KL: Hypogammaglobulinemia predisposing to infection in foals, *J Am Vet Med Assoc* 166(1):71-75, 1975.

McGuire TC, Poppie, MS, Bank KL: Combined (B- and T-lymphocyte immunodeficiency: a fatal genetic disease in Arabian fools, *J Am Vet Met Assoc* 164(1): 70–76, 1973.

Miller JM, Miller LD, Olson C, and others: Virus-like particles in phylohemagglutinin stimulated lymphocyte cultures with reference to bovine lymphosarcoma, *J Natl Cancer Inst* 43:1297-1305, 1969.

Moore PF: Systemic histiocytosis of Bernese mountain dogs, *Vet Pathol* 21:554-563, 1984.

Moore PF, and Rosin A: Malignant histiocytosis of Bernese mountain dogs, *Vet Pathol* 23:1-10, 1986.

Moroff SD, Harvitz AI, Peterson ME, and others: IgA deficiency in SharPei dogs, *Vet Immunol Immunopathol* 13:181-188, 1986.

Nazerian K, Sharma JM: Brief communication: detection of T-cell surface antigens in a Marek's Disease lymphoblastoid cell line, *J Natl Cancer Inst* 54:277-279, 1975.

Okazaki E, Purchase HG, Burmester BR: Protection against Marek's disease by vaccinations with a herpesvirus of turkeys, *Avian Dis* 14:413-429, 1970.

Olson C, Baumgartener LE: Pathology of lymphosarcoma in sheep induced with bovine leukemia virus, *Cancer Res* 36:2365-2373, 1976.

Osborne CA, Perman V, Sautter JH, and others: Multiple myeloma in the dog, *J Am Vet Med Assoc* 153:1300-1319, 1968.

Perryman LE, McGuire TC, Hilbert BJ: Selective immunoglobulin M deficiency in foals, *J Am Vet Med Assoc* 170(2):212-215, 1977.

Perryman LE, Boreson CR, Conaway MW, and others: Combined immunodeficiency in an Appaloosa foal, *Vet Patol* 21:547-548, 1984.

Pinder M, Whithey K, Roelants G: *Theileria parva* parasites transform a subpopulation of T-lymphocytes, *J Immunol* 127:389-390, 1981.

Potter M: The plasma cell tumors and myeloma proteins of mice. In Busch H, editor: *Methods in cancer research*, vol 2, New York, 1967, Academic Press.

Raich PC, Takashima I, Olson C: Cytochemical reactions in bovine and ovine lymphosarcoma, *Vet Pathol* 20:322-329, 1983.

Renshaw HW, Chatborn C, Bryan GM, and others: Canine granulocytopathy syndrome: neutrophil dysfunction in a dog with recurrent infections, *JAVMA*, 166:443-447, 1975.

Renshaw HW, Davis WC, Renshaw SJ: Canine granulocytopathy syndrome: defective bactericidal capacity of neutrophils from a dog with recurrent infections, *Clin Immunol Immunopathol* 8:384-395, 1977.

Renshaw HW, Davis WC: Canine granulocytopathy syndrome, *Am J Pathol*, 95:731-744, 1979.

Roth JA, Lomas LG, Altszuler N: Thymic abnormalities and growth hormone deficiency in dogs, *Am J Vet Res* 41:1256-1262, 1980.

Roth JA, Kaeberle ML, Grier RL, and others: Improvement in clinical condition and thymus morphologic features associated with growth hormone treatment of immunodeficient dwarf dogs, *Am J Vet Res* 45:1151-1155, 1984.

Scott RE, Dale DE, Rosenthal, and others: Cyclic neutropenia in grey collie dogs, *Lab Invest* 28:514-425 1973.

Shephard VJ, Dudds-Laffin J, Laffin RJ: Gamma A myeloma in a dog with defective hemostasis, *J Am Vet Med Assoc* 160:1121-1127, 1972.

Stevens DR, Osburn BL: Immune deficiency in a dog with distemper, *J Am Vet Med Assoc* 168(6):493-498, 1976.

Theis GA: Effects of lymphocytes from Marek's disease-infected chickens on mitogen responses of syngenic normal chicken spleen cells, *J Immunol* 118:887-893, 1977.

Virella G, Slappendel RJ, Goudswaard J: Multiple myeloma IgA cryoglobulinemia and serum hyperviscosity in a dog, *Int Arch Allergy Appl Immunol* 55:537-541, 1977.

Whitbread TJ, Batt RM, Garthwaite G: Relative deficiency of serum IgA in the German shepherd dog: a breed abnormality, *Res Vet Sci* 37:350-352, 1984.

Winkelstein JA, Cork LC, Griffin DE, and others: Generically determined deficiency of the third component of complement in the dog, *Science* 212:1169-1170, 1981.

Winkelstein JA, Johnson JP, Swift AJ, and others: Genetically determined deficiency to the third component of complement in the dog: in vitro studies on the complement system and complement-mediated serum activities, *J Immunol* 129:2598-2602, 1982.

Yohn DS: Oncogenic DNA viruses of primates, *Med Primatology*, Proc 3rd Conf Exp Med-Surg-Primates, Lyon, 1972, Pt III, 197-214 (Karger, Basel 1972).

Zolla-Pazner S, Sullivan B, Richardson D: Cellular specificity of plasmacytoma-induced immunosuppression, *J Immunol* 117:563-568, 1976.

13 Immunologic Mechanisms in Immune-Mediated Diseases

The immune system is designed to protect the host from a myriad of pathogenic agents. This same immune system can cause detrimental effects resulting in the development of disease. Such immune-mediated diseases are often the result of either a misdirected or an exuberant immune response. The concept of altered reactivity to antigen was originally developed by von Pirquet and termed allergy. The terms *allergy* and *hypersensitivity* are frequently used synonymously. Hypersensitivity describes a variety of reactions that produce tissue injury. Gell and Coombs developed a classification scheme for hypersensitivity reactions based on the immunologic mechanism involved. In this system, Types I to III have antibody as the important initiating reactant and Type IV is mediated by T lymphocytes. The antibody class that initiates Type I hypersensitivity is IgE, which is also called reaginic antibody or homocytotropic antibody. Type II hypersensitivity is caused by an IgG or IgM antibody that is specific for a cell-associated antigen, such as an erythrocyte antigen. Immune complexes formed by antigen, IgG, and complement cause the reactions characteristic of Type III hypersensitivity.

MECHANISMS OF HYPERSENSITIVITY REACTIONS

Type I hypersensitivity

Type I hypersensitivity is mediated by the IgE class of antibody. IgE antibodies are synthesized following exposure to antigens, which are referred to as allergens when they induce an IgE response. Allergens are often environmental in origin, consisting of substances such as pollens, molds, dusts, and parasites. *IgE* has the unique ability to bind tightly to receptors on the membrane of mast cells in skin and connective tissue and basophils in the blood. These receptors bind to the Fc piece of IgE, leaving the Fab parts of the immunoglobulin available for antigen binding. When these sensitized *mast cells* are exposed to the allergen that caused production of the IgE, degranulation of the mast cell with mediator release occurs. The mast cell mediators cause physiologic reactions, such as smooth muscle contraction, which initiate the clinical signs seen with Type I reactions, such as the bronchoconstriction in asthma. Type I reactions will be discussed in greater detail later in this chapter (Figure 13-1, A)

Type II hypersensitivity

The mechanism involved in this type of hypersensitivity results in cell lysis or damage. Antibody of the *IgG* and/or *IgM* class and *complement* are the important reactants. The antibodies bind to *cell surface epitopes*, fix complement, and initiate cell destruction by one of several methods. These methods include the lytic complement cycle or opsonization followed by destruction by phagocytosis and removal by the reticuloendothelial system (Figure 13-1, B). Two examples of a Type II reaction are the transfusion reaction, in which antibodies against erythrocyte determinants bind and facilitate erythrocyte destruction, and neonatal isoerythrolysis of newborn foals. Removal of erythrocytes from the circulation by opsonization with antibody and phagocytosis by macrophages or lysis of these cells by complement results in anemia.

The presence of antierythrocyte antibodies in other forms of Type II disease may be the result of antibody production to self-antigens. This also occurs in autoimmune hemolytic anemia (see Chapter 15) or in response to a drug metabolite adsorbed to an erythrocyte membrane.

Type III hypersensitivity

Type III hypersensitivity occurs when both antibody and antigen are present and *immune complexes* form as a result of antigen and antibody binding in vivo. Sometimes the antigen is produced by a pathogenic agent that is infecting the host; other times the antigen is a self-antigen, such as nucleic acid (see Chapter 14). Immune complexes large enough to lodge in small blood vessels and the glomerulus of the kidney evoke a reaction that results in inflammation; this is called Type III hypersensitivity. When the antibody-antigen complex becomes lodged in a small vessel, it initiates the complement cascade. Complement fixation causes the production of chemotactic factors (C5a), that attract neutrophilic leukocytes to the area. These *neutrophils*, in their attempt to engulf and digest the immune complexes, spill their lysosomal contents into the area. The enzymes include collagenase, elastase, lysozyme, and toxic oxygen intermediates. The result is inflammation and tissue destruction, which leads to glomerulonephritis, arthritis, or skin lesions (depending on the site involved) (Figure 13-1, **C**). This mechanism occurs in equine infectious anemia (EIA) in which persistent viremia allows for immune complex development, and in systemic lupus erythematosus (SLE) in which the antigens involved are self-antigens, such as DNA. The same mechanisms are involved in the Arthus reaction and serum sickness (see Chapter 14).

Type IV hypersensitivity

Historic descriptions of hypersensitivity divided the reactions into immediate and delayed, based on the amount of time it took a lesion to develop after introduction of antigen. In that simple classification scheme, Types I through III are immediate, that is, the reaction occurs within minutes or hours of antigen contact. The Type IV reaction differs in that it takes several days (24 to 48 hours) after antigen exposure for the sensitized host to exhibit the reaction. Another important difference is that the Type IV reaction is mediated not by antibody, but by sensitized *T lymphocytes*.

A frequently cited example of Type IV hypersensitivity is the skin reaction to tuberculin. When an animal that is sensitized to and/or infected with *Mycobacterium tuberculosis* is injected with 0.1 μg of a purified protein derivative (PPD) of the organism intradermally, an erythematous, indurated swelling appears at the site of injection after 48 hours. The pathogenic mechanism that causes this lesion begins with the uptake of antigen by dendritic cells and presentation to CD4+ T lymphocytes that recognize the antigen presented by the macrophage in association with MHC Class II antigens. Binding of antigen initiates a series of reactions that result in the production of interleukin 1 (IL-1) and interleukin 6 (IL-6). A variety of lymphokines are then produced by T lymphocytes. Macrophage inhibition factor (MIF) prevents macrophages from leaving the area of the reaction. Gamma interferon (IFN-γ) activates macrophages so that there is increased toxic oxygen radical production, membrane activity, and metabolic reactivity. These changes prepare the macrophage to more effectively kill the invading organisms. Also produced by activated macrophages in small but pharmacologically active amounts is a molecule called tumor necrosis factor (TNF) alpha. This cytotoxic protein can kill susceptible cells after binding to high-affinity receptors on the surface. Lymphotoxin, a similar cytotoxic protein, is also produced by activated CD4+ lymphocytes and participates in the reaction. The resultant delayed-type hypersensitivity (DTH)-lesion in the skin is indurated as a result of the accumulation of mononuclear cells and often contains areas of necrosis (Figure 13-1, **D**).

TYPE I IMMEDIATE TYPE HYPERSENSITIVITY: IMMUNOGLOBULIN E

IgE binds to Fc receptors on mast cells and basophils. The concentration of IgE in serum is in very low (nanogram) amounts, although severely allergic or parasitized animals have elevated serum concentrations. Once bound to Fc receptors on mast cells, IgE remains attached for weeks to months.

IgE has been identified and characterized in humans, monkeys, mice, rats, rabbits, cattle, horses, dogs, and sheep. IgE-like activity is reported for the cat, but the isolation and characterization of the molecule has yet to be definitively reported.

Early methods of quantitating for IgE relied on its ability to sensitize mast cells. Thus the passive cutaneous anaphylaxis test (PCA) and the Prausnitz-Küstner (PK) test are performed by injecting 0.1 to 0.2 ml of test serum into the skin of a healthy animal of the same species as the test serum. After a latent period of at least 24 hours, the healthy animal is injected with the antigen for which the test serum IgE reactivity is being evaluated. In the PCA test the antigen is injected intravenously with Evans blue dye. In the PK test the antigen is injected intradermally in the site of the sensitizing injection. In both tests a positive reaction is indicated by the development of a weal within 30 minutes. If the test serum is heated to 56°C for at least 30 minutes before intradermal injection, the Fc piece of the IgE antibody is altered such that it is no longer able to bind to cutaneous mast-cell receptors.

Another method used to test for the presence of allergen-specific IgE in the patient is the direct skin test. In this skin test, allergen is injected directly into the skin, where it reacts with IgE on sensitized mast cells and elicits the Type I reaction and consequent wheal and erythema development. The direct skin test and the modification, called the scratch test, are widely used in clinical allergy and veterinary dermatology. In vitro tests to measure IgE are based on solid-phase binding such as the radioimmunoassay or enzyme-linked immunosorbent-assay (ELISA). The radioallergosorbent test (RAST) is performed using antigen coupled to an inert substrate such as a filter paper

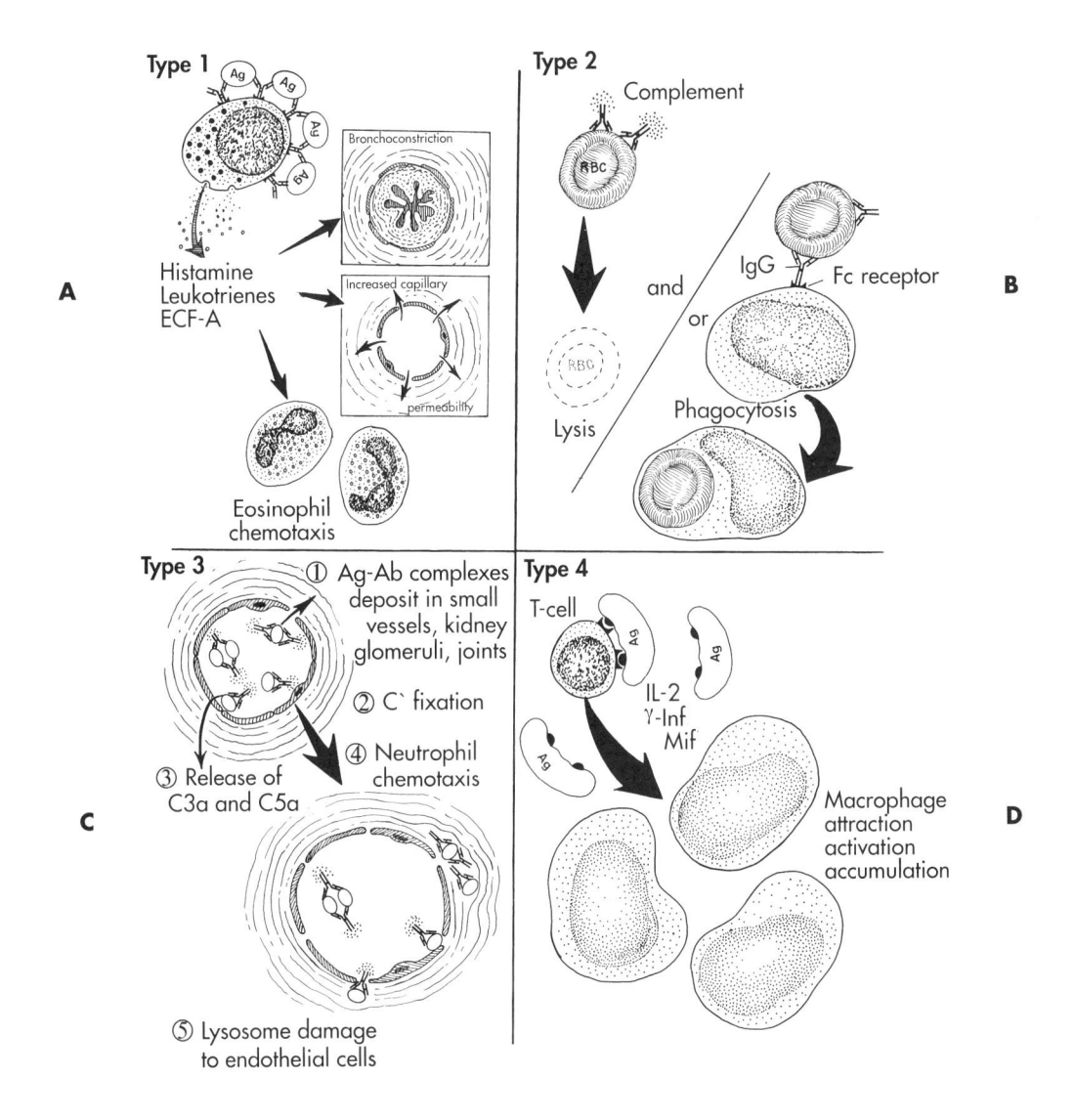

Figure 13-1 Gell and Coombs' four types of hypersensitivity. **A,** Type I involves mast-cell bound IgE cross-linked by multivalent antigen, triggering the release of vasoactive mediators. **B,** Type II is caused by antibody binding to cell-surface epitopes and initiating complement fixation and cell lysis or opsonization. **C,** Type III is caused by deposition of antigen-antibody complexes in blood vessel walls and tissue damage resulting from complement-induced neutrophil chemotaxis. **D,** Type IV reactions occur as a result of sensitized T lymphocytes reacting with antigen, releasing cytokines, and activating macrophages.

or sepharose bead. Test serum is incubated with this solid phase, and after washing to remove unbound antibody, it is incubated with anti-IgE serum labeled with a radioisotope. The amount of radioactivity bound is proportional to the amount of IgE in the patient's serum that has bound to the allergen on the solid support (bead, filter, or microtiter well). The ELISA method is similar but it involves substitution of the isotope with an enzyme conjugate.

REGULATION OF IgE PRODUCTION

The low serum levels of IgE indicate a tightly regulated system. In humans, cattle, and dogs, plasma cells that produce IgE have been found in high number in mucosal sites in the respiratory tract and intestine, in tonsils, and especially in mesenteric lymph nodes. IgE-specific immunoperoxidase staining of mesenteric lymph nodes of cattle with moderate levels of intestinal parasitism reveals percentages of IgE-containing cells as high as 27%. This means that mesenteric lymph nodes are an important site for IgE synthesis.

IgE production is T-cell dependent, as demonstrated by the lack of IgE production in nude (athymic) mice, which lack T lymphocytes. Although regulation of IgE responses has not been studied at the cell or molecular level in domestic animal species, it is likely that the studies performed in mice and verified in human beings will have at least some similarity to IgE control mechanisms in domestic animal species. Studies in mice have shown there are two types of CD4+ helper T lymphocytes. Helper T Type I cells produce IFN-γ response to antigenic stimulation, while helper T Type II cells produce Il-4. Under the influence of Il-4, B lymphocytes change from IgM to IgE production. When helper T Type I cells are predominant, there is an inhibitory effect on IgE production because of the blocking of the Il-4 effect by IFN-γ.

Studies in mice have demonstrated that IgE production is kept under control by suppressor T cells. Experiments have been performed in which suppressor T lymphocytes from genetically low-responder mice were removed by irradiation or cyclophosphamide treatment; the IgE responses of the treated mice increased. This demonstrated that in the absence of T suppressor cells, mice normally considered low IgE producers become high producers.

A low-affinity Fc receptor for IgE is present on human B lymphocytes. Synthesis of this receptor is enhanced by Il-4, and soluble fragments are released into the extracellular fluid. Current theories credit this fragment with a regulatory role in receptor synthesis.

The tendency to develop IgE antibodies in response to environmental antigens is heritable. Individuals with the "high IgE responder" phenotype are called atopic. *Atopy* is described in certain breeds of dogs such as the dalmatian and West Highland white terrier, which show increased incidences of allergy. Allergic reactions to vaccine components have been observed within certain inbred herds of holstein cows; the same vaccine has not elicited any adverse effects in genetically different cattle. Thus evidence exists for genetic control of IgE production in domestic animals, as well as for humans and mice.

SYSTEMIC ANAPHYLAXIS: THE PROTOTYPE IgE-MEDIATED REACTION

The Type I hypersensitivity reaction has three essential steps: sensitization, latent period, and reexposure. These steps are necessary for the elicitation of the pathologic process. Sensitization involves the entrance of antigen into the body. Entrance of antigen is often by inhalation but can be by ingestion or injection either by syringe or biting insect. Introduction of the antigen initiates the production of antibodies of the IgE class. IgE is a homocytotropic or reaginic antibody, characterized by its ability to bind tightly to Fc receptors on mast cells present in the skin and along mucous membranes, and to similar receptors on blood basophils.

The latent period between initial introduction of the antigen and elicitation of an allergic reaction includes the period of time during which the IgE response is initiated through the production of the IgE antibodies and their attachment to receptors.

Reexposure to the antigen causes degranulation of the sensitized mast cells when the multivalent antigen cross-links the Fc receptors on the mast cells. Aggregation of the IgE receptors causes an influx of calcium ions, which is followed by a rapid rise in intracellular cAMP levels. This initiates membrane reactions that cause mast cell granules to release preformed mediators such as histamine and serotonin and to begin synthesis of eciosanoids, including the leukotrienes, formerly known as the slow-reacting substance of anaphylaxis. Pharmacologic effects of these mediators, including smooth muscle contraction, vasodilation, and increased capillary permeability, account for the clinical signs of anaphylaxis.

MEDIATORS OF ANAPHYLACTIC TYPE REACTIONS

There are two kinds of mediators that are released following mast cell activation. The first group is preformed and the second requires synthesis.

Mediators present in mast cell granules that are secreted preformed include *histamine, basic pro-*

teases, and *proteoglycan*, either *heparin* (mast cells) or chrondroin sulfate (basophils), *chemotactic factor for eosinophils* (ECF-A), and *chemotactic factor for neutrophis*. There are some species differences in the amount and kind of mast-cell mediators.

There are four important effects of histamine acting on H_1 receptors. Histamine causes constriction of smooth muscle of the bronchi and the gastrointestinal tract, increases permeability of small blood vessels, stimulates nasal mucous secretion, and causes pruritus and vasodilation in the skin. Antihistamines are effective in alleviating these effects because of the H_1 receptor antagonist function. However, antihistamine drugs are not effective in controlling effects of other, more potent mediators of anaphylaxis.

The proteases present in mast-cell granules include tryptase and chymase. They are extruded in stable complex with proteoglycan and are active in the extracellular environment.

The preformed ECF-A in the mast-cell granules consists of two tetrapeptides. Eosinophils play an important role in the allergic reaction as a negative feedback by releasing histaminase and arylsulfatase, which destroy histamine and leukotrienes, respectively. These chemotactic factors attract eosinophils to the site of the inflammatory reaction.

Mediators that are generated after activation of the mast cell are products of lipid metabolism. These are the ecisonoids, produced from metabolism of arachidonic acid in membrane phospholipids by the lipooxygenase and cyclooxygenase pathways (Figure 13-2). *Prostaglandin D_2*, produced by the cyclooxygenase pathway, is important in causing bronchospasm and increased vasopermeability. Previously called *slow-reacting substance of anaphylaxis* (SRS-A) because of the time required for their synthesis, the leukotrienes are produced by the lipooxygenase pathway. *Leukotriene (LTR) C_4, D_4, and E_4* produce increased vascular permeability and vasoconstriction; LTR B_4 attracts and stimulates neutrophils. The leukotrienes, prostaglandins, and thromboxane can be quantitated in plasma and secretions using a radioimmunoassay. Counteraction of the effects of the leukotrienes can be accomplished by administration of epinephrine.

Platelet activating factor (PAF) is produced by mast cells and causes smooth muscle contraction, increased vascular permeability, platelet aggregation, and chemotaxis of neutrophils.

Late-phase allergic reactions in type I hypersensitivity

IgE-mediated reactions have traditionally been thought to be of the immediate type, that is, occurring within minutes and lasting no longer than several hours. Recently the late-phase allergic reaction has been well described. Reaction to antigen can elicit a dual response: the traditional immediate reaction and the late phase reaction. The late-phase reaction peaks between 4 and 8 hours after antigen challenge and subsides after 12 to 72 hours. Experimental work has proven that this late-phase reaction requires mast cells, allergen, and specific IgE. Furthermore, late-phase reaction cannot be reproduced by administering histamine or bradykinin, but it can be duplicated with leukotrienes C_4, B_4, and D_4.

The late-phase reaction in humans can occur in the skin (late cutaneous reaction), the bronchial system (as in asthma), and the nasal mucosa. The late-phase bronchial reaction has been described in sheep that have IgE antibodies specific for *Ascaris suum*. Sheep sensitive to *A. suum* antigen and subjected to its inhalation develop increased lung resistance within minutes of this allergen inhalation. Resistance remains elevated for 4 hours. After it decreases to baseline, resistance again increases 8 hours after the allergen challenge. This phenomenon is similar to the dual response seen in allergic humans. The leukotrienes generated by arachidonic acid metabolism during the initial mast cell-IgE-allergen interaction are important mediators of the late-phase reaction.

TYPE I HYPERSENSITIVITY: CLINICAL SYNDROME

The mechanism of Type I hypersensitivity, in which mast cells sensitized with specific IgE are triggered to degranulate by binding antigen to Fab fragments of IgE, is responsible for a variety of clinical syndromes. The type of syndrome that occurs depends on several factors such as, the genetic composition of the host, the type and quantity of antigen, and the route of exposure to the antigen. The following are some examples of the clinical manifestations of Type I hypersensitivity in veterinary medicine. More comprehensive coverage can be found in several clinical veterinary immunology texts; see the Suggested Readings section at the end of this chapter.

Systemic anaphylaxis (all species)

When antigen is presented to the host by a route that facilitates rapid and wide distribution in the body and sensitized mast cells are present, the result is likely to be systemic anaphylactic shock. Although intravenous administration of antigen is the surest way to induce anaphylaxis in a sensitive host, other routes of injection are capable of causing the syndrome in highly sensitized animals. Vaccines have elicited anaphylactic shock in cattle, horses, and dogs. Anaphylactic shock is also a

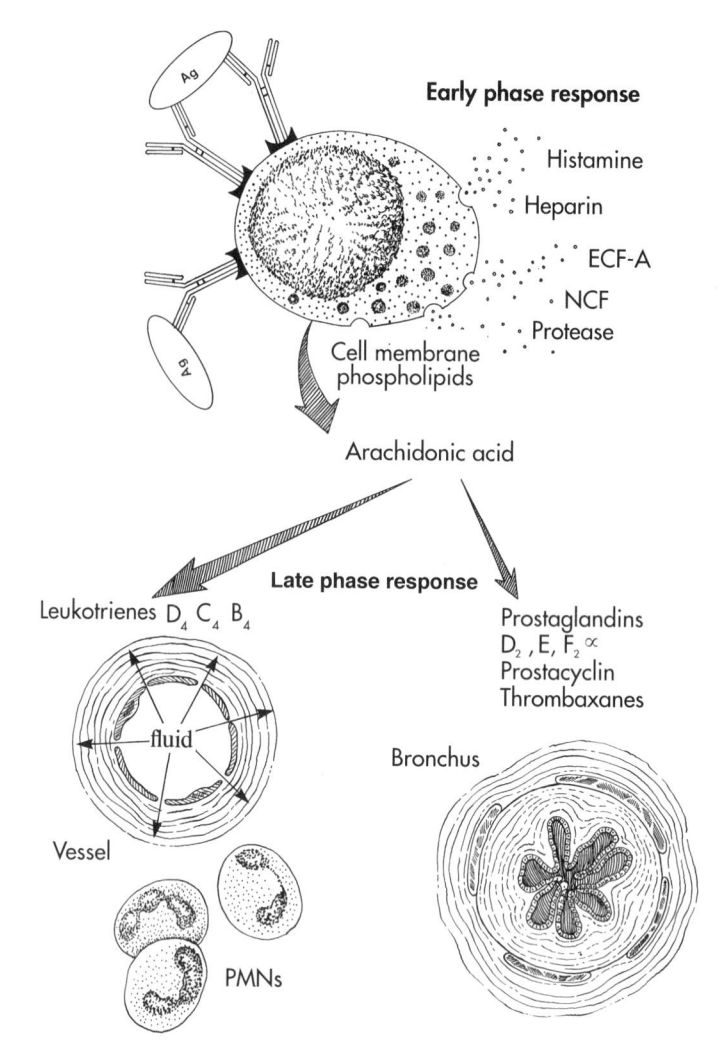

Figure 13-2 Type I hypersensitivity involves the release of preformed mediators that cause an immediate physiologic effect, as well as the initiation of the arachidonic acid metabolism through the cyclooxygenase pathway and the lipooxygenase pathway. This process produces prostaglandins and leukotrienes, respectively, the mediators responsible for the late-phase reaction.

potential result of hyposensitization therapy for allergic skin disease. Anaphylaxis is brought about by massive degranulation of mast cells with mediator release.

The clinical and pathologic appearance of anaphylactic shock varies from species to species because the shock organ differs (Table 13-1). Two contrasting species are cattle and dogs. In cattle the principle organ system affected is the lung, giving rise to clinical signs of dyspnea and cough. In severe cases collapse and death follow unless an injection of epinephrine is made to reverse the process. The dog manifests anaphylaxis differently with signs referable to circulatory shock because of pooling of blood in the hepatic vasculature.

Canine allergic dermatitis

Certain dogs are genetically programmed to be "high-IgE responders." These dogs are atopic. They develop pruritic lesions that usually begin around the feet, face, and axillary region. A syndrome known as *allergic inhalant dermatitis* results from inhalation of one or more environmental allergens. Identification of the offending allergens from a battery of extracts of molds, pollens, dust, and mites is accomplished by intradermal skin testing with extracts of the allergens (as described earlier). In vitro assays to measure circulating allergen-specific IgE can also be performed.

Identification of the offending allergen(s) is the first step to hyposensitization therapy. This form

Table 13-1 Systemic anaphylaxis: species differences

Species	Shock organ	Predominant clinical signs
Bovine	Respiratory tract	Dyspnea, cough
Canine	Hepatic veins	Shock-induced collapse, preceded by vomiting and diarrhea
Equine	Respiratory tract	Dyspnea
	Intestinal tract	Diarrhea
Feline	Respiratory tract	Dyspnea, cough
	Intestinal tract	Vomiting, diarrhea
Human	Respiratory tract	Laryngeal edema, dyspnea
Ovine	Respiratory tract	Dyspnea, cough

of therapy for allergy, which had been used for years in humans, is currently performed with increasing frequency by veterinarians. Hyposensitization therapy requires that the patient be injected on a regular basis with gradually increasing doses of the allergen(s) to which it is allergic. It is unknown exactly how hyposensitization therapy works. Blocking antibodies of the IgG class are induced and as their titer rises, IgE titers fall. The improvement in clinical signs is not directly related to the production of IgG. Current theory is that hyposensitization therapy also causes an increase in suppressor T-cell activity, such that specific IgE production is decreased.

Canine respiratory allergy

Although allergy to inhalants is more commonly manifested as dermatitis in dogs, *allergic rhinitis* occurs infrequently from inhalation of allergens, such as pollens. Seasonal episodes of sneezing are characteristic of allergic rhinitis.

Allergic bronchitis is described in some dogs and results from the inhalation of allergens. The disease is manifested by a chronic cough, which is a result of a chronic low-grade antigenic stimulation. Chronic exposure to allergen, such as mold or dust, rather than seasonal pollens, is often implicated in cases of allergic bronchitis.

Allergenic pneumonitis is a less common sequela of inhalent allergy in dogs. It is manifested as an allergic alveolitis and bronchiolitis, which is accompanied by eosinophilia. Similar pulmonary symptomatology can occur as a result of inhalation of allergens and as a result of parasite migration. In both instances an IgE-mediated Type I hypersensitivity reaction is implicated in the pathogenesis. Affected dogs show dyspnea and exercise intolerance, usually accompanied by a cough.

Canine and feline gastrointestinal allergy

Allergic gastritis occurs with moderate frequency in dogs and cats as a result of ingestion of food to which the dog has developed IgE antibodies. Affected dogs and cats vomit several hours after eating. The vomitus usually consists predominately of bile-tinged mucus. Gastric allergy is best diagnosed with the use of a hypoallergenic diet. Recent research in this area has shown that in dogs, diagnostic endoscopy using locally applied food extracts yields useful information because of the formation of local Type I responses on gastric mucosa at sites of application of the offending food.

Allergy to dietary components can also be manifested as *allergic enteritis*. In affected dogs and cats there is a loose, fetid stool and chronic weight loss. Dietary elimination is the best means of diagnosis. Intradermal skin testing is not useful in detecting allergy to food components.

Feline asthma

A syndrome in cats that resembles asthma in humans occurs with moderate frequency. The disease is quite similar clinically with transient attacks of wheezing and dyspnea. Just as in human asthmatics, there is a sudden onset of bronchoconstriction accompanied by the production of a thick tenacious mucus. The relationship between IgE-mediated allergy and feline asthma has not been delineated. Genetic factors may also be important in the determination of why certain cats develop asthma; genetic predisposition is definitely a factor in the determination of which humans develop asthma.

Bovine IgE-mediated disease

There are several syndromes in cattle that appear to have an atopic etiology. Jersey cows in high milk production sometimes develop an allergic reaction to their own milk proteins. This is called *milk allergy*. This often occurs in heavy producers whose milk is allowed to accumulate in the udder, thus creating pressure that allows some milk protein seepage into the circulation. This predisposes the animal for antibody production and subsequent IgE-mediated reactions.

Recent studies on bovine respiratory syncytial virus infection have implicated virus-specific IgE antibodies in pathogenesis of the disease. A similar observation has been made in human infants, in which atopic children develop more severe disease with respiratory syncytial virus infection than nonatopic children. IgE antibodies specific for the virus and increased histamine concentrations in nasopharyngeal exudate show a positive correlation with increased clinical severity.

Allergic rhinitis has been described in cattle, and a variety of inhalant allergens are, implicated. Usually the cattle are at pasture during the spring when grass, weeds and pollens are particularly prevalent. Direct skin testing demonstrates reactivity to grass pollens in affected cattle and sometimes in asymptomatic cattle as well.

Equine IgE-mediated disease

Horses develop *urticaria*, also called hives or allergic wheals, as a result of an exposure to a variety of allergenic substances. Feeds, bedding, fly sprays, and vitamin preparations are a few such initiators of the reaction. Treatment with antihistamines and avoidance of the offending allergen is usually sufficient to correct the problem.

Chronic obstructive pulmonary disease (COPD), also known as "heaves," thought to be a bronchopulmonary mold allergy with a strong component of Type I hypersensitivity as its cause. The analogous disease in humans, allergic asthma, is known to have a major late phase component of reactivity. This leukotriene-mediated reaction results in sustained smooth muscle contraction. The ineffectiveness of antihistamines for treatment of this disease is easily explained by a such a late phase reactivity. While skin tests with mold and dust allergens yield positive results in affected horses, these same tests are often positive in horses without clinical signs of respiratory disease.

The syndrome known as *Queensland Itch* is an allergic dermatitis that affects horses. They are primarily affected in the summer months when the Culicoides gnat is biting. Affected horses have intense pruritis, which is often most severe at night. A hypersensitivity to the Culicoides gnat has been suggested by elevated plasma histamine levels and positive skin test results with gnat antigen.

IgE-MEDIATED REACTIONS IN PARASITIC DISEASE

Production of IgE is readily elicited by antigens of parasites; it is also noteworthy that eosinophils are stimulated to accumulate in greater numbers in the blood of parasite-infected animals. "Self cure" is described in sheep parasitized with Ostertagia; local IgE-mediated degranulation of mast cells with resultant increased capillary permeability and smooth muscle contraction has been cited as the cause of a parasite purge from the gastrointestinal tract.

Infection of dogs with *Dirofilaria immitis*, or heartworm, has been shown to elicit an IgE response to several stages of the nematode, including microfilaria, third and fourth stage larvae, and adults of both sexes. The IgE response appears as early as 2 weeks after infection and may prove to be an important indicator of early infection.

Although demonstration of a role for IgE in parasite killing has not been well studied in most veterinary infestations, a larval form (schistosomula) of the human nematode, *Schistosoma mansona*, is readily killed by IgE, eosinophils, and macrophages in a form of antibody-dependent cytotoxicity (ADCC). The effector cell has low-affinity IgE receptors (CD23) that bind the Fc portion of the IgE, leaving the Fab portion available to bind to antigenic determinants on the schistosomula membrane. This process creates a bridge allowing the eosinophil to cause membrane damage by degranulation on the schistosomula membrane (Figure 13-3). It is likely that such killing is involved in other parasitic diseases.

TYPE II HYPERSENSITIVITY: CYTOTOXIC ANTIBODY REACTIONS

As described earlier, Type II reactions are mediated by complement-fixing antibodies directed to cell-surface–associated antigens and their effect is exerted on those cells. The clinical conditions that are caused by Type II reactions include autoimmune and other types of reactions. Autoimmune Type II disease is caused by the effect of antibodies that are directed against self-antigens; these will be discussed in Chapter 15. Other reactions include hemolytic disease of the newborn (*neonatal isoerythrolysis* in foals and calves), hemolytic anemia as a result of the production of antibodies to red cell contaminants of anaplasmosis vaccine in cattle, and as a sequela to repeated blood transfusion.

Neonatal isoerythrolysis occurs in horses when the dam contains antibodies in her serum (often from exposure to alloantigens from previous pregnancies) that react with antigens on the foal's erythrocytes. The most frequent blood group determinants causing this reactivity are A and Q. Acute hemolysis occurs within several hours after the neonatal foal suckles the colostrum. Prevention can be achieved if the mare and stallion are blood typed and crossmatched before the foaling date. If the mare has antibodies reactive with dominant antigens on the stallion's erythrocytes, then the foal must be removed before nursing and fed an alternate source of colostrum.

MIXED IMMUNOLOGIC MECHANISM IN DISEASE

Types I, II, III, and IV hypersensitivity define a specific immunologic reaction that is responsible for the pathophysiologic outcome. For each type of hypersensitivity there is a prototype reaction (as described earlier and in Chapter 14). However,

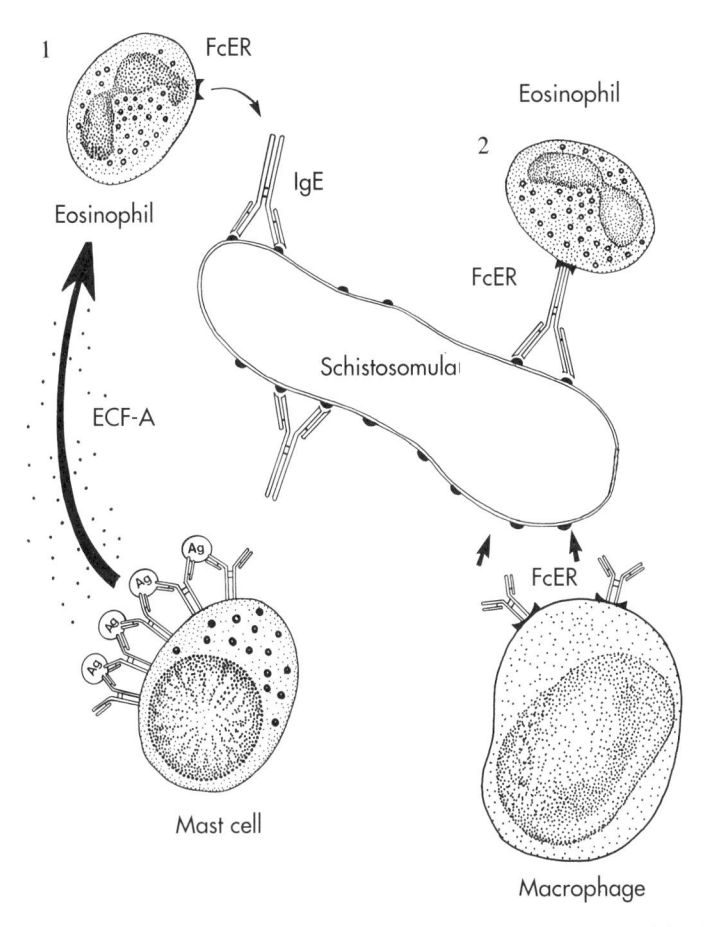

Figure 13-3 The participation by IgE in antibody-dependent cellular cytotoxicity (ADCC) involves binding of the IgE to low-affinity epsilon receptors (CD23) on eosinophils and macrophages. When the IgE is specific for parasite antigens, ADCC is initiated by bridging of the target and effector cell by the IgE.

some interactions between host and antigen involve more than one of the Gell and Coomb's type reactivities.

Canine flea allergy dermatitis

Flea bite dermatitis in dogs is described as having elements of both Type I and Type IV hypersensitivity. There are several allergens in flea saliva. The low molecular weight protein <1000 daltons (**D**) binds to dermal proteins and induces a Type IV reaction as a hapten. Larger multivalent antigens induce an IgE response and bind with mast-cell or basophil-bound IgE to elicit a Type I response. In most affected dogs, both a Type I and Type IV reaction occur, in either order. In fact, a late-phase IgE reaction may also occur in addition to the immediate weal and flare reaction characteristic of Type I. Examination of biopsy specimens from skin of dogs allergic to flea bites shows a combination of edema with eosinophil infiltration and mononuclear cell infiltration (characteristic of Type IV). Sometimes a preponderance of basophils is observed; this is called *cutaneous basophil hypersensitivity* and is sometimes seen in flea allergy. When flea-allergic dogs are skin tested by intradermal injection with flea saliva extract, most dogs show an immediate weal reaction and some show the indurated later reaction recognized as a Type IV response.

Chronic obstructive pulmonary disease in horses

This disease was mentioned earlier under Type I reactions. For some horses there is evidence for an additional component, Type III hypersensitivity, in the immunologic pathogenesis. Common to most horses with COPD is exposure to and consequent development of an immune response to inhaled allergens such as molds, pollens, and dusts. Intradermal skin testing of affected horses usually reveals the development of a localized immediate weal at the injection site, characteristic of a Type I response as well as a Type III reaction, at 4 to 6 hours after intradermal injection. In affected horses inhalation challenge elicits increased respiratory resistance. Lung histopathology can indicate chronic bronchiolitis with eosinophilia and/or signs of complement activation.

SUGGESTED READINGS

Baker DG, Gershwin LJ: Immunoglobulin E and Type I hypersensitivity in bovine ostertagiosis, *Vet Parasitol* 46:93-102, 1993.

Baker E: *Small animal allergy: a practical guide*, ed 1, Philadephia, London, 1990, Lea & Febiger.

Capron A, Dessaint JP: From protective immunity to allergy: the cellular partners of IgE, *Chem Immunol* 49:236-244, 1990.

Eyre P, Lewis AJ: Acute systemic anaphylaxis in the horse, *Br J Pharmacol* 48:426-437, 1973.

Gershwin LJ, Dygert BS: Development of a semiautomated microassay for bovine immunoglobulin E: definition and standardization, *Am J Vet Res* 44:891-895, 1983.

Gershwin LJ, Gershwin ME: The regulation of the IgE response, *Immunol Today* 7:328-329, 1986.

Halliwell REW, Gorman NT: Nonatopic allergic skin diseases. In *Veterinary clinical immunology*, 1989, WB Saunders.

Hammer KK, Kirchhofen B, Schmid T: Detection of homocytotropic antibody associated with a unique immunoglobulin class in the bovine species, *J Immunol* 1:249-257, 1971.

Kleinbeck ML, Hites MJ, Loker JL, and other: Enzyme linked immunosorbent assay for measurement of allergen-specific IgE antibodies in canine serum, *Am J Vet Res* 50:1831-1839, 1989.

Leiferman KM, Gleich GJ: The role of inflammatory cells in LPR. Drosch W, editor: *Late phase allergic reactions*, Boston, 1990, CRC Press.

Lemanske RF Jr: Mast cell-derived mediators. In Dorsch W, editor: *Late phase allergic reactions*, Boston, 1990, CRC Press.

Lewis RM, and Picut CA: *Veterinary clinical immunology: from classroom to clinics*, Philadelphia, 1989, Lea & Febiger.

Russi EW: Late phase bronchial reaction in sheep. In Dorsch W, editor: *Late phase allergic reactions*, Boston, 1990, CRC Press.

Yamagata GR, Gershwin LJ, Wong MM: Immunoglobulin E recognition of *Dirofilaria immitis* antigens is more specific than immunoglobulin G, *Vet Parasitol* 44:231-245, 1992.

14 Immune Complex Diseases

The immunologic principles that explain immune complex disease were originally demonstrated by Maurice Arthus in 1903. Arthus observed that when rabbits were injected at weekly intervals with milligram quantities of horse serum by the intradermal route, initially there was no effect on the rabbits. But as the antibody titer to the horse serum proteins increased, dermal inflammatory reactions were observed from 3 to 8 hours after injection. These lesions were characterized by edema, hemorrhage, and necrosis. As the number of immunizations with horse serum increased, so did the intensity of the skin reactions.

The Arthus phenomenon (Figure 14-1) is a Type III hypersensitivity reaction, which differs from the Type I hypersensitivity response in the following important aspects: (1) the primary cell type involved in Arthus is the polymorphonuclear leukocyte, whereas mast cells and eosinophils are the major effector cells in the Type I response; (2) the Type I response occurs within minutes, compared with the 3 to 8 hour lag period for development of the Arthus reaction; (3) the dose of antigen required to elicit an Arthus reaction is milligram amounts, whereas the Type I response can be elicited with microgram quantities of antigen; and (4) the major antibody class that elicits Arthus is IgG, whereas IgE causes the Type I response.

Formation of immune complexes occurs in the body whenever there is both circulating soluble antigen and antibody specific for that antigen. Although this mechanism serves as a method of elimination of antigen, it can also become a mechanism for the induction of a Type III hypersensitivity reaction. The size of the immune complexes is a pivotal fact in determining whether a hypersensitivity reaction or mere antigen elimination results from the antigen-antibody binding. The larger complexes that are insoluble are readily removed by phagocytes; it is the smaller insoluble complexes that lodge in various tissues and organs, initiating an inflammatory response. The sources of antigen for immune complex formation include virus, bacteria, parasites, and self-antigens such as DNA. Disease manifestations of immune complex formation include arthritis, vasculitis in skin, and glomerulonephritis.

The mechanism of initiation of the Type III hypersensitivity reaction and its continuation is described in Chapter 13. In brief, the complexes are deposited in small blood vessels, whereupon complement is fixed and chemotactic factors are produced (Table 14-1). The subsequent egress of neutrophils from local blood vessels and their migration along the chemotactic gradient toward the site of antigen-antibody complex deposition involves a complex array of adhesin molecules on the endothelial cells of the blood vessels and on the surfaces of the leukocytes. Once arrived at the site of deposition, the neutrophils begin a process that has been described as "frustrated phagocytosis," whereby they proceed to spill their granule contents on and around the tissue wherein the complexes are lodged. These granules contain proteolytic enzymes such as collagenase and protease, which digest the tissue. Hemorrhage and leakage of fluid are immediate sequelae, followed later by scarring and a resulting decrease in function.

Although the Arthus reaction is an excellent prototype for a localized Type III reaction, the natural occurrence of immune complex disease can be grouped into the following three main categories; (1) low-grade, persistent infection with bacteria, virus, or parasite in the presence of a relatively weak antibody response leading to immune complex formation; (2) autoimmune disease in which there is persistence of a soluble autoantigen and an antibody response to that antigen; and (3) development of IgG antibodies to inhaled antigens resulting in a Type III reaction in the lung.

Pathologic mechanism of tissue damage induced by immune complex deposition

An important factor that governs the fate of an antigen-antibody complex is its size. The larger complexes are removed by the reticuloendothelial system, including hepatic Kupffer cells. These phagocytic cells use the IgG Fc receptor to adsorb the complexes or, in the case of those species that have complement receptors called CRI receptors

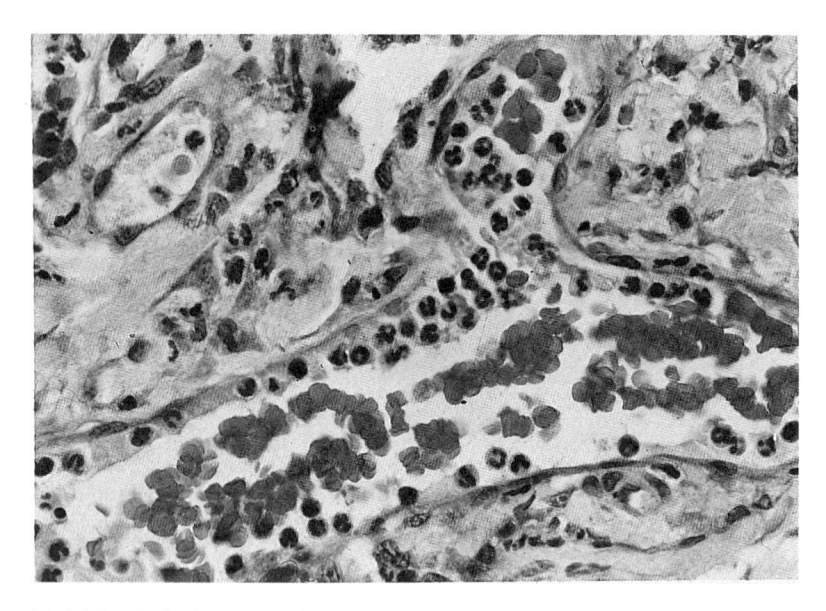

Figure 14-1 Histologic features of the cutaneous Arthus reaction. Note the margination and emigration of neutrophils in the lumen of the venule. Platelet activation and fibrin deposition have occurred and are visible as amorphous eosinophilic debris. Stained with hematoxylin and eosin. (× 168.)

Table 14-1 Inflammatory mechanisms identified for immune complex disease

Source	Active intermediates	Biologic effects
Complement	C3a, C5a	Anaphylatoxin chemotactic for leukocytes
Complement	C1q activation	Binds endothelium, producing increased permeability
Complement	C5-C9 (membrane attack complex)	Cytolysis; indirect by induced secretion of inflammatory mediators
Mast cells basophils	Histamine, seratonin	Increased vascular permeability
Platelets	Platelet aggregation	Vascular occlusion (thrombosis)
Neutrophils	Lysosomal enzymes	Tissue digestion, necrosis

on erythrocytes, the erythrocyte can adsorb complexes prior to removal by phagocytes. The small soluble complexes are readily taken up by the macrophages. It is important to point out that formation of immune complexes alone does not cause disease; it is their deposition and the subsequent inflammatory response that causes disease. Deposition depends on several factors, including increases in vascular permeability and blood pressure. Not all tissues are equally susceptible to immune complex deposition. Deposition tends to occur in tissues with a rapid drop in arterial blood pressure over a short distance (as in the renal glomerulus); in areas of vascular turbulence, such as vessel walls, or in filtration areas such as the uvea, choroid plexus, and renal glomerulus.

The immediate cause of tissue deposition is immune complex–mediated increases in local vascular permeability. These increases are accomplished by release of vasoactive amines from mast cells, basophils, and platelets by immune complexes by the action of complement components (e.g., C3a, C5a) to induce liberation of histamine and other vasoactive mediators. These same complement components have chemotactic function for polymorphonuclear leukocytes. Cytokines such as interleukin-1 and tumor necrosis factor are released from local macrophages, and they exert neutrophil recruitment effects by increasing neutrophil–endothelial cell adhesion. Adherence of platelets and neutrophils to endothelium facilitate the formation of microthrombi and fibrin accumulation. Neutrophils marginate and then emigrate through vessel walls into surrounding tissue spaces (Figure 14-1). The neutrophils are often referred to as "frustrated phagocytes" in this situation because they attempt to engulf the immune complexes that are lodged in tissue. Unable to engulf the complexes, they degranulate in the area. Neutrophil degranulation releases lysosomal enzymes that include proteases and collagenases and a variety of other destructive enzymes. Tissue damage ensues. Hemorrhage and edema follow segmental necrosis of arterioles and venules. By 24 hours to 48 hours after introduction of the antigen a repair process has begun, and mononuclear cells are found in the area.

The sites of immune complex deposition vary with different diseases. The kidney is a frequent site of complex deposition in disease caused by infectious organisms and in systemic lupus erythematosus, (SLE), an autoimmune disease. In the renal glomerulus the site of complex deposition depends on the size of the complex. Large complexes cannot cross the glomerular basement membrane and remain between the endothelium and the basement membrane or the mesangium. Whereas the smaller complexes go all the way through the basement membrane and are deposited on the epithelial side of the glomerulus. In SLE, deposition can occur in blood vessels, kidneys, joints, skin, and brain. This broad distribution of complex distribution accounts for the multisystemic nature of SLE (see Chapter 15).

Serum sickness: a model of systemic immune complex disease

Administration of passive antibody as therapy or prevention of certain infectious diseases has been used since the turn of the century. During wartime, the use of hyperimmune horse serum to treat gunshot victims with incipient tetanus was standard procedure. Some patients treated with the antisera became febrile 10 to 14 days after injection, and glomerulonephritis, vasculitis, and arthritis developed. The first person to identify and characterize this phenomenon was von Pirquet. This disease became known as serum sickness and was considered a rarely fatal but necessary risk of treatment.

In the 1950s the pathogenesis of serum sickness was further defined by Dixon and colleagues. Using a rabbit experimental model system, they successfully reproduced acute serum sickness with the intravenous administration of bovine serum albumin (BSA). The immunokinetics of the disease were followed by means of quantitation of radiolabeled BSA in serum of treated rabbits. A schematic illustration of the Dixon group's findings is presented in Figure 14-2.

After the infusion of BSA, a short equilibration phase occurred. It was followed by a gradual decline in the amount of BSA in serum, lasting from 1 to 10 days and corresponding to the expected half-life of normal serum albumin. Seven to 10 days after injection, a precipitous decline in radiolabeled BSA occurred, with nearly 100% clearance by day 14. Accelerated clearance correlated with the onset of fever and other signs of serum sickness. Total serum complement levels decreased

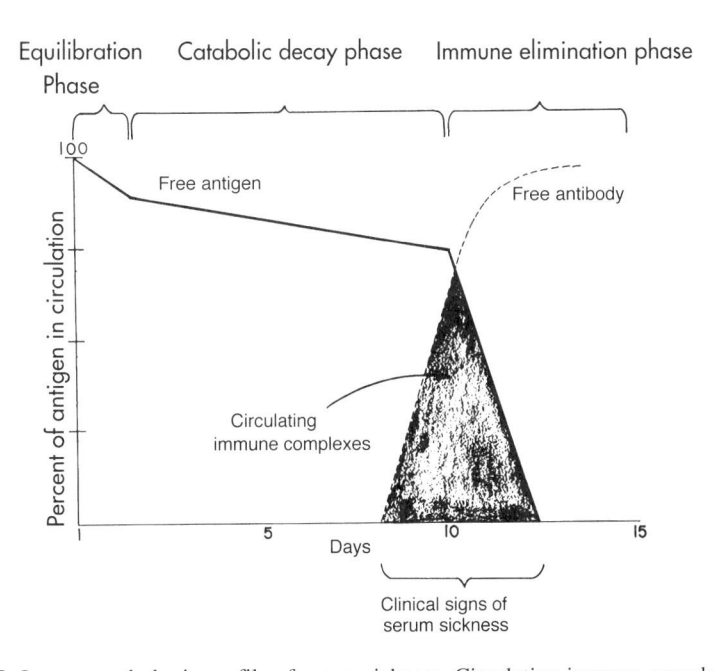

Figure 14-2 Immunopathologic profile of serum sickness. Circulating immune complexes are found when antibodies bind to circulating antigens; clinical signs occur during this time.

dramatically. During this phase, no free BSA antibodies could be demonstrated in serum. This period was called the *immune clearance phase*.

Free antibody was observed in the serum on day 14 after injection. The antibody titer increased to maximum levels within 1 to 2 weeks. During this time, the complement levels in serum returned to normal. The rabbits showed lesions compatible with those seen in human serum sickness, including deposition of immune complexes in joints, renal glomeruli, and blood vessels.

The heterogeneity of the response in rabbits increased our understanding of the pathogenesis of serum sickness. It was observed that the disease did not develop in all rabbits so treated. Upon further analysis it became evident that the rabbits could be sorted into the following three groups: (1) nonresponders producing no antibody response, (2) responders that cleared the antigen without development of disease, and (3) responders that produced only moderate levels of antibody. The last group was most susceptible to development of immune complex disease.

Two very important requirements for the development of immune complex disease are illustrated by this rabbit experiment. The first is the genetics of the animal, which determines the inherent ability of the body to respond to antigen by antibody production. The second point concerns the physicochemical nature of the toxic immune complexes. Maximum pathogenic effects are produced with complexes in moderate antigen excess. Complexes with molar antibody-antigen ratios higher than 1:2 or 1:3 are soluble and thus escape physiologic clearance by the reticuloendothelial system. Complexes in high antibody excess are large and relatively insoluble and thus are easily eliminated from the circulation by normal physiologic means. This concept has been confirmed with complexes of varying sizes and ratios in vitro and subsequent testing for pathogenic effect in vivo.

Serum sickness is a disease of declining importance since the discovery of antibiotics and improved vaccines. It is still useful as a model for the study of the pathogenesis of immune complex disease. Several applications still exist for passive administration of heteroantisera, such as antivenoms and antitoxins.

GLOMERULONEPHRITIS MEDIATED BY IMMUNE MECHANISMS

The renal glomerulus is an important blood filtration system. Approximately one quarter of the volume of cardiac blood output passes through the kidneys. All renal arterial blood passes through the renal glomerulus and is filtered, removing low–molecular-weight compounds. This filtration process occurs as a result of osmotic pressure gradients and hydrostatic pressure in the afferent arteriole of the glomerulus. It is apparent that glomerular filtrate must pass through capillary endothelium, through basement membrane, and probably between glomerular epithelium on its way to the formation of urine.

This filtration mechanism is occasionally the site of a disease process. Large molecules may become trapped in this filtration apparatus, interfering with glomerular function (Figure 14-3). Potentially pathogenic circulating antigen-antibody complexes in the usual circumstances are removed from the bloodstream by the reticuloendothelial system in the spleen and liver. As with serum sickness, only certain types of complexes, particularly those with slight antigen excess, are soluble enough to be trapped in glomeruli.

The most common type of glomerulonephritis encountered in veterinary medicine is that mediated by preformed soluble immune complexes. It is important to realize that the site of formation of these complexes may be distant from and unrelated to their immediate pathogenic effects on the kidneys and other tissues. Efficiency of trapping of these complexes in glomeruli depends on several factors, including size, net charge, mesangial clearing apparatus, and hemodynamics.

It was formerly believed that glomerulonephritis was caused exclusively by the deposition of preformed complexes. Currently it is recognized that some antigens preferentially localize in the glomerular basement membrane, independent of antibody. For example, native DNA has a strong binding affinity for collagen of the glomerular basement membrane (GBM). Thus glomerulonephritis associated with SLE (in which DNA antibodies are produced) may be explained by this antigen-mediated selection process. Perfusion studies have revealed that antigen binding to GBM is mediated largely by net electric charge. Thus cationic antigens preferentially bind to the anionic proteoglycan component of the GBM.

Simple mechanical trapping of complexes or free antigens in the kidneys is not, however, the whole story. Of significant importance in the development of immunologically mediated glomerulonephritis is a change in microvascular permeability. Vasoactive amines and peptides released from basophils or aggregated platelets are important components in the reaction. The reaction of circulating immune complexes with platelets and basophils is thought to result in the release of histamine, serotonin, and other vasoactive substances. These mediators increase vascular permeability in the glomeruli, thereby increasing access to the basement membrane (Figure 14-4).

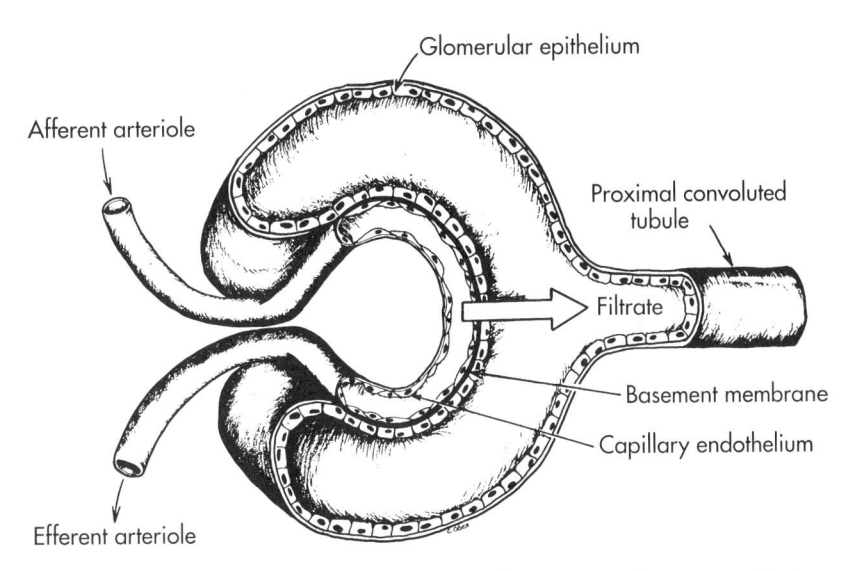

Figure 14-3 The renal glomerular filtration apparatus. Immune complexes are unable to pass through the filter and become trapped in the basement membrane.

1. Normal
2. Release of vasoactive amines from platelets and basophils by immune complexes
3. Increased capillary permeability
4. Deposition of immune complexes and complement in glomerular basement membrane
5. Attraction of neutrophils, damage to glomerular basement membranes, and leakage of serum proteins into the glomerular lumen

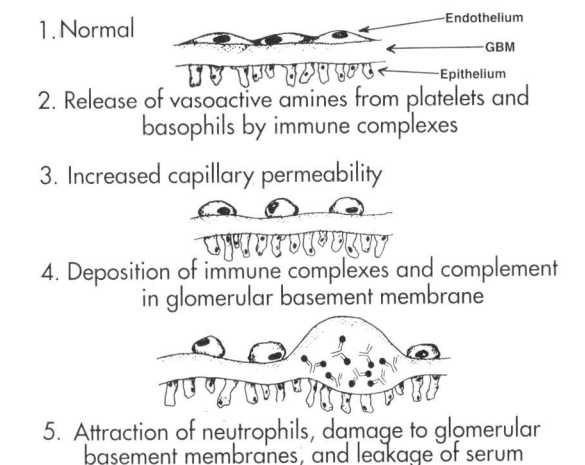

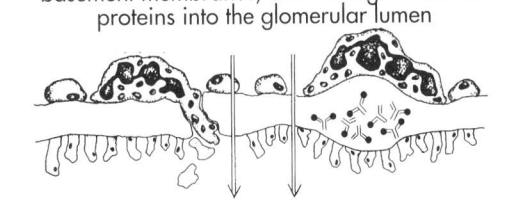

Figure 14-4 The sequence of events that leads to the deposition of immune complexes in the glomerular basement membrane (GBM).

Several mechanisms antagonize the tendency for immune complexes to be deposited glomeruli. One is the presence of mesangial cells, pluripotential phagocytic cells at the base of the glomerular tuft. When complexes are small or of limited quantity, they are cleared from the glomerular interstitium by phagocytosis and digestion. The second mechanism is actually complement. Complement delays the formation of complexes by intercalating in the lattice of the antigen-antibody complex, effectively decreasing the number of epitopes available for binding and resulting in a smaller complex. Complement can also participate in the resolubilization of immune complexes, by way of the alternate pathway. Apparently the mechanism for this solubilization is the insertion of C3b and C3d into the complex. This property explains why, in dogs with inherited C3 deficiency, life-shortening glomerular immune complex disease develops (see Chapter 12).

The pathogenesis of the lesion in the glomerulus initially involves the deposition of immune complexes or free antigen, with subsequent binding by antibody in glomerular basement membranes, providing a focus for the accumulation of inflammatory cells, chiefly neutrophils. Subsequent damage to tissues is mediated by secretion of lysosomal enzymes, vasoactive amines, leukotrienes, and prostaglandins and the reactive oxygen species generated by the respiratory burst in neutrophils. These are antagonized in situ by many physiologic factors, including cellular desensitization and decay (prostaglandins), enzyme—based inhibitors (histaminase, carboxypeptidase, and arylsulfatase) and tissue-based scavengers of free radicals (glutathione, ascorbate, alpha tocopherol, and enzymatic inactivation of superoxide and hydrogen peroxidase). If the inflammatory episode is transient or mild, repair and return to normal structure/function is likely. If, however, the inflammatory stimulus is prolonged, then fibrous connective tissue is produced, resulting in glomerular sclerosis. In the usual case, animals are presented in frank kidney failure. Retrogressive changes (i.e., fibrosis and atrophy) are evident in glomeruli. Often secondary tubular or interstitial involvement complicates the clinical presentation. Diagnosis is difficult in veterinary medicine because of the veterinarian's inability to detect early glomerular disease clinically.

GLOMERULONEPHRITIS MEDIATED BY AUTOANTIBODIES TO GLOMERULAR BASEMENT MEMBRANE

The second major type of glomerulonephritis distinct from that induced by circulating or in situ–produced immune complexes is that caused by basement membrane antibodies. This is an example of a Type II hypersensitivity reaction. Other synonyms for this disease are nephrotoxic serum nephritis and Masugis nephritis. Immune complexes are not involved. This type of nephritis is mainly an immunologic model for autoimmunity. In the usual circumstance, animals are immunized with kidney tissue or, more specifically, glomerular basement membrane. Both homologous and heterologous basement membranes are effective immunogens. The sequence of events is as follows. Basement membrane antibodies are generated as a result of immunization and appear in the circulation. As they pass the glomerular apparatus, contact with the basement membrane is made, the antibody is deposited along it, and the inflammatory response is initiated.

The deposition of complement or antibody can be evaluated by immunolabeling or electron microscopic methods. A linear pattern of deposition of antibody or complement coinciding with the convolutions of the basement membrane is evident. On electronic microscopy, immunoglobulin and complement are visualized as linear, electron-dense deposits on the capillary endothelial side of the basement membrane.

Proof that membrane antibody causes the glomerular lesions was obtained by successful passive transfer of nephrotoxic serum from one animal to another. Furthermore, antibody can be eluted from renal tissue, and its specificity for basement membranes can be established by reaction and localization as on normal renal glomeruli.

In human beings, this form of glomerulonephritis is recognized in somewhat less than 5% of the cases of glomerulonephritis examined. Only one report exists of spontaneous basement membrane nephritis in domestic animals. In that study, 3 of 53 horses studied had linear deposition of gamma-globulin and complement in glomeruli. The reason for basement membrane antibody induction was not established. Thus, although the mechanism of injury is well understood, the nature and the source of the antigens, or even the sequence of events leading to autologous immunization of basement membrane, under natural circumstances, is unknown. Basement membrane antigen is continually shed into urine. It is possible that exposure of this material to immunoreactive lymphocytes results in the generation of autoimmune disease. Once the response is initiated, it is easy to visualize the self-perpetuating nature of the injury. That is, as more tissue is damaged more immunogen is released, resulting in more immunogenic stimulation.

The second possible means of acquiring basement membrane antibodies concerns immunogenic exposure to cross-reacting antigenic determinants on microbes and other environmental contaminants. Several investigators have demonstrated serologic cross-reactions between streptococcal cell wall antigens and GMBs. However, the correlation between streptococcal infection and this type of glomerulonephritis is low. Thus, although the immunopathogenesis of this form of glomerulonephritis is well understood, there is little if any clinical significance in veterinary medicine to incriminate this form of injury as a widespread cause of glomerulonephritis in domestic animals.

IMMUNE COMPLEX GLOMERULONEPHRITIS IN DOMESTIC ANIMALS
Canine

Primary glomerulonephritis in dogs is considered a relatively rare disease. The incidence, however, may be higher than suspected as a result of a tendency to overdiagnose chronic interstitial nephritis in a dog with clinical signs of kidney failure. It is found that most if not all instances of chronic interstitial nephritis have attendant and often severe glomerular involvement. In such "end-stage" kidneys, widespread fibrosis, parenchymal degeneration, and necrosis preclude accurate interpretation of the inciting pathogenesis.

Immune complex glomerulonephritis has been reported in dogs in conjunction with a variety of diseases, including mastocytomas, streptococcal tonsillitis, canine SLE and pyometra. Both infectious canine hepatitis and canine distemper, two important canine viral diseases, have been implicated, but much more work is necessary before these viral diseases can be established as entities in immune complex disease. A recent study provided evidence that canine distemper virus immune complexes are capable of inducing oligodendrocyte degeneration in the brain, presumable through Fc receptor–mediated macrophage stimulation.

Glomerulonephritis is commonly associated with infection of dogs with *Dirofilaria immitis*, the canine heartworm. Granular and linear deposits of IgG have been reported along the GMB, and antibody eluted from affected kidneys has been shown to be reactive with adult heartworm antigens, not with autologous tissue. Experimental studies in dogs infused by the renal interarterial route with *D. immitis* antigen have demonstrated that parasite antigens can bind to the glomerular tissue, thereby causing the formation of immune complexes in situ. This adherence of antigen to the glomerulus can be caused by charge interactions, affinity of the antigen for carbohydrate moieties of the capillary wall glycoproteins, or both. Once adhered, the antigen can react in situ with antibody to form immune complexes.

Another infectious disease associated with immune complex glomerulonephritis is canine brucellosis. The persistence of this bacterial antigen is compatible with the development of immune complexes; the organism has been isolated from blood and bone marrow from dogs for up to 36 months after infection. Deposited immunoglobulins have been found in kidney glomeruli of infected dogs.

As mentioned previously, immune complex glomerulonephritis regularly develops in homozygous C3-deficient dogs (Figure 14-5).

Equine and bovine

Glomerulonephritis has been described as a result of both viral and bacterial disease in horses. Equine infectious anemia (EIA) is a persistent viral infection of horses characterized by hemolytic anemia, hypergammaglobulinemia, hepatitis, glomerulitis, and widespread lymphoproliferative lesions. Horses once infected remain viremic for life despite the presence of neutralizing, complement-fixing, and precipitating antibodies in serum. Glomerulus-bound complexes can be demonstrated as early as 3 weeks after infection. Histologically, the glomerular lesion is of the mesangioproliferative type; both proliferative and infiltrative (mainly neutrophils) lesions are noted in EIA-infected horses. Interestingly, despite convincing physical evidence of glomerular damage mediated by immune complexes, few if any horses infected with EIA have clinical or biochemical evidence of kidney failure.

Equine glomerulonephritis with kidney failure was described in a 12-year-old thoroughbred gelding. Immunofluorescence staining of the renal cortex revealed a heavy accumulation of dense coarse granular deposits, which stained for both IgG and C3. Antiserum to streptococcal R antigen produced strongly positive staining on immuno-

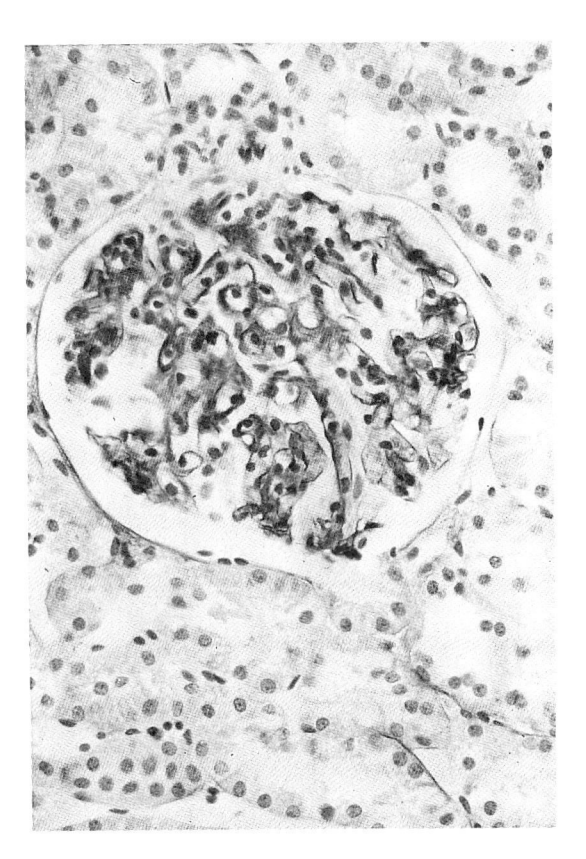

Figure 14-5 Immunoperoxidase labeling for renal glomerular-bound IgG in a dog with inherited C3 deficiency. Stained with rabbit anti-dog IgG conjugated to horseradish peroxidase, hematoxylin counterstain.

fluorescence study. Antibody eluted from the kidney of this horse reacted with the M protein and a common protein antigen of *Streptococcus equi* and *Streptococcus zooepidemicus*. It was found that there was less intense reactivity with the R antigen from group C streptococci. In human beings, poststreptococcal glomerulonephritis is seen frequently in association with recent exposure to group A streptococcus.

Feline

There have been a few reported cases of immune complex glomerulonephritis in cats. In one case a cat reported with a diagnosis of membranous glomerulonephritis showed complex deposition by electron microscopic evaluation. In another case, four cats reported to have nephrotic syndrome had electron-dense deposits in the basement membrane.

Two serious viral infectious diseases of cats, feline leukemia virus infection and feline infectious peritonitis infection, have been known to cause immune complex disease. However, extrarenal manifestations of disease are more important in the overall disease pathogenesis.

Other species

Chronic hog cholera infection in swine has been implicated as a cause of immune complex glomerulitis in this species. Immune complex disease in sheep has also been reported. A peculiar form of immune complex disease has been described in Cheviot lambs in Scotland. Not only do they have renal involvement they also exhibit choroiditis and attendant central nervous system signs that are immune complex mediated. The antigen or assumed underlying infectious process is unidentified.

DIAGNOSIS OF IMMUNE COMPLEX DISEASE

Detection of circulating immune complexes

Circulating immune complexes are not routinely quantitated in individual patients by the veterinary diagnostic laboratory. However, several studies have used assays to evaluate circulating immune complex formation in experimental studies or in particular groups of patients. The assay most commonly used is the C1q-binding assay. This method is based on one described for human sera by Zubler in 1976. The immune complexes are detected with radioiodinated human C1q. There are several variations to the assay: One method uses precipitation of ^{125}I-C1q–bound complexes with polyethylene glycol, whereas another uses a solid phase binding assay (ELISA). In one study, circulating immune complexes were detected in dogs infected with the protozoan parasite *Leishmania*. In another study immune complexes were detected in both serum and synovial fluid of dogs with rheumatoid arthritis, infectious arthritis, and arthritis resulting from rupture of the cruciate ligament.

DETECTION OF IMMUNE COMPLEXES IN RENAL GLOMERULI

The clinicopathologic hallmark of renal glomerular disease in both animals and human beings is persistent or intermittent proteinuria. This occurs as a result of damage of GBM and subsequent leakage of low-molecular-weight proteins (chiefly albumins) from the blood vascular system into the glomerular filtrate. Detection of protein in urine may also be the result of inflammatory disease of the lower urinary tract. In this instance, other evidence of inflammation (e.g., neutrophils in urine cytosediment) will differentiate this cause of proteinuria from glomerular origin. The reader is referred to any modern textbook on veterinary internal medicine for clinical signs and appearance of renal glomerular disease.

The diagnosis of immune complex glomerulonephritis is confirmed by demonstration of the complexes (Figure 14-5). Biopsy means of specimens or tissue sections may be examined for bound antibody or complement by immunolabeling techniques (see Chapter 10). One convenient approach, suitable for use in formalin-fixed tissues and thus compatible with histopathologic examination, is outlined in Chapter 10. Snap-frozen sections have been traditionally employed, and this is still the method of choice for detecting complement because the method used on formalin-fixed tissues has not yet been successful for demonstration of C3. The pattern of IgG deposition is substantially different from the autoimmune nephritis syndrome. In immune complex disease the deposition is discontinuous and beaded in appearance. This pattern is spoken of as "lumpy-bumpy." Electron microscopy has also been used. Ultrastructurally, complexes appear as electron-dense deposits located on both the capillary and the glomerular epithelial sides of the basement membrane. Ideally, the antigen should be identified; however, in most cases the origin and nature of the antigens involved are unknown.

Caution should be used to avoid overinterpretation of the results obtained with immunolabeling technique. Kidney tissue from clinically normal animals may have morphologic evidence of immune complex disease. Animals with primary renal tubular or interstitial disease may be erroneously said to have immune complex glomerulonephritis. For example, dogs affected with chronic interstitial nephritis have immunoglobulin deposits in damaged glomeruli. In this instance, a primary role for immune complexes in the initiation of this lesion is difficult to assign; serum proteins are entrapped in damaged tissues as a secondary event. Also, primary glomerular viral disease caused by canine adenovirus type I (infectious canine hepatitis) can be erroneously diagnosed as the immune complex type of glomerulonephritis. In the convalescent phases of the infection, adenovirus antibodies bind to virus-infected glomerular endothelial cells and thus appear to be an immune complex disease by immunofluorescence. Glomerulosclerosis secondary to *D. immitis* (heartworm) infestation is common. Although immune complexes are generated during this disease it is thought that the glomerular lesion evolves from direct damage to glomeruli mediated by motile circulating microfilariae.

One of the major pathologic manifestations of diabetes mellitus is systemic thickening of vascular basement membranes. The deficiency is metabolic in origin and results in GMB deficient in proteoglycan content. As a consequence, serum proteins including albumin and IgG adhere to the diabetic GMB. This adherence may result in glomerular disease superficially resembling that mediated by immune complexes.

OTHER CLINICAL FORMS OF IMMUNE COMPLEX DISEASE

Hypersensitivity pneumonitis

Another site for the occurrence of immune complex disease is the lung. In human beings many lung diseases result from the inhalation of a variety of antigens, usually organic dusts, which evoke an IgG response and form immune complexes in the lung. These diseases have a variety of common names, derived from the antigenic exposure that resulted in the condition. Some examples are mushroom worker's disease (from chronic exposure to *Thermoactinomyces vulgaris*), pigeon breeder's disease (from chronic exposure to bird excreta), and farmer's lung disease (from chronic exposure to *Micropolyspora faeni* a contaminant of moldy hay). The largest group of hypersensitivity pneumonitis diseases are caused by thermophilic actinomyces, but other fungi, animal proteins, and protein from thermotolerant bacteria (*Bacillus cereus* causes humidifier lung) are also implicated in immune complex lung disease.

The pulmonary lesions observed are mediated by formation of immune complexes in the alveoli. The disease usually appears in an acute form, with symptoms of disease developing 4 to 12 hours after antigen exposure. Precipitating antibody reactive with the offending antigen can usually be found in the serum of the patient. These antibodies are of the IgG and IgM classes and are detectable on immunodiffusion study. In acute cases, within a day of exposure, biopsy and immunofluorescence staining reveals immune complex deposition and vasculitis. In cases of chronic farmer's lung disease a lung biopsy reveals diffuse interstitial pneumonitis with an infiltrate of inflammatory cells (primarily mononuclear cells) in the alveolar walls. Staining of sections with anti-IgG, anti-IgM, and anti-IgA reveals plasma cells and lymphocytes containing these antibodies. The continued exposure of a sensitized individual to aerosolized antigen causes chronic lung damage with irreversible fibrosis and emphysema.

Bovine extrinsic allergic alveolitis, which closely resembles the farmer's lung disease of human beings has been reported in Switzerland as "Urner pneumoniae" and in England and Scotland as "fog fever." In herds with a high incidence of this disease, precipitin antibodies to extracts of moldy hay and extracts of *Micropolyspora* spp. occur in nearly 50% of affected animals. Although hypersensitivity is a cause of interstitial pneumonia, the clinical signs are easily confused with toxicity from 3-methyl indole, which is a metabolite of L-tryptophan that is produced in the rumen during digestion of certain lush foodstuffs. Toxicity produced by this compound on bronchiolar epithelial cells can result in cell destruction and interstitial changes.

In horses, the condition known as "heaves" is thought by some to be a hypersensitivity pneumonitis. This disease, chronic obstructive pulmonary disease, is characterized by an increase in respiratory resistance and is accompanied by clinical signs of decreased exercise tolerance and a chronic cough. When bronchoscopy is performed on these horses, neutrophils and eosinophils are commonly found. Intradermal skin testing with environmental allergens has been performed in several studies, but the degree of reactivity in nonsymptomatic horses obscures the importance of this test as a diagnostic aid. Reactions indicative of a Type I response occur at 30 minutes, and reactions occur at 4 to 6 hours indicative of a Type III response. Whether this disease is a Type I or a Type III disease is the subject of much debate. Most likely a combination of these two disease mechanisms are involved, with one or the other assuming the greater role in different individuals, perhaps dependent on the genetic makeup of the patient.

Anterior uveitis

A common sequel to infectious canine hepatitis caused by canine adenovirus I (CAV-1) is anterior uveitis with concomitant corneal edema or "blue eye" (Figure 14-6). This reaction is observed in the convalescent stages of the disease or following vaccination. The lesion is characterized histologically as a nongranulomatous iridocyclitis. The ocular lesions are mediated by local production of immune complexes.

The virus replicates in vascular endothelial cells, with production of viral antigens in the anterior chamber of the eye. Antibody production in response to these antigens results in immune complex formation. Complement-derived chemotactic factors attract neutrophils and monocytes to the area, with eventual phagocytosis of the complexes. A by-product of this reaction is corneal edema.

Anterior uveitis can be diagnosed on clinical examination in combination with clinical history. The cornea is opaque, primarily because of the inflammation-mediated accumulation of fluid within it. The ocular lesion is self-limiting, usually lasting only 4 to 5 days. Topical treatment with anti-inflammatory agents is contraindicated

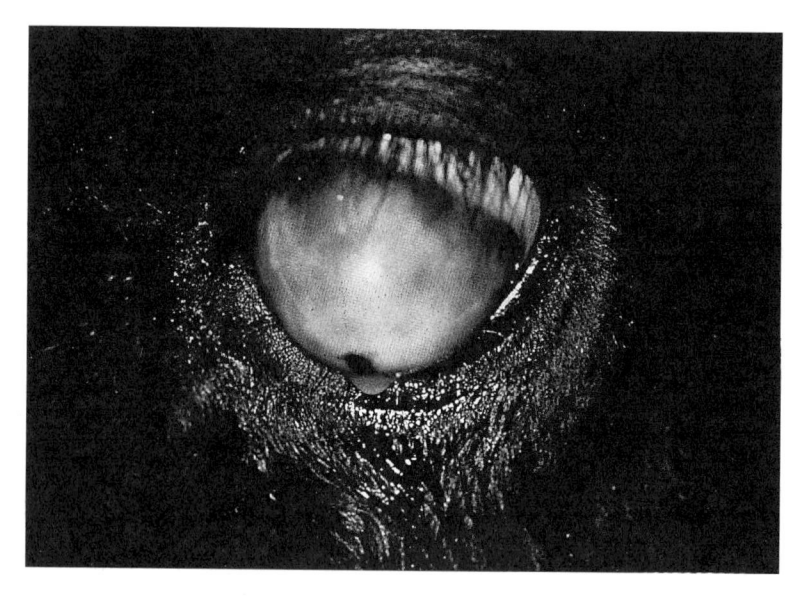

Figure 14-6 Corneal edema and ulceration in a dog with canine adenovirus 1 (infectious canine hepatitis)-induced anterior uveitis.

and may in fact aggravate the condition. This clinical condition is rare in today's veterinary practice, chiefly because of widespread vaccination of the population with formulations containing CAV-II an innocuous pathogen of the respiratory tract which is serologically similar to CAV-I.

Immunologically mediated dermatitis

A variety of immune-mediated diseases affecting the skin have been recognized in recent years. Some of these, such as the bullous diseases called pemphigus, are considered primarily Type II hypersensitivity. However, the cutaneous manifestations of SLE is characterized by demonstration of immune complexes along the basal laminae in the skin. These autoimmune disorders are discussed in greater detail in Chapter 15. Other skin lesions are recognized in which immune complex–mediated vasculitis can be demonstrated in the dermis with immunofluorescence study.

SUGGESTED READINGS

Abrahamson DR: Recent studies on the structure and pathology of basement membranes, *J Pathol* 149:257-278, 1986.

Anderson LJ, and Jarrett WFH: Membranous glomerulonephritis associated with leukemia in cats, *Res Vet Sci* 12:179-180, 1971.

Banks KL, Henson JB, McGuire TG: Immunologically mediated glomerulitis of horses. I. Pathogenesis in persistent infection by equine infectious anemia virus, *Lab Invest* 26:701-707, 1972.

Brown P: A case of feline membranous glomerulonephritis, *Vet Rec* 50:100-116, 1971.

Burkholder PM, Oberley LD, Barber TA, & others: Immune adherence in renal glomeruli, *Am J Pathol* 86:633-651, 1977.

Botteron C. Zurbiggen A, Griot C, & others: Canine distemper virus immune complexes induce bystander degeneration of oligodendrocytes, *Acta Neuropathol* 83:402-407,1992.

Brandonisio O, Carelli G, Altamura M, & others: Circulating immune complexes and autoantibodies in canine Leishmaniasis, *Parasitologia* 32:275-281, 1990.

Cameron JS: Platelets and glomerulonephritis, *Nephron* 18:253-258, 1977.

Carmichael KE, Medic BLS, Bistner SI, & others: Viral-antibody complexes in canine adenovirus Type I (CAV-I) ocular lesions: leukocyte chemotaxis and enzyme release, *Cornell Vet* 65:331-351, 1975.

Carter SD, Bell SC, Bari ASM, & others: Immune complexes and rheumatoid factors in canine arthritides, *Ann Rheum Dis* 48:986-991, 1989.

Cheville NF: *Cell Pathology*, Ames, IA 1976, Iowa State University Press.

Cheville NF, Mengelin WL, Zinober MR: Ultrastructure and immunofluorescent studies of glomerulonephritis in chronic hog cholera, *Lab Invest* 22:458-469, 1970.

Couser WG: In situ formation of immune complexes and the role of complement activation in glomerulonephritis, *Clin Immuno Allergy* 6:267-286,1986.

Divers TJ, Timoney JF, Lewis RM, & others: Equine glomerulonephritis and renal failure associated with complexes of group-C streptococcal antigen and IgG antibody, *Vet Immunol Immunopathol* 32:93-102, 1992.

Dixon FJ, Cochrane CC, Theofilopoulos AN: Immune complex injury. In: Samter M, Talmage DJW, Frank MM & others, editors: *Immunological diseases*, Boxton 1988, Little, Brown.

Emancipater SM, Lanin ME: Pathways of tissue injury initiated by humoral immune mechanisms, *Lab Invest* 54:475-478, 1986.

Farrow BRH, Huxtable CR, McGovern VJ: Nephrotic syndrome in the cat due to diffuse membranous glomerulonephritis, *Pathology* 1:67-72,1969.

Grauer GF, Culham CA, Dubielzig RR, & others: Experimental *Dirofilaria immitis*–associated glomerulonephritis induced in part by in situ formation of immune complexes in the glomerular capillary wall, *J Parasitol* 75:585-593, 1989.

Hensen JB, McGuire GC: Immunopathology of equine infectious anemia, *Am J Clin Pathol* 56:306-314, 1971.

Kim JCS: Immunologic injury in "shipping fever" pneumonia of cattle, *Vet Rec* 100:109-111, 1977

Lerner RA, Dixon FJ: Spontaneous glomerulonephritis in sheep, *Lab Invest* 15:1279, 1966.

Lerner RA, Dixon RJ, Lee S: Spontaneous glomerulonephritis in sheep. II. Studies on natural history, occurrence in other species, and pathogenesis, *Am J. Pathol* 53:501, 1968.

McCluskey RT, Klassen J: Immunologically mediated glomerular, tubular, and interstitial renal disease, *N Engl J Med* 288:564-569, 1973.

Merrill JP: Glomerulonephritis, *N Engl J Med* 290:257-266, 1974.

Morrison WI, Wright NG: Detection of immune complexes in the serum of dogs infected with canine adenovirus, *Rec Vet Sci* 21:119-121, 1976.

Oldstone MBA: Virus neutralization and virus-induced immune complex disease, *Prog Med Virol* 19:84-119, 1975.

Olenchock SA: Animal models of hypersensitivity pneumonitis: a review, *Ann Allergy* 38:119-126, 1977.

Osborne CA, Vernier RR: Glomerulonephritis in the dog and cat: a comparative review, *J Am Animal Hog Assoc* 9:101-127, 1973.

Renking EM, Robinson RR: Glomerular filtration, *N Engl J Med* 290:785-792, 1974.

Roitt I, Brostoff J, Male D: Immunology, ed St. Louis, 1993, Mosby.

Sabnis SG, Gunson DE, Antonovych TT: Some unusual features of mesangioproliferative glomerulonephritis in horses, *Vet Pathol* 21:574-581, 1984.

Scott DW, Wolfe MJ, Smith CA, & others: The comparative pathology of non-viral bullous skin disease in domestic animals, *Vet Pathol* 17:257-281, 1980.

Slauson DO, Russel SW, Schechter RD: Naturally occurring immune complex glomerulonephritis in the cat, *J Pathol* 103:131-133, 1971.

Virella G: Immune complex diseases. In Varella G, Gouse JM, Fudenberg HH, and others, editors: *Introduction to medical immunology*, New York, 1986, Marcel Dekker.

Wright NG, Eisher EW, Morrison WI, and others: Chronic renal failure in dogs: a comparative clinical and morphological study of chronic glomerulonephritis and chronic interstitial nephritis, *Vet Rec* 98:288-293, 1976.

15 Autoimmunity

DEFINITION AND THEORIES

The ability to recognize self and to distinguish self from nonself is critical to normal function of the immune system. This is accomplished by recognition early in fetal life of the major histocompatibility complex (MHC) antigens unique to the individual and purging of clones of lymphocytes that would specifically recognize these self antigens as foreign. Recognition of foreign antigens is accomplished in the context of self. For example, a cytotoxic T cell must recognize a self Class I MHC antigen in conjunction with a viral antigen to effectively kill that virus-infected cell. The tremendous diversity generated by the codominant MHC alleles at multiple loci provide for a large number of cell surface molecules and create a unique MHC type for each individual.

Despite the uniqueness of the individual that allows for immune recognition of all other antigens as foreign, occasionally there is a breakdown in this "self tolerance," and an individual makes an immune response to his or her own antigens. This phenomenon is called *autoimmunity*. It is important to note that the mere presence of autoreactive antibodies or effector cells does not necessarily constitute autoimmune disease. Although they are a hallmark of autoimmune disease, autoantibodies can be present in healthy members of the species without the occurrence of disease. Other factors thought to be involved in the initiation of autoimmune disease include immune defects, hormonal levels, genetic background, and environmental factors (such as exposure to ultraviolet light, drugs, and infections).

Natural autoantibodies against a number of self antigens have been described in human beings and in animals. These autoantibodies are generally specific for highly conserved structures such as myelin basic protein, nucleic acids, and cytoskeletal proteins. Some of the determinants with which the antibodies react are protected in their sites by lack of vascularization, others by histochemical barriers. The present of these natural antibodies and the notable fact that they share a conserved recurrent idiotype with pathologic autoantibodies found in such diseases as systemic lupus erythematosus indicate the potential for both a physiologic role in immune regulation and a potential pathologic role.

Several theories describe how the autoimmune reaction develops. *Sequestered antigens* are contained in tissues that are present in the body of a mature animal that were not exposed to the immune system during development. These include the lens of the eye, the central nervous tissue, and spermatozoa. Normally the immune system does not make contact with these tissues; they are sequestered. However, on occasion—as a result of injury or inflammation resulting from infection—the barrier is broken and the sequestered antigens are exposed to the cells of the immune system. T cells recognize these antigens as foreign and respond accordingly. Thus an immune response is directed against host antigens. Trauma to the central nervous system or lens of the eye is sometimes accompanied by the development of cytotoxic T lymphocytes, antibodies directed against central nervous system antigens, or both. In neuritis of the cauda equina in horses, antibodies are directed to the P2 protein of myelin. Another example of the presence of autoantibodies to myelin is canine distemper encephalitis. The infection of the central nervous system by virus in this disease interrupts the integrity of the blood-brain barrier and permits immunization of the host with the previously sequestered antigens.

Crossreaction with environmental antigens is another cause of autoantibody development. A small percentage of human patients with group A streptococcal pharyngitis develop a syndrome known as rheumatic carditis. This disease results from an apparent cross-reaction between host cardiac antigens and group A streptococcal antigens. The response appears to be associated with a B-cell alloantigen detected with increased frequency in patients with acute rheumatic carditis.

Another explanation for the initiation of autoimmune disease is based on the *presence of natural antibodies* and their reaction with the autologous antigen. An example of such a natural antibody is the gal antibody that constitutes 1% of circulating IgG in human beings but is not present in the serum of nonprimate mammals and New World monkeys. The epitope recognized by this antibody (alpha-galactosyl) is not present on human cells but is present on bacteria (*Salmonella*, *Klebsiella*, *Escherichia coli*) and other disease agents such as *Trypanosoma cruzi* and *Leishmania mexicana*. The gene coding for the enzyme alpha-1-3 galactosyltransferase has been found in the human genome. It normally exists in a suppressed form. Activation of this gene and the de novo expression of alpha-galactosyl epitopes has been suggested as a potential cause of autoimmune reactivity.

Loss of suppressor T cells, which have presumably been keeping potentially autoreactive B cells from responding to autoantigens, can be another cause of autoimmune reactivity. There is some evidence for this in the New Zealand mouse model, in which the autoimmune disease systemic lupus erythematosus (SLE) occurs spontaneously.

Many drugs and toxins can induce autoimmune reactivity in animals and in human beings. For example, mercuric chloride has been associated with the development of autoimmune disease in experimentally exposed rats and rabbits. D-Penicillamine has been associated with development of antibodies to intracellular cement substance of the skin in the disease pemphigus, autoantibodies to the acetylcholine receptor resulting in myasthenia gravis, and antibodies to nuclear components with resultant lupus-like disease. Procainamide has been associated with antibodies to red blood cells and autoimmune hemolytic anemia. In cats receiving propylthiouracil, an autoimmune disease characterized by native DNA antibodies developed.

Mechanisms proposed for drug-induced autoimmunity include a toxin or drug metabolite becomes stuck on an autoantigen, such as an erythrocyte membrane, which then becomes an "innocent bystander" to the antidrug response. This mechanism may also account for the immunogenicity of small drug metabolites; the autoantigen would act as a carrier and the drug as a hapten.

The idea that an infectious agent has a role in causing SLE has been frequently entertained. Some evidence for the existence of a retrovirus in mice and dogs with SLE has been presented.

ORGAN-SPECIFIC AUTOIMMUNE DISEASES
Hematopoietic system

Autoimmune hemolytic anemia

Autoimmune hemolytic anemia (AIHA) is a disease characterized by the occurrence of autoantibodies against erythrocytes. The binding of these antibodies to the surfaces of the erythrocytes causes increase destruction and resulting anemia. The disease occurs in several species, including the dog, cat, horse, and cow. Pathogenesis can involve intravascular erythrocyte destruction or extravascular hemolysis. There are several types of disease, dependent on the class of autoantibody, the temperature at which it reacts, its ability to fix complement, and the role of phagocytes in erythrocyte destruction. Intravascular agglutination can occur when high-titer IgG or low-titer IgM crosslinks antigenic determinants on erythrocytes causing their aggregation. When complement is activated (most efficiently done by IgM) intravascular hemolysis occurs. The third potential outcome is extravascular erythrocyte destruction by phagocytes. The last mechanism of destruction is most commonly seen in canine patients.

Cryopathic immune mediated hemolytic anemia
Cryopathic immune mediated hemolytic anemia is a disease that occurs in dogs and cats in which there is an IgM antibody reactive with the patient's erythrocytes at temperatures less than $32°C$. Erythrocytes agglutinate in small blood vessels in the periphery of the body, where the temperature is cool. Necrotic lesions are found in such sites as the tip of the tail, footpads, and tips of the ears. These lesions are the result of vascular occlusion by erythrocyte aggregates.

Direct Coombs antiglobulin test
The presence of antierythrocyte antibodies is detected by means of the *direct Coombs antiglobulin test*, which tests for the presence of antibody on the patient's erythrocytes. In this test, a sample of the patient's blood is taken in heparin or ethylenediamine tetraacetate (EDTA), and the erythrocytes are washed three times in phosphate-buffered saline solution. The erythrocytes of the patient are incubated with the antiglobulin reagent and are observed for agglutination as an indication of the presence of autoantibody on the erythrocyte surface membrane. The indirect antiglobulin test evaluates the presence of circulating erythrocyte antibodies in the patient's serum. In this test, the patient's serum is incubated with normal canine erythrocytes; after the addition of the antiglobulin reagent, agglutination indicates a positive test.

Coombs positive autoimmune hemolytic anemia
Coombs positive autoimmune hemolytic anemia can occur as a single disease or along with involvement of other body systems in SLE. Some cases of immune-mediated hemolytic anemia are caused by

antibodies directed toward drug or microbial antigens that adhere to the erythrocyte membrane. In other cases there is a true autoantibody directed toward erythrocyte antigens. The resulting erythrocyte destruction occurs by means of a Type II hypersensitivity reaction in either case.

Autoimmune thrombocytopenia

Immune-mediated thrombocytopenia (AITP) is recognized in dogs as a distinct disease entity and in conjunction with other immune-mediated diseases such as autoimmune hemolytic anemia and SLE. Although thrombocyte counts of less than 200,000/mm^3 are indicative of disease, clinical signs of bleeding often are not visible until the platelet count falls to less than 30,000/mm^3. The decrease in platelets is caused by elimination of platelet-antibody complexes by phagocytes of the reticuloendothelial system or by decreased production due to antibody-mediated or antibody complement-mediated destruction of megakaryocytes. Clinical signs are referable to a bleeding disorder (epistaxis, petechia, ecchymosis, lethargy, weakness, and anemia if bleeding is sufficiently prolonged).

Diagnosis involves the performance of a *platelet factor 3 test, immunofluorescence detection of megakaryocyte antibodies*, or both. In the platelet factor III test, heat-inactivated serum from the patient is added to freshly isolated platelets from a healthy dog and allowed to incubate. Then activated clotting factors XI and XII and calcium are added. In the presence of antiplatelet antibody the clotting time will be accelerated by at least 10 seconds, compared with the result of a test performed with serum from a healthy dog. The immunofluorescence test is performed on a bone marrow aspirate in which megakaryocytes that have canine antibody bound to the surface are stained with antiglobulin tagged with fluorescein.

Immune-mediated arthritides

Several forms of immune-mediated arthritis are recognized in small animals. Deforming or erosive arthritis of dogs is most similar to rheumatoid arthritis in human beings. The pathogenesis of rheumatoid arthritis in human beings and the similar disease entity described in dogs is still not clear. A commonly accepted hypothesis states than an unknown antigen—bacterial, viral, or mycoplasmal—is deposited in a joint during a systemic infection. In most individuals, such an infection would be easily cleared by the immune system. However, in some individuals (perhaps genetically predisposed), an acute inflammatory response occurs and develops into an autoimmune response. The eventual outcome of this localized response is a chronic inflammation resulting in proliferative and erosive synovitis with subsequent joint destruction.

Most recently, lymphokines have been implicated as mediators that act on the synovial cells. As these cells proliferate, they degrade the extracellular matrix. Prostaglandin E$_2$ (PGE$_2$) and collagenases are important in stimulating joint breakdown. Recent research has shown that the production of interleukin-1 (Il-1) by mononuclear cells in the joint stimulates the growth of synovial cells and fibroblasts, but also elicits collagenase and PGE$_2$ production by synovial cells. There is also a role for gamma interferon (IFN-y) produced by T lymphocytes. IFN-y can stimulate macrophages to produce Il-1. Tumor necrosis factor is also thought to play a role in joint inflammation because it induces cartilage breakdown, bone resorption, and release of collagenase and PGE$_2$ from synoviocytes.

B lymphocytes accumulate in the inflamed joints of rheumatoid arthritis patients; B-cell and plasma cell numbers are increased in synovial membranes and fluid. These B cells actively produce immunoglobulin, including the rheumatoid factors, which are the major autoantibody present in rheumatoid arthritis. *Rheumatoid factor* (RF)—usually IgM, reactive with IgG in the joint—forms immune complexes. These RFs are found in the sera of 70% to 90% of human patients with rheumatoid arthritis but in only about 25% of canine patients with the disease. RF is detected with a passive agglutination test using "altered" IgG-coated latex particles. A kit is available for this test in the canine patient. The original test for RF is the Rose-Waller test, which uses rabbit IgG bound to sheep erythrocytes. The results of this test must be interpreted with some caution because it has a low predictive value for rheumatoid arthritis. In human beings, the test of a positive reaction in rheumatoid arthritis is 90%, but the assay has a 35% positive frequency for SLE.

Another form of immune-mediated arthritis is *idiopathic nondeforming arthritis*. It occurs in dogs and less commonly in cats; it is more common than rheumatoid arthritis. Analysis of joint fluid reveals a sterile joint with large numbers of leukocytes in the synovial fluid. Negative results are obtained for antinuclear antibody (ANA), LE cells, and RF. The arthritis that is seen in conjunction with SLE in dogs and cats is similar to idiopathic nondeforming arthritis; a positive ANA titer and clinical signs relative to other body systems allow differentiation of SLE from the former disease.

Antibodies are sometimes induced in response to drugs (particularly antibiotics, such as sulfa drugs, cephalosporins, and penicillin) that have adhered to host tissue components. These create immune complexes that accumulate in small blood vessels and joints, where an inflammatory response develops. Joint fluid from affected joints shows increased numbers of neutrophilic polymorphonuclear leukocytes.

Neuromuscular system

Polymyositis is a generalized inflammatory disease of the muscles, generally affecting large-breed dogs such as the German shepherd. The pathogenesis is thought to be immune-mediated, with antibodies reactive with the sarcolemma detectable in about half of the cases. ANA tests are likewise positive in some cases. Polymyositis occurs alone and as a part of the systemic autoimmune disease SLE.

Myasthenia gravis

Myasthenia gravis, a disease characterized by muscle weakness and fatigability with sustained effort, is an autoimmune disease caused by the destruction of post-synaptic regions of neuromuscular junctions. Acquired autoimmune myasthenia gravis occurs in human beings, dogs, and cats. It is characterized by the demonstration of autoantibodies reactive with acetylcholine receptors. These autoantibodies induce postsynaptic membrane damage through complement activation and receptor destruction through the membrane attack complex (type 2 reaction). Antibodies can also initiate destruction by crosslinking receptors on the motor end plate, thereby causing their internalization and destruction by cellular lysosomes. The number of acetylcholine receptors remaining after autoimmune attack varies from patient to patient; in human patients studied there are usually only 30% to 50% of the normal number. The treatment strategy of administering antiacetylcholine esterase is effective because it preserves acetylcholine so that it can react with more than one receptor.

The diagnosis of myasthenia gravis is accomplished by detection of serum antibodies specific for acetylcholine receptors by means of indirect immunofluorescence. Treatment with prednisolone causes receptor-specific serum titers to decrease. In both human and canine myasthenia gravis, association with thymoma has been noted in up to a third of the patients. Thymectomy is a controversial form of therapy for such cases.

Endocrine system—thyroid gland

Autoimmune thyroiditis

Autoimmune disease involving endocrine organs is well recognized in human beings. Antibodies to antigens of the thyroid gland were first detected in the 1950s. These early studies used thyroglobulin as antigen. It is now established that there are five main antigen-antibody systems involving different components of the thyroid gland. The antigens involved include thyroglobulin, "microsomal antigen," the second antigen of colloid, a cell surface antigen, an antigen related to the thyrotropin receptor, and thyroxine and triiodothyronine. At one time it was thought that thyroglobulin was a "sequestered" antigen—that is, one that is not "seen" by the immune system until tissue damage released it to the circulation. It is known that thyroglobulin actually begins to leak into the circulation in utero. Thyroglobulin-reactive B cells have been identified in the fetal circulation.

Patients with *Grave's disease* and *Hashimoto's thyroiditis* often have antibodies reactive with thyroglobulin, microsomal antigen, and cell surface antigen. Antibodies to T3 and T4 can also occur and can interfere with the quantitation of plasma levels of T3 and T4 depending on the type of assay used. In Grave's disease the antibody response to an antigen closely related to the thyroid-stimulating hormone receptor has been called *thyroid stimulating immunoglobulin*, also known as the *long-acting thyroid stimulator*. This antibody produces stimulation by interacting with the thyroid-stimulating immunoglobulin receptor.

In dogs, lymphocytic thryoiditis develops. It is identified histologically by the infiltration of lymphocytes, plasma cells, and macrophages into the gland. Follicles are destroyed, and the gland becomes fibrotic. These changes result in hypothyroidism when more than 75% of the gland is destroyed. The demonstration of antigen-antibody complexes in affected glands, as well as the presence of antibodies to thyroglobulin, indicate that lymphocytic thyroiditis is an autoimmune disease. Antibodies to T3 and T4 are often found in the plasma of dogs whose samples have been submitted for analysis of T3 and T4 levels. These antibodies are not thought to have clinical significance, but they can interfere with T3 and T4 level quantitation as a result of interference.

In cats, hyperthyroidism develops; however, antibodies similar to thyroid-stimulating immunoglobulin have not been detected in such cats. However some affected cats have positive ANA tests and lymphocytic infiltration in the thyroid. Hyperthyroidism in dogs is usually associated with neoplasia.

Pancreas

Diabetes mellitus

Diabetes mellitus is a disease that results in an inability of the body to use glucose. Several forms of this disease are recognized in human beings;

they have been classified as type 1 and type 2 disease. Type 1 diabetes mellitus includes insulin-dependent diabetes; this is the form most frequently seen in dogs. In both human subjects and dogs, diabetes mellitus has a familial pattern of inheritance. In human beings a relationship between certain human leukocyte antigens (HLAs) and type 1 diabetes has been recognized. The pathogenesis of type 1 diabetes mellitis involves destruction of the beta cells in the pancreas and a failure to regenerate those cells. Autoantibodies reactive with the beta cells are found in the serum of patients, often years before the onset of clinical signs. It has been suggested that some of the type 1 diabetes mellitus cases are initiated by a viral infection.

The demonstration of islet cell antibodies in sera of type 1 diabetes mellitus by means of immunofluorescence techniques in 1974 was preceded by the recognition that the mononuclear cell infiltration of the islets of Langerhans seen in terminal patients with diabetes was suggestive of an immunologic reaction. The antibodies are reactive with cytoplasmic antigens in alpha, beta, and delta cells of the islets of Langerhans. In canine insulin-dependent diabetes mellitus, islet cell antibodies have also been demonstrated.

Additional studies in human patients with diabetes mellitus have shown that autoreactive T-cell responses also occur. A depression in nonspecific suppressor cell function indicates a possible defect in immunoregulation in these patients.

Adrenal gland

Addison's disease

Hypoadrenalcortism (adrenal insufficiency), or Addison's disease, results from lack of sufficient cortisol production. In many human patients with idiopathic hypoadrenalcortism there is strong evidence of an autoimmune pathogenesis. Infiltration of the adrenal glands of such patients with lymphocytes and plasma cells is common. This type of histopathologic lesion is also most commonly seen in dogs with hypoadrenalcortism. In affected human patients low-titer cytoplasmic adrenal autoantibodies are seen in 70% of patients. Other antibodies reactive with the cell surface are also seen in 86% of the patients with antibodies reactive with cytoplasmic antigens. With a leukocyte migration test, cell-mediated immune reactions to adrenal antigens have been demonstrated in 46% to 80% of human patients with Addison's disease, indicating that cell-mediated immune responses may have a role in gland destruction. The presence of circulating antibodies reactive with the cells of the adrenal cortex has been demonstrated by indirect immunofluorescence in dogs.

Dermatologic immune-mediated disorders

Pemphigus diseases

Immune-mediated skin diseases include the bullous disorders, collectively termed the *pemphigus complex*. The most severe of these and the first discovered in a domestic animal species is *pemphigus vulgaris*. Other varieties, such as *pemphigus foliaceous, pemphigus vegetans*, and *pemphigus erythematosus* are variants, generally of less severe nature. These variants can be differentiated by their histopathologic diagnosis with reference to the site of vesicle formation.

Pemphigus vulgaris and its variants cause blisterlike lesions, which easily ulcerate after self-trauma by scratching to form ulcerous lesions that, when biopsied and stained with fluorescein-conjugated anti-IgG or anti-C3, reveal the deposition of immunoglobulin and complement in an intercellular pattern in the epidermis. In these diseases an autoantibody is formed that reacts with the keratinocyte cell-surface glycoprotein. Pathogenesis of the disease is thought to involve a circulating autoantibody, which penetrates the basal laminae and attaches to the keratinocytes within the epidermis (Figure 15-1). This reaction precipitates an enzymatic release by the targeted keratinocyte, resulting in dissolution of the intercellular cohesiveness and acantholysis. The ulcerative lesions of pemphigus are prominent along mucocutaneous junctions.

A related disease, *bullous pemphigoid*, has been described in dogs, cats, and horses. In this disorder there is the production of an autoantibody, which binds to antigen the dermal-epidermal basement membrane. Direct immunofluorescence

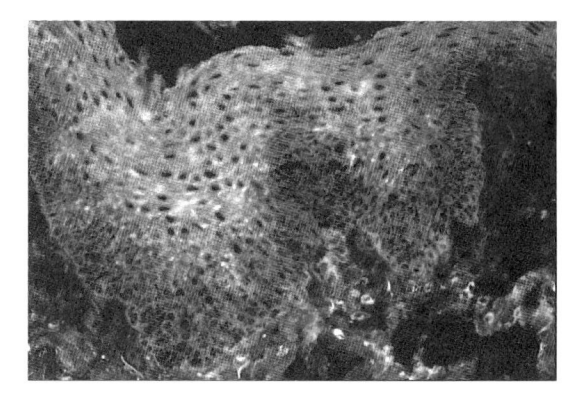

Figure 15-1 Intercellular fluorescence is demonstrated on a frozen skin section from a dog with *Pemphigus vulgaris*. Stained with fluorescein-conjugated anti-IgG ($\times$ 160).

staining shows fluorescence at the dermal-epidermal junction rather than an intercellular epidermal fluorescence. Like pemphigus vulgaris, bullous pemphigoid is characterized by blisters and ulcers on the skin and mucous membranes. The principal mechanism for differentiating these diseases is direct immunoflourescence study to identify the site and pattern of immunoglobulin deposition in the skin.

Discoid lupus

Discoid lupus is a dermatologic condition resulting from a Type III hypersensitivity reaction in the skin. The deposition of antigen-antibody complexes at the basal laminae, with resultant influx of inflammatory cells, creates a vesicular, erythematous lesion that must be distinguished from the pemphigus diseases. Direct immunofluorescence reveals granular deposits at the dermal-epidermal junction.

Systemic autoimmunity

SLE

The systemic autoimmune disease SLE is a severe, debilitating disease of human beings and domestic animals. The underlying defect in this disease is the production of both tissue- or cell-specific autoantibodies and antibodies to broadly reactive nuclear antigens. Thus the interaction of these autoantibodies with their respective antigens initiates a Type III hypersensitivity reaction. Formation of immune complexes containing autoantibodies and their soluble antigens is followed by deposition of these complexes in the walls of small blood vessels, resulting in initiation of the complement cascade and neutrophil influx with resulting tissue damage and vasculitis. One of the most commonly affected organs is the kidney, where glomerular capillaries are damaged. Because of the widespread nature of these antigens, many body systems can be affected.

Clinical diagnosis of SLE relies heavily on the ANA test. The ANA test, performed on a patient serum sample, measures the presence and titer of antibodies reactive with nuclear antigens. These antigens are not restricted to a particular cell type but are ubiquitous. They include double-stranded DNA, nucleoproteins, histones and single-stranded DNA. The ANA is an indirect immunofluorescence test. Some of these antinuclear antibodies participate in pathogenesis of the disease by forming immune complexes, which circulate and localize in sites such as kidney glomeruli, where they cause a Type III hypersensitivity reaction with subsequent tissue damage and resulting glomerulonephritis. Deposition of such complexes in joints can cause immune-mediated arthritis, and deposition in the skin cause the dermatologic form of SLE, with immune complex deposition at the dermal-epidermal junction. This observed deposition demonstrated by direct immunofluorescence, is sometimes referred to as the *lupus band* (Figure 15-2). Autoantibodies reactive with other nuclear antigens may not be pathogenic but, rather, indicators of disease.

Organ-specific disease is caused by the production of autoantibodies reactive with tissue-specific antigens, such as erythrocyte membrane antigens and platelet surface antigens; AIHA and AITP may occur as part of SLE. Type II hypersensitivity reactions are important mechanisms of pathogenesis when AIHA and AITP are a part of the disease picture.

Clinically SLE is a severe disease; however, it can be controlled with large doses of prednisone and other immunosuppressive drugs.

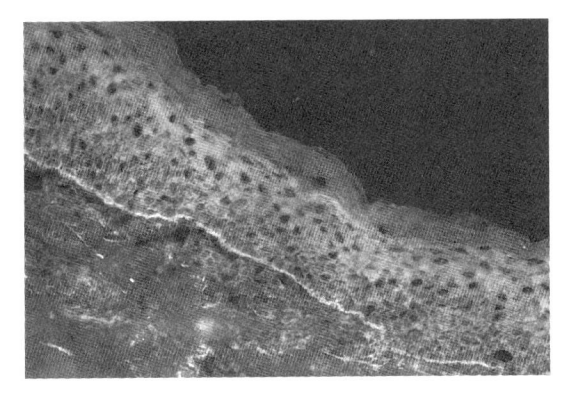

Figure 15-2 A "lupus band" is present at the dermal-epidermal junction of this frozen skin section from a dog with systemic lupus erythematosus (SLE). Stained with fluorescein-conjugated anti-IgG ($\times$ 160).

MHC class II association with autoimmune disease

Most autoimmune diseases recognized in human beings are associated with one or another HLA Class II antigen. In domestic animals, these associations have not been well worked out, but increased incidence of autoimmune disease in certain dog breeds is a strong indication that similar associations will be found with canine autoimmune disease. Both the MHC Class II molecule and the helper T-cell are important in initiation of the autoimmune process. In murine and human disease, Class II variants in the alpha and beta chains have been linked to development of type 1 diabetes. Similarly certain T-cell–receptor gene segments have been linked to development of autoimmune encephalitis in murine models, and the contribution of T-cell–receptor genes to development of myasthenia gravis is recognized in human beings.

SELECTED REFERENCES

Bigazzi PE: Autoimmunity in diabetes mellitus and polyendocrine syndromes: current concepts of pathogenesis and etiology. In Bagazzi PE, Wick G, Wicher K, editors: *Organ-specific autoimmunity*, Immunology series, vol 52, New York, 1990 Marcel Dekker.

Firestein GS, Zvaifler NJ: Immunopathogenesis of rheumatoid arthritis. In Bagazzi PE, Reichlin M, editors: *Systemic autoimmunity*, New York, 1991 Marcel Dekker.

Kumar V, Kono DH, Urban JL, & others: The T cell receptor repertoire and autoimmune diseases, *Annu Rev Immunol* 7:657, 1989.

Lopate G, Pestronk A: Autoimmune myasthenia gravis, *Hosp Prac* 28:109-131, 1993.

Volpe R: Autoimmunity in thyroid disease. In Volpe R, editor: *Autoimmunity in the endocrine system: monographs on endocrinology*, Berlin, 1981, Springer-Verlag.

Rossini A, Mordes J, and Like A: Immunology of insulin-dependent diabetes mellitus, *Annu Rev Immuno* 3:269, 1988.

Theophilopoulos A, Dixon F: Murine models of systemic lupus erythematosus, *Adv Immunol* 37:269, 1988.

PART FOUR

Principles of Immunoprophylaxis

16 Immune Response and Infectious Disease

The study of infectious diseases forms the base on which the modern science of immunology has evolved. Long before immunologists realized the importance of helper T cells or even that there was more than one kind of lymphocyte, it was recognized that recovery from disease was often accompanied by resistance to reinfection. The germ theory of disease was definitively proven by Koch, whose well-known postulates describe the process required to prove that a given disease is caused by a particular organism. In this process, the organism must be isolated from an animal that suffers from the disease and put into a healthy animal; if it causes the same disease, the etiology is confirmed.

Host-pathogen relationships are not all alike. For example, disease can result from a seemingly commensal organism such as the bacteria *Pasteurella haemolytica* that often resides in mucous membranes of normal cattle with no ill effect. It is a change in conditions, such as stress, that can trigger disease. Different still is the development of tetanus, in which the growth of the tetanus organisms, accompanied by toxin production in the host tissues, invariably induces severe disease in the nonimmune animal. Another type of host-pathogen relationship exists between the cat and the feline infectious peritonitis virus (FIP). In this disease the immune response to the virus causes exacerbation of the disease. Feline immunodeficiency virus demonstrates that a pathogen is capable of essentially shutting down the immune system thereby enabling it as well as a variety of normally less-virulent organisms to replicate. Thus the relationship between the host's immune system, and the pathogen is complex and variable, depending on both hosts- and pathogen-related factors. In this chapter we will examine some examples of veterinary disease and how the immune system responds.

GENERAL CHARACTERISTICS OF INFECTIOUS DISEASES

Infectious diseases are caused by the replication of living organisms (e.g., bacteria, viruses, protozoa, fungi, metazoon parasites) in host tissues. Toxins, products of microbial replication, are the direct cause of clinical disease in some infections, but in other infections it is the organism itself that causes most of the damage. Infection can be generalized, involving many tissues and organs, or localized. Transmission of agents from host to host may be horizontal, through direct contact with excretions or secretions, or vertical, from mother to fetus. Means of horizontal disease spread may be by aerosol, by fomites, or in food and water.

Local infections are the simplest form of microbial infection. Examples of local infections are epitheliotropic viruses such as pox and Influenza virus, bacteria like *Staphylococcus* and *Streptococcus* spp., and fungi like *Trichophyton* or *Microsporum* spp. The innate mechanism of immunity (described in Chapter 1) details the host defenses that must be overcome before development of local infection.

Systemic infection implies two things—a method to transverse epithelial barriers and a method of spread by lymph or blood to distant tissues. Bacteria such as *Salmonella* can penetrate through intestinal epithelial cells and gain systemic access through subsequent infection of mononuclear phagocytes. Other bacteria secrete enzymes such as hyaluronidase or collagenase that attack intercellular cementing substances and permit easy access to underlying tissues between cells. Most systemic viral infections use leukocytes to facilitate systemic spread. A few viruses, such as porcine enteroviruses, remain free in plasma. Members of the herpesvirus group use monocytes. Neutrophils from cats infected with the feline leukemia virus (FeLV) contain viral antigen. Feline panleukopenia virus replicates in neutrophilic precursor cells in the bone marrow and may be disseminated in that manner. Erythrocytes facilitate the spread of Newcastle disease virus of chickens, as well as other members of the parainfluenza/influenza groups. Platelets are involved in the spread of FeLV.

An example of a true intravascular bacterial septicemia is the disease anthrax, in which phagocytosis is inhibited by the presence of the capsule surrounding the bacteria. Bacteria that reside in the intracellular environment have developed mechanisms to resist lysosomal degradation. It is the presence of a T-cell response, production of gamma interferon (INF-γ), and macrophage activation, that provides for the eventual demise of these facultative intracellular organisms, although persistent infection and the development of a carrier state sometimes occur. Examples of this type of infection are the tubercle bacilli, *Brucella* spp., and *Salmonella* spp.

Interaction of microbes with components of the immune system

Mononuclear phagocytes

Phagocytes, including monocytes, are important as the first line of defense against microbes following transepithelial invasion. The digestive and killing properties of these cells are nonspecific, yet the macrophage is also an integral part of developing immunity, as discussed in previous chapters. A number of different monocyte-microbe intersections have been found that subvert the extraordinary killing abilities of phagocytic cells.

Virulence of some microbes is enhanced by microbial factors that kill the monocyte. Staphylococcal leukocidin and streptococcal hemolysin are examples of extracellular cytotoxic substances. Some microbial products inhibit monocyte response to chemoattractants. Other organisms resist phagocytosis with polysaccharide capsules. The M protein of *Streptococcus* spp. facilitates attachment to epithelial cells and prevents attachment by monocytes. Classic examples of the microbial cell wall hindering phagocytosis are the polysaccharide walls of pneumococci and anthrax bacilli. Bacterial colonies that are smooth when grown on agar are more virulent than are rough-colony variants. Virulence is related to the nature of cell-wall polysaccharides.

The mechanism of virulence associated with intracellular survival of some (facultative intracellular) bacteria inside monocytes can involve prevention of phagosome-lysosome fusion, as occurs with *Mycobacteriaum* and *Brucella* spp. Another escape mechanism is to leave the phagosome and exist in the cytoplasm; this is one tactic that *Listeria* uses to remain viable within the macrophage. *Salmonella typhimurium* is resistant to digestion by virtue of its lipopolysaccharide cell wall. Once a strong cell-mediated immune response is evoked, sensitized T cells release INF-γ, which is able to activate the macrophages and allow them to kill these previously-resistant organisms.

Neutrophil phagocytes

The other important phagocytic cell is the neutrophil. Like macrophages, neutrophil killing is subject to evasion. Several different bacteria are able to depress phagocytosis and/or chemotaxis by secreting substances that interfere with these functions. *Pseudomonas aeruginosa,* a common cause of secondary burn infections, is one such organism. Pneumonic pasteurellosis, an important respiratory disease of cattle involves the production by *P. haemolytica* of a leukotoxin that kills bovine leukocytes, thus enabling the organisms to divide and grow in the presence of weakened defenses. Another method of neutrophil evasion is the inactivation of the respiratory burst, an ability of Listeria.

Lymphoid cells

Successful microbes have developed several different methods to avoid or subvert developing immune responses. Some infections are tolerogenic. These infections are usually associated with massive doses of antigen released from a generalized infectious process. Generalized fungal diseases such as histoplasmosis and coccidioidomycosis exhibit split tolerance; although antifungal antibodies are formed, no cell-mediated immunity (CMI) is observed. A similar situation exists in congenital infection with rubella virus (German measles) in children. Affected children do not have a cell-mediated response to the virus or antiviral antibody of the IgG type, yet they possess circulating antivirus IgM antibodies.

A more general mechanism of immunologic dysfunction is microbe-mediated immunodepression. Suppressive effects of primary infection permit tissue invasion by secondary organisms, which often cause equally severe disease. Transient depression of tuberculin hypersensitivity during measles virus infection was first noted by von Pirquet in 1908. Suppression of T-lymphocyte responses in animals during viral infection is a common phenomenon. Although it has long been recognized in canine distemper virus (CDV), FeLV, feline panleukopenia, Newcastle disease virus, and equine herpesvirus infection, the emergence of acquired immuno-deficiency syndrome (AIDS), simian aquired immuno-deficiency syndrome (SAIDS), and FIV infection has created the best examples of viral-induced immunosuppression. Anergy of infection is seen with chronic generalized microbial diseases, such as generalized demodicosis in dogs. Malarial infections have associated suppression of humoral, not cell-mediated, responses. Trypanosomiasis inhibits both humoral and cellular response, but animals with leishmaniasis show decreased antibody responses to soluble antigens.

The mechanisms of suppression vary with each disease. With CDV, a direct cytolytic viral effect on cells of T & B lineage is operable early during the viremic phase; hyporesponsiveness of lymphocytes to mitogens persists into the convalescence stage, when viral antigens can no longer be found. The retroviral immunodeficiency viruses are very specific in their effect. The human immunodeficiency virus (HIV) has developed the unique ability to use the CD4 determinant on helper T lymphocytes as its site of entry into the cell. By selectively infecting and killing the helper T cell subpopulation of the immune system, the virus prevents effective immune responses against all pathogens. Cats infected with FeLV show a loss of both CD4 and CD8 positive lymphocytes. Depressed CMI and thymic atrophy are commonly seen in affected cats. Depression of immune function is generally associated with a viral protein, p15E. FeLV also causes immunosuppression, and with this virus the loss of CD4 cells is greater than the loss of CD8 cells.

Other methods of avoiding immunologic defenses

Another method in which microbes avoid contact with immune cells or antibody is by replicating or residing in areas inaccessible to defense mechanisms. Viruses, being obligate intracellular parasites are best able to do this. Viruses are susceptible to antibody only during release into the extracellular environment. Furthermore, viruses such as the herpesvirus group spread from cell to cell by fusion, without ever being exposed to developing immunity. Anatomic exclusion of parasites and bacteria in extravascular tissues or glandular lumens, such as in the mammary gland, may shield these organisms from specific antibodies.

Certain persistent parasitic and viral agents have the capacity to survive and replicate within immunologically-competent hosts in the face of an apparently effective immune response. These agents are able to do this by the process of antigenic variation. This mechanism is particularly suited to antigenically-complex parasitic protozoal infections such as trypanosomiasis. Following primary trypanosome infection there is an immune response to surface antigens, and a crisis is observed following an antibody-mediated decrease in parasitemia. Thereafter, a new generation of antigenically-distinct trypanosomes begins to replicate and multiply until terminated again by one variant-specific antibody. This process continues, with the parasite being one antigenic "tap" ahead until the death of the host.

A similar phenomenon has been described in horses that are persistently infected with equine infectious anemia (EIA) virus. This viral disease is characterized by persistent lifelong viremia, concurrent antibody response, and manifestations of immune complex disease. Sera collected from these horses is only capable of neutralizing EIA viruses isolated from these horses at the same time. Sera collected early in the infection do not neutralize viruses isolated later in the disease, and vice versa. The mechanism of antigenic variation remains elusive because it cannot be determined whether new serotypes are selected by immunologic pressures from spontaneous mutation or by individual parasitic adaption. Thus the capacity to develop different serotypes within the host enables these parasites to evade the host's immune response.

Finally, some infectious agents avoid host-immune mechanisms by being completely nonimmugenic. Diseases caused by unconventional agents such as scrapie, kuru, and transmissible mink encephalopathy are characterized by the absence of an immune response capable of neutralizing or inhibiting the infective principle.

General characteristics of the immune response in infectious disease

Primary natural infection by invading organisms is characterized initially by a small, subimmunogenic, antigenic mass. Replication increases antigenic load to threshold levels and then continues as the immune response is initiated. Consequently, the classic division of response into primary and secondary bursts of antibody production merge into one. As with nonreplicating immunogens, IgM antibody appears first, followed by IgG. Presence of IgM antibody can be used diagnostically to indicate recent infection. For example, cattle vaccinated with a virulent Brucella 19 strain develop antibodies only of the IgM type, whereas naturally-infected cows have IgG antibodies. Thus reactors can be distinguished from vaccinates by testing for bacterial agglutinins before and after treatment of serum with reducing agents (e.g., 2-mercaptoethanol) that preferentially destroy IgM.

Specific antibodies diffuse from the site of formation and are most effective against bacteria and their products. Antimicrobial actions of antibodies include opsonin activity, neutralization of toxins or viruses (by binding to surface receptors), complement-mediated microbial lysis, complement activation with subsequent activation of inflammation, and immobilization of motile bacterial or protozoa; all of which increase the chances of phagocytic killing. Antibody is the chief means of terminating viremia. Specific IgA antibody, along with interferon, is also an effective mechanism for terminating infections on mucosal surfaces. Finally, anaphylactic properties of immunoglobulins (IgE) in intestinal helminth infections are thought to cause worm expulsion from the intestine by inducing histamine-associated diarrhea and smooth muscle contraction (intestinal peristalsis).

Cellular or T-lymphocyte–mediated immunity depends on direct contact of cytotoxic lymphocytes with the microbe in tissues for immunologic effects. Functions of CMI include assistance in production of antibodies, generation of lymphokines to attract and activate phagocytes, recruitment of potentially immunocompetent cells, and cytolysis mediated by specific T cells. Intact CMI is the chief immunologic defense against intracellular microbes including tuberculosis and brucellosis, and viruses such as herpesviruses, poxviruses, and paramyxoviruses such as measles and CDV. In the case of many enveloped RNA viruses, T-cell–mediated cytotoxic phenomena appear to be directed chiefly at internal core or nucleocapsid proteins and not at envelope antigens. Cells are destroyed by the process of immunocytolysis, mediated directly by T cells and indirectly through antibody and complement-dependent cellular mechanisms.

Phagocytes and the complement system assist specific immunity by acting together with antibody and T cells as effectors in destroying or immobilizing invading microbes.

True recovery from infection is characterized by the disappearance of microbes from host tissues and the specific retention of long-lived immunity to reinfection, which is mediated chiefly by IgG and/or memory T cells. A persistent infection remains in the host following development of specific immunity. Persistent infections are epidemiologically important in that affected animals may serve as a reservoir for infection within the population. In addition, persistent infections in individuals may be accentuated by immunosuppressive treatments or environmental stress, resulting in renewed clinical disease. Furthermore, persistent infections promote secondary immune-mediated diseases such as immune complex glomerulonephritis and, in the case of feline and bovine leukemia viruses, neoplastic transformation.

Examples of persistent bacterial infections of public health significance are tuberculosis and brucellosis. Viral infections such as EIA, Aleutien mink disease, infectious canine hepatitis, and hog cholera are examples of diseases in which the carrier state has been established.

EXAMPLES OF IMMUNITY TO SPECIFIC INFECTIOUS DISEASES IN VETERINARY MEDICINE

In this section a detailed analysis of the immune responses to several different types of infectious diseases encountered in veterinary medicine is presented (Table 16-1). Obviously, a complete review of all diseases is impossible. Nonetheless, the principles of immunity illustrated by these infections indicate the wide variety of immunologic defense mechanisms available to the host.

Table 16-1 Immunologic mechanisms in infectious disease

Disease/organism	Protective immune/response
Extracellular bacteria:	
Staphylococcus	Phagocytes, antibody
Facultative intracellular bacteria:	
Listeria	T cell, macrophage activation
Viral:	
Influenza	Antibody and CMI
Herpes	CMI
Fungal:	
Cryptococcus	CMI
Aspergillus	Alternate complement pathway (initial), CMI
Parasitic:	
Nematode	Antibody (IgG, IgE), ADCC
Protozoa (intracellular)	CMI
Protozoa (extracellular)	Antibody

Tetanus toxin-antitoxin reaction

The immune response to bacterial toxins or toxoids is the simplest type of response to an infectious process. Tetanus is caused by the action of the neurotoxin tetanospasmin, which is produced by *Clostridium tetani*, a gram-positive, spore-forming, anaerobic bacterium. The toxin attaches to ganglioside receptors of motor nerve terminals and prevents the release of afferent inhibitory messengers. The tetanic seizure is characterized by generalized contraction of muscle groups. No loss of consciousness occurs, and the convulsions are extremely painful.

Infection by the bacterium itself is relatively innocuous. Thus an effective immune response must be made against the toxin. Adequate defense against the effects of the toxin requires antibody-mediated neutralization of the toxin as it is produced. Antibody is less effective in neutralizing the toxin once the toxin is fixed in tissue. Thus the immunologic principle for prophylaxis is that antitoxin antibody induced by active immunization or acquired by passive immune therapy must be present at the onset of infection.

The toxoid is prepared from bacteria-free culture fluids rendered nontoxic by treatment with formalin. Active immunization is achieved by incorporating the toxoid into an aluminum hydroxide adjuvant.

Immune serum for passive protection is made in horses and is used for treating contaminated wounds or following surgical procedures such as castration, when immediate toxin-neutralizing effects are needed. The potency of equine-origin antitoxin is measured by an *in vivo* mouse protection test. Measured amounts of toxin are mixed with dilutions of antitoxin, and the mixture is then inoculated into mice. Protection is assessed by comparing mortality rates in mice given toxin only; antiserum potency or titer is compared to a biologic standard and assigned a value in international units. The dose of antitoxin necessary to afford protection is given by the manufacturer.

Local immunity: transmissible gastroenteritis of piglets

Transmissible gastroenteritis (TGE) is a coronavirus infection of pigs that is transmitted orally. In vivo, the target cells for viral replication are the intestinal absorptive cells in the duodenum and jejunum. The virus buds from the Golgi apparatuses of these cells and is a cytolytic type of infection. During the infection, undifferentiated crypt epithelial cells undergo hypertrophy and hyperplasia in an attempt to cover denuded villi. Pigs of all ages are susceptible to TGE, but fatal clinical disease is seen only in piglets less than 10 days of age. The cause of death is malabsorptive diarrhea and dehydration secondary to loss of intestinal absorptive cells. In piglets the regenerative capacity of crypt cells is not sufficient to repair the defect. Mortality rates in piglets approach 100%.

Sows that have been exposed to TGE transmit complete immunity to their offspring through colostrum. Early attempts to stimulate immunity in some sows by parenteral inoculation of the agent were unsuccessful. Subsequently, herdsmen discovered that simply feeding infected intestines to pregnant sows was a successful method of preventing TGE in piglets. Thus active or passive immunity is achieved only by the oral route and, more specifically, only by providing immune IgA antibodies.

Subsequent work on the disease has confirmed the protective role of IgA. For vaccination purposes, only cross-reactive strains of TGE that induce IgA antibody can be used as oral immunogens. Parenteral immunization with TGE produces only partial protection as a result of preferential production of IgG over IgA. Two other intestinal diseases of swine, hemorrhagic jejunitis caused by *Clostridium perfringens type C* and swine dysentery caused by *Treponema hyodysenteriae*, are superficially similar to TGE. However, in both instances parenteral immunization or systemic administration of immune IgG prevents clinical disease. Thus with TGE, local immunity mediated by IgA is the immunologic factor that confers resistance to the disease.

Tuberculosis recovery depends on cell-mediated immunity

Tuberculosis is an ancient malady caused by three related species of tubercle bacilli, *Mycobacterium tuberculosis, Mycobacterium bovis,* and *Mycobacterium avis*. As pathogens they are primarily intracellular residents in the host, with chronicity or latency being characteristic features of infection. Of great interest is the apparently innocuous relationship between bacilli and monocytes/macrophages. The organisms produce neither exotoxins nor endotoxins and do not appear to cause cellular death.

What, then, is the mechanism hereby the lesions (i.e., granulomas, caseation, and necrosis) of tuberculosis are produced? Tuberculosis is characterized by development of delayed-type hypersensitivity (DTH) to a protein fraction of the organism. T-lymphocyte–mediated sensitization induces a chronic inflammatory response around the organisms, and the tissue damage observed is a consequence of this "anergy of infection." Once sensitized to tuberculin, this process persists indefinitely even if the infection that induced it remains localized or is eliminated. Reinfection is prevented chiefly by T-lymphocyte–mediated activation of macrophages that acquire enhanced bactericidal capability following recontact with mycobacteria.

Studies in laboratory animals have confirmed the role of cellular immunity in protection against tuberculosis. Antibodies are produced to both the protein and carbohydrate components of the bacterium, but all attempts to protect animals with passively-transferred immune serum have failed. Transfer of histocompatible immune cells creates resistance.

Diagnosis of occult tuberculoses is accomplished by skin tests with tuberculin, a bacteria-free concentrate of broth cultures, or purified protein derivative (PPD), a protein extracted from suspension cultures of mycobacteria by ammonium sulfate trichloroacetic acid precipitation. A localized reaction of lymphocyte and macrophage infiltration at the skin test site 48-72 hours later is considered presumptive evidence for tuberculosis. Unfortunately, a number of different saprophytic myobacteria can induce similar reactions; today this is the major source of reactor cows without lesions of tuberculosis.

In many countries tuberculosis is controlled through vaccination of animals and humans with an avirulent strain of mycobacteria called bacilli Calmette-Guerin (BCG). BCG is a strong stimulator of CMI; however, it does render recipients' skin tests positive to tuberculin. Thus screening populations for tuberculosis by skin testing cannot be performed if animals have been vaccinated with BGC.

Tuberculosis is the protype infection for a number of different obligate intracellular bacterial and fungal infections in which CMI is the sole immunologic means of resistance.

Canine distemper virus infection

CDV a systemic infection with recovery as a result of humoral and cellular immune mechanisms, is a generalized, viral, infectious disease (e.g., Paramyxoviridae, genus morbillivirus) of canids and their relatives. The pathogenesis of acute infection in a fully-susceptible host is probably identical regardless of species. There is general agreement that, under natural conditions, the most likely, obvious, and important route of infection is by infective aerosols droplets. Thus transmission of the virus is facilitated by coughing, sneezing, and close confinement in a warm, human, closed environment. The initial events in the pathogenesis of distemper in ferrets and dogs are similar. Infective aerosols are inhaled. Tissue macrophages and monocytes located in or along respiratory epithelium and tonsils appear to be the first cell type to pick up and replicate CDV. Following a local burst of virus production in these sites, the virus is then spread by lymph and blood to distant lymphoreticular tissues. This is accomplished by leukocyte-associated viremia and occurs anywhere from 2 to 4 days after the initial infection. Significant quantities of free infectious virus appear in the plasma of CDV-infected dogs. Between 8 and 9 days after infection, the virus will spread beyond lymphoreticular tissues to involve epithelial and mesenchymal cell elements. This probably occurs in every animal regardless of the outcome of the disease process. It is at this stage of the process that specific host immune responses to viral antigens influence the outcome. At least one of three possible clinical syndromes can result from infection. The acute fatal or fulminant form is characterized by unrestricted viral spread to virtually every tissue in the body. Virus can be found in every excretion and secretion and, by appropriate tracing techniques, antigen can be demonstrated in virtually every cell type within the body. In most of these animals, uncomplicated by secondary bacterial infection, the most likely proximate cause of death is fulminant fatal neurologic involvement. A second group of animals exhibits clinically-delayed progression of disease and modest convalescent immune responses. If present, clinical signs are subtle early in the disease and are a reflection of viral persistence within the central nervous system. Subsequent development of overt central nervous system disease is variable. The third group of animals exhibits no overt clinical signs of disease and is recognized as convalescent, clinically normal animals.

The actual mechanism of viral spread from the portal of entry to distant sites within the body is controversial. As mentioned previously, the spread of virus is thought to occur by a leukocyte-associated viremia. Virus can be detected as early as 2 to 3 days after infection in the blood of animals. Using very sensitive immunocytochemical viral antigen–tracing techniques, it has been shown that the first component of the central nervous system that experiences rival infection is the cerebrovascular endothelium and not the choroid plexus as previously thought. Infection of endothelium is likely achieved by contact with cell-free or platelet-IgG virus complexes. As a result of this platelet-virus-endothelium or virus-endothelial interaction, the subadjacent tissues, whether they be brain or other tissues, acquire the infection. This occurs by one of two mechanisms. Either virus-infected endothelial cells fuse with adjacent uninfected parenchymal cells and transmit the infection, or infected endothelial cells contract, thereby producing localized areas of enhanced vascular permeability. Subsequent to this increased vascular permeability, virus-infected leukocytes adhere to damaged endothelium or subendothelial collagen and then emigrate into extravascular locations.

As mentioned previously, transmission from dog to dog is principally by infective aerosols. Other routes of transmission are possible. Transplacental transmission of the virus has been documented. The sequence of events in pups injected in utero presumably occurs by the same pathways as outlined earlier.

Other than age at the time of infection, the protective effect of the developing immune response is the chief determinant of recovery. This was shown conclusively in studies where pretreatment with immunodepressive drugs such as cyclophosphamide induced fatal CDV infection in dogs subsequently given avirulent vaccine strains of CDV.

Both humoral and cellular immune responses are thought to play roles in recovery of dogs or ferrets from CDV infection. In addition, there are nonspecific host defenses, including intact mucosal surfaces, an active phagocytic system, high plane of nutrition, etc., that also contribute to resolution of the disease process. Fortunately all laboratory and wind strains of CDV appear to share common envelope and core antigens and are thus extensively cross-reactive. This feature of CDV facilitates serologic studies and simplifies the development of safe and effective vaccine products.

Quantitative and temporal aspects of the humoral antiviral response correlate with eventual recovery from clinical disease. Dogs that recover develop virus-neutralizing antibodies rapidly (9 to 10 days after infection), and titers rise to a ratio of >1:100. The viremia declines coincidentally with the appearance of free antibodies in serum. Low or absent virus-neutralizing antibody levels along with a constant viremia characterize those dogs that eventually die from infection. Exceptions are those dogs that develop a persistent often subclinical infection, chiefly involving the brain. Virus-neutralizing antibodies appear in serum and cerebrospinal fluid late in the course of the disease. Recently, distemper virus antibodies may also be measured using enzyme-linked immunosorbent assays (ELISA). These test procedures have the advantages of being rapid, economical, reproducible, and can provide the investigator or the diagnostic laboratory with the ability to process large numbers of samples at one time. Further, with ELISA it is possible to determine class-specific immune responses to distemper virus antigen, and thus get an indication of time of exposure to CDV infection.

Regardless of the method used to measure humoral immunity, it is clear that an animal, once vaccinated or subclinically infected, recovers from the infection and develops a lifelong immunity. Of course, the exact role of this antibody in protection of animals to subsequent exposure to CDV has not yet been determined in great detail. However, it is thought that antibody neutralizes extracellular virus, alone or with complement. This opsonizing function prevents widespread reinfection within the immune host and thus is a mechanism of immediate protection to external reinfection.

The role of virus-specific activated T cells in recovery/resistance to CDV infection is unclear. Lymphocyte-associated (presumably T-cell) virus-specific immune responses have been measured and correlated to outcome of disease. Lymphocytes from immune dogs (but not controls) were capable of inhibiting the formation of virus-specific cytopathic effect, namely syncytia formation on a monolayer within a 24-hour incubation period. This syncytia inhibition response was rapid, dependent on viable effector cells, independent of circulating antibody, and was not histocompatibility or DLA (dog leukocyte antigen)-restricted. Dogs expressing this syncytia inhibition response, when challenged with virulent CDV, demonstrated a rapid rise to high levels of activity in convalescence; this response persisted for at least 45 days after rechallenge. In a related assay, autologous and heterologous CDV-infected target cells labeled with ^{51}-chromium, were incubated with effector T cells, and cells functioning in antibody-directed cellular cytotoxicity (ADCC) reactions in various lymphocytetarget/cell ratios. Essentially the same results were obtained; specifically that the cytotoxic T-cell response following vaccination with a modified live product was short-lived (approximately 1 to 3 weeks). Recall is rapid, and the cytotoxic response in dogs convalescing from virulent CDV infection was much more dramatic and prolonged. These investigations concluded that cytotoxic T cells do play a role in recovery from CDV production. It is likely that cytotoxic T cells kill, lyse, or otherwise inactivate CDV-infected target cells in vivo, thereby decreasing the internal source of viral infection.

Both assays described earlier noted preexistent (e.g. nonimmune) cell-associated antiviral effects, tentatively attributed to canine natural killer (NK) cell activity. Further work is needed to define the sale of NK cells and other nonimmune defense mechanisms and CDV disease.

A major manifestation of CDV disease is virus-associated immunosuppression. Many of the signs of acute systemic CDV (e.g., diarrhea, fever, and malaise) are attributable to secondary and/or concurrent infection with various secondary bacterial, mycotic, and viral pathogens. Many of the systemic manifestations of CDV can be controlled by appropriate antibiotic or supportive therapy, and nonneurologic signs are completely absent in CDV-infected gnotobiotic dogs. Clinically, veterinarians have spoken for years of the anergy of infection associated with this disease. Probably the main and most important bacterial pathogens associated with disease in dogs are the pneumonic bacterial species including *Bordetella bronchiseptica* and *Pasterurella* spp., and of course, *Staphylococcus* and *Streptococcus* spp. These agents are responsible for the purulent conjunctivitis, rhinitis, and bronchopneumonia noted in CDV-infected dogs. Mixed viral infections, chiefly of the respiratory type, are also common. In addition to canine adenovirus type 2 infection, reovirus, canine parainfluenza virus, and presumably other viruses such as canine herpesvirus are all involved in this dual or multiple mixed-infection problem.

The virus readily replicates in all lymphoreticular tissues with a particular early tropism for monocytes/macrophages. In fatally-infected dogs, lesions observed include systemic lymphoid depletion, focal necrosis, and syncytium formation. In vivo, serum immunoglobulin production is also suppressed. In convalescent animals, repopulation of lymphoid tissues is evident 17 to 20 days after infection and germinal-center formation in the thymus as a residual lesion has been noted. During the viremic phases of the disease, allograft skin rejection time may be delayed and the intradermal skin test response to PHA-P is suppressed. Lymphocytes from viremic dogs are unresponsive to phytomitogens; this unresponsiveness persists for several months after virus can no longer be demonstrated in lymphocytes. The latter has been tentatively attributed to CDV-activation of a suppressor mononuclear cell.

Lymphocytes from CDV-infected dogs are poorly responsive in pokeweed mitogen (PWA)-driven B-cell differentiation assays, yet T cells collected from the same animals are still capable of producing measurable quantities of interleukin-2 (IL-2). In contrast, monocytes collected from viremic dogs are defiant in their ability to produce IL-1 and release significant quantities of immunosuppressive prostaglandin E_2 (PGE_2). Paradoxically, the effect of CDV NK-cell responses to various target cell systems, including CDV-infected target cells, appears not to be affected by acute viral disease.

The most important factor for suppression in virus-infected dogs is undoubtedly a direct viral effect on the responding cellular population(s). Immunologic paralysis is a logical consequence of infection because, CDV, like other viruses, subverts host cell protein and nucleic acid synthesis toward replication of virus-coded materials. Unresponsiveness is reflected in depressed blastogenesis, depressed capacity to synthesize and release immunoglobulin, and failure to respond to added lymphokines. Indirect effects appear to be more prominent in the monocyte/macrophage system in that IL-1 production is reduced and PGE_2 synthesis is enhanced.

Gastrointestinal nematode parasites and mucosal immunity

Immunity to helminth infection is of particular interest for several reasons. First, an effective parasite does not want to kill its host; the parasitic relationship demands that the host be alive and able to supply nutrients to the parasite. Secondly, unlike bacterial or viral infections, most helminths (with several exceptions) reside in the extracellular environment of the intestinal lumen. These nematodes are relatively resistant to developing host immunologic defenses. Nonetheless, several different specific effects of host immune response to helminth parasites have been delineated.

These parasites must establish themselves in the host by attachment/penetration of intestinal mucosa. However, most of these parasites also have a migration phase of their lifecycle during which they trigger an immune response to which they are quite susceptible. Gastrointestinal immune responses may eliminate infective larvae and/or may trigger expulsion of adult worms. Besides these effector mechanisms, additional effects on parasites may include stunting, inhibition of larval growth, and reduced reproductive capacity in adults. IgE antibodies are commonly associated with nematode infections. Such responses have been documented in dogs infected with *Drofilaria immitis* early after infection, when the third-stage larvae are migrating through the tissues. Similarly, IgE responses have been identified in bovine ostertagiosis, wherein the IgE response is associated with production of leukotrienes and prostaglandins. These specific antibodies and mediators of inflammation are thought to damage worms and/or assist in their expulsion.

Self-cure is seen in sheep infected with *Haemonchus contortus*. Haemonchosis is one of the few examples of gastrointestinal parasitism that is likely to result In death. The worm burrows into the abdominal mucosa and consumes blood, resulting in hypochromic anemia.

Self-cure is characterized by a sudden and massive expulsion of living worms from the abomasum. It occurs most frequently in sheep exposed to gradually-increasing parasite loads rather than one massive dose, and is initiated by larvae as they molt from the third to fourth stages of development. Self-cure is an immediate-type allergic reaction, occurring in the abomasum, that is induced only by living larvae. Worm expulsion follows abomasal edema and increased peristaltic movements. Self-cure can be prevented by antihistamines and anti-5-hydroxytryptamine and is associated with rising titers of skin-sensitizing antibodies (IgE).

Dissection of the various immunologic components involved in self-cure has been accomplished in rats infected with *Nippostronglylus braziliensis*. In this model system, self-cure is regularly observed 10 to 12 days after infection. The sequence of events that occurs is as follows:

1. Primary infection with the helminth parasite
2. Induction of humoral and cellular immune response 9 to 10 days after infection
3. Binding of IgE to intestinal mast cells, with release of pharmacologic mediators of immediate-type hypersensitivity
4. Increased gut and blood-vascular permeability, with leakage of serum and cells into the intestinal lumen
5. IgM and IgG antibody-mediated metabolic and structural damage of worms without expulsion
6. Expulsion of antibody-damaged worms by the action of mediators, causing smooth muscle contraction and the effect of T-cell cytokines

Thus in this infection, conventional antibodies, allergic antibodies of the IgE type, and specifically-sensitive T lymphocytes cooperative in effecting worm expulsion. Further, abrogation of any of these three steps through thymectomy, cytostatic drugs, or histamine antagonists interferes with expulsion.

Equine infectious anemia

EIA is a viral disease of horses characterized by cyclic episodes of fever, depression, anemia, lifelong persistent viral infection, and immune-mediated host-tissue damage. The disease is transmitted from horse to horse by surgical instruments or syringes that have been contaminated by blood or blood-sucking insect vectors.

The causative agent is a nononcogenic lentivirus in the Retroviridae family. Viral reverse transcriptase is present. All viral isolates tested have a common core antigen that can be measured by complement fixation or precipitation in agar gel. Precipitating antibody response to this core antigen is the basis for the use of the Coggin's test for EIA. The main site of viral replication in vivo is macrophages.

Because the disease is lifelong and characterized by the continuous presence of infectious virus in plasma and serum, early workers suggested that infected horses were tolerant to the infection and no antiviral antibodies were produced. In the mid 1960s, virus-specific antibodies were discovered. Complement-fixing (CF) IgG antibody to EIA core antigen appears 20 to 40 days after inoculation and fluctuates on and off throughout the life to the animal. Complement fixation inhibiting (CFI) antibodies of the IgG(T) class are also found; these levels vary inversely with CF. These antibodies are distinct from virus-neutralizing antibodies (IgG and IgG[T]) that appear in serum by 40 days after inoculation and persist throughout the clinical course.

The coincident presence of infectious virus and antiviral antibodies suggests that circulating immune complexes are produced. This is the case, in that greater than 99% of infectious virus in plasma is complexed with antibody. The mechanism of viral persistence in the presence of vigorous antiviral immune response is that the virus is always changing. A horse that recovers from one episode of infection will seem fine until it relapses. The relapse is caused by a variant that is not recognized by the neutralizing antibodies evoked by the first infection. Once neutralizing antibodies are produced to the new variant, the virus is eliminated and viremia ends until the next variant arises. This antigenic drift is similar to that seen in trypanosomiasis, discussed earlier in this chapter.

Lesions seen in EIA-infected horses are immune-mediated, and the severity of these lesions correlates with the clinical findings. Cyclic episodes of anemia are immune-mediated with erythrocyte hemolysis occurring in intravascular and extravascular locations. Erythrocytes are damaged by viral antigen-antibody-complement reactions on the red cell surface. A viral subunit with hemagglutinating properties attaches to the red cell, and antibody and complement subsequently react with it. True immune complex glomerulonephritis is a constant feature of EIA, though the severity varies from case to case in individuals. Immune complex vasculitis is also seen, but this is not a constant feature of EIA.

Thus EIA is an example of an infectious disease that stimulates an ineffective immune response. Lesions and clinical signs are a consequence of this immune response and not a direct effect of the virus on the host tissues.

Feline leukemia virus

FeLV is a contagious viral disease of domestic cats caused by a retrovirus. It has been implicated as the major etiologic agent of lymphosarcoma, thymoma, leukemia, fibrosarcoma, and aplastic anemia. Viral infection usually occurs through infected salivary secretions; the virus then makes its way into oral lymphoid tissues, where it gains access to the blood-vascular system and undergoes viremia. The outcome of exposure of FeLV is varied, with less than half of exposed cats becoming infected. Of those that do become infected a little more than half develop an immune response, clear the virus, and do not become viremic. Of those that do become persistently viremic, most develop one of several FeLV-related diseases and die within several years. FeLV-related diseases involve two pathogenic events—virus infection that culminates into a viremia and the induction of neoplastic cells. One of the sequelae to persistent infection is the development of tumors. Lymphosarcoma, thymoma, and leukemias are frequently associated with FeLV infection.

The dynamics that occur between the FeLV and the immune system vary between cats and the ultimate result of infection. Some cats that become viremic sequester the virus in the bone marrow and no longer have the virus circulating in the blood. More commonly, viral antigen is detectable in the blood of infected cats. The original test (developed by Hardy) uses immunofluorescence to detect group-specific viral antigen in circulating leukocytes. Infection of kittens commonly results in persistent viremia.

Another antigen that has been the target of test development is the FOCMA antigen (feline oncornavirus-associated cell membrane antigen).

This antigen is found on tumor cells of infected cats, and the production of antibodies against this antigen is associated with resistance to tumor formation. Cats that develop antibodies to the group-specific viral antigen but not the FOCMA antigen usually develop FeLV-related disease.

SUGGESTED READINGS

General
Tizare I: *Veterinary immunology: an introduction,* ed 4, Philadelphia, 1992, WB Saunders.

Mims CA: *The pathogenesis of infectious disease,* London, 1976, Academic Press.

Olsen RG, Krakowka S: Immune dysfunction associated with viral infection, *Comp Continuing Education* 6:422-430, 1984.

Transmissible gastroenteritis
Bohl EH, Gupta RKP, McCloskey LW, and others: Immunology of transmissible gastroenteritis, *J Am Vet Med Assoc* 160:543-549, 1972.

Frederick GT, Bohl EH: Local and systemic cell-mediated immunity against transmissible gastroenteritis, and intestinal viral infection of swine, *J Immunol* 116:1000-1004, 1976.

Canine distemper virus
Appel MJG, Gillespie JJ: Canine distemper virus, *Virology Monographs* 11:1-67, 1972.

McCullough B, Krakowka S, Koestner A: Experimental canine distemper virus-induced lymphoid depletion, *Am J Path* 74:155-166, 1974.

Krakowka S, Confer A, Koestner A: Evidence for transplacental transmission of canine distemper virus: two case reports, *Am J Vet Res* 35:1251-1253, 1974.

Krakowka S, Olsen RG, Confer AW, and others: Serologic response to canine distemper viral antigens in gnotobiotic dogs infected with R252 canine distemper virus, *J Infect Dis* 132:384-392, 1975.

Krakowka S, Cockerell G, Koestner A: Effects of canine distemper virus on lymphoid function *in vitro* and *in vivo*, *J Infect Immun* 11:1069-1078, 1975.

Krakowka S, Wallace A, Koestner A: Syncytia inhibition by immune lymphocytes: an *in vitro* test for immunity to canine distemper, *J Clin Micro* 7:292-297, 1978.

Krakowka KS, Higgins, RG, Koestner A: Canine distemper virus: A review of structural and functional modulation in lymphoid tissues, *Am J Vet Res* 41:284-292, 1980.

Krakowka S, Higgins, RG, Metzler AE: Plasma phase viremia in canine distemper virus infection, *Am J Vet Res* 41:144-146, 1980.

Winters KG, Mathes LE, Krakowka SW, and others: Immunoglobulin class response to canine distemper virus in gnotobiotic dogs, *Vet Imunol Immunopathol* 5:209-215, 1983.

Krakowka S, Axthelm MK, Johnson G: Canine distemper virus. In Olsen RG, Krakowka S, Blakeslee J, editors: *Pathobiology of viral diseases,* Boca Raton, Fla. 1985, CRC Press.

Ringler SS, Krakowka S: The effects of canine distemper virus upon natural killer (NK) cell activity of canine peripheral blood leukocytes, *Am J Vet Res* 46:1781-1786, 1985.

Krakowka S, Ringler SS, Lewis M, and others: Immunosuppression by canine distemper virus: modulation of *in vitro* immunoglobulin synthesis, interleukin release and prostaglandin E2 production, *Vet Imunol Immunopathol* 15:181-201, 1987.

Gastrointestinal helminths and immunity
Baker DG, Gershwin LJ: Immunoglobulin E and Type I hypersensitivity in bovine Ostertagiosis, *Vet Parasitol* 46:93-102, 1993.

Kelly JD: Mechanism of immunity to intestinal helminth, *Aust Vet J* 49:91-97, 1973.

Dinein JK, Oglivie, BM, Kelly JD: Expulsion of *Nippostrongylus brasiliensis* from the intestine of rats: collaboratory between humoral and cellular components of the immune response, *Immunology* 24:457-475, 1973.

Jarrett EEE: Reaginic antibodies and helminth infection, *Vet Rec* 93:480-483, 1973.

Miller HRP: The protective mucosal response against gastrointestinal nematodes in ruminants and laboratory animals, *Vet Imunol Immunopathol* 6:167-259, 1984.

Yamagata GR, Gershwin LJ, Wong MM: Immunoglobulin E recognition of microfilarial, larval, and adult *Dirofilaria immitis* antigens is more specific than Immunoglobulin G, *Vet Parasitol* 44:211-221, 1992.

Equine infectious anemia
Evermann JG: Comparative features of retroviral infection of livestock, *Comp Immunol Microbiol Infect Dis* 13:127-136, 1990.

Hensen JB, Gorham JR, Kobayashi K, and others: Immunity to equine infectious anemia, *J Am Vet Med Assoc* 155:336-343, 1969

McGuire TC, O'Rourke KI, Perryman LE: Immunopathogenesis of equine infectious anemia lentivirus disease, *Dev Biol Standard* 72:31-37, 1990.

Kono T, Kobayashi K, Eukunaga Y: Antigenic drug of equine infectious anemia virus in chronically infected horses, *Arch Gesamie Virusforsch* 41:1-10, 1973.

Sellon DE: Equine infectious anemia: veterinary clinics of North America, *Equine Prac* 9:321-336, 1993.

17 Vaccines, Vaccination, and Immunomodulators

In spite of its widespread application to all fields of biology and medicine, the essence of immunology is centered around mechanisms that promote recovery from infectious diseases through induction of the specific immune response. The principles of specificity, memory, and activation of host cellular defenses following invasion by pathogens can be mimicked, usually without harmful effects, through the active process of vaccination. Additionally, short-term immunity can be acquired by the administration of antibody by passive transfer techniques—naturally, through colostrum, or artificially, by oral, intravenous, or subcutaneous injection.

PASSIVE IMMUNE PROTECTION

Transfer of antibody to the neonate by the ingestion of colostrum or milk is a natural process designed to confer a measure of protection to the neonate during the vulnerable postnatal period. In certain circumstances infusions of immune serum or IgG into young adult or adult animals will accomplish the same goal.

Immune functions in the neonate are suboptimal when compared to similar responses in adults. This period of relative immunodeficiency is somewhat species-dependent. As a general rule, acquisition of adult immunocompetency is achieved at approximately the same time as adult thermoregulating mechanisms develop. Neonates and fetuses are immunocompetent, however. Because the induction of active immunity in the postpartum world takes 7 to 10 days, acquisition of maternal immunoglobulin through the placenta or colostrum provides passive protection to the newborn throughout this critical period.

Unlike primates, domestic animals receive essentially all maternal immunoglobulin (Ig) through ingestion of colostrum in the immediate postpartum (12 to 24 hour) period. Less than 5% of maternal immunoglobulin is acquired transplacentally in dogs and cats. The values are even less for calves, foals, and piglets. Selective transfer of IgG into the mammary gland accounts for the predominance of this immunoglobulin in colostrum and hence, serum of calves. For pigs, IgA is the dominant colostral Ig species. For equines, IgG and IgG(T) are most prominent. Transport of immunoglobulin across the neonatal small intestine is limited to the first 12 to 24 hours of life in most species. After this period, intestinal closure is observed; orally associated immunoglobulins are not absorbed into the circulation but are degraded by proteolytic enzymes. The process of absorption is an active pinocytotic event that occurs at the level of the intestinal epithelial cell.

Passive acquisition of antibodies is an important survival mechanism for the newborn. Protection is afforded rapidly, without the requirement for immunologic "work" on the part of the neonate. The rate of decay of these antibodies in serum varies with the immunoglobulin (Ig) class. For IgG, the half-life is 9 to 21 days; for the IgM it is 3 to 5 days. Failure of passive transfer (FPT) of maternal immunoglobulin is the most important immunologic deficit in veterinary medicine because it is significantly correlated to heightened susceptibility to numerous microbial infections in the postnatal period. Transfer of maternal immunoglobulin from serum, to colostrum, to the intestinal tract, and, finally, to the neonatal vascular system is a complex process with many potential sites for disruption. Some dams fail to produce sufficient quantities of colostral immunoglobulin premature lactation or agalactia may reduce the total available immunoglobulin for ingestion. The inability of the neonate to physically suckle and/or rejection by the dam are obvious causes of FPT. Finally, some neonates experience FPT even in the face of ingestion of adequate amounts of colostral immunoglobulin. This malabsorption syndrome is thought to be the result of premature closure of intestinal epithelia, possibly mediated by cortisol secreted by the neonatal adrenal gland.

Passive immunity has several distinct disadvantages compared to active immunity. Protection is limited to antibody specificities developed in the dam. Thus new pathogens acquired postnatally are not hindered by preexisting antibodies. Furthermore, passively acquired antibodies may interfere with the induction of active immunity induced by subclinical infection or vaccination. Finally, acquired maternal immunoglobulins can have specificity for fetal erythrocytes and/or platelets, resulting in immunologically mediated neonatal isoerythrolysis or thrombocytopenia (see Chapter 10).

Therapeutic administration of immunoglobulin to provide protection against selected pathogens does have a place in veterinary medicine. Thus far, those agents most amenable to immune therapy are those restricted to the gastrointestinal lumens. Successful treatment of neonatal diarrhea, induced by *Escherichia coli* is achieved by oral administration of monoclonal antibody specific to the K-88 antigen of the organism. Similarly, enteric viruses such as rotavirus and transmissible gastroenteritis (TGE) of piglets are amenable to oral treatment with polyclonal immune serum.

ACTIVE IMMUNITY: CURRENT PRINCIPLES OF VACCINATION

The process of inducing a specific immune response in an animal by controlled introduction to an immunogen, using the appropriate dose and route, is referred to as active immunization or vaccination. Unlike passive immunity, induced active immunity is long-lived and anamnestic in nature and involves both humoral and cellular immune mechanisms.

Successful vaccines are predicated on the optimal functions of a basic biologic principle—the ability of all life forms to distinguish self from nonself, thereby limiting the effects of a hostile environment on vital processes. Even bacteria, by virtue of the intact cell wall, reflect this concept. In higher life forms, this self-nonself discrimination is achieved by specialized living tissue or organs such as skin and mucosal membranes, and internally by recognition, effector, and memory responses of the lymphoreticular (immune) systems. The vaccination process is based on the observation that animals (or humans) that recover from an infectious disease are resistant to that same disease when exposed (challenged) at some future time. At its most elementary level, vaccination is controlled exposure of susceptible animals to the agent in a form that will not produce clinical disease. Because immunity is an acquired property and takes time (days to weeks), introduction of vaccine before the exposure represents the most important practical approach to disease prophylaxis. Considering its impact on the health of both human and animal populations, the process of vaccination probably represents the most significant biologic advance of medicine in the last 100 years.

The goal of any vaccination procedure is disease prevention, not cure. The same rules of antigenic specificity and memory apply. Insofar as vaccines are concerned, three different categories of disease-causing entities exist. One category consists of practical vaccines that work under field conditions. Examples of these are canine distemper, feline panleukopenia, and clostridial infections of food animals. Experimental vaccines constitute the second category. In this instance the number of practical vaccines increases as vaccination procedures move from experimental laboratory products to commercial production. The third type of agent is one in which little prospect for successful vaccination exists at this time. Examples of this type are most parasitic diseases, viruses such as equine infectious anemia, organisms with multiple antigenic serotypes like *Salmonella* spp. or upper respiratory viruses (rhinoviruses), and unconventional infectious agents such as scrapie or transmissible mink encephalopathy.

Vaccines are prepared from microorganisms or their products. The chief goal of any vaccine is to incorporate the immunogen that stimulates protection into a dose that stimulates an immediate immune response when administered. Bacterial biologics may consist of whole, killed organisms or fractions thereof (bacterins), chemically-inactivated bacterial products (toxoids), or occasionally, live, attenuated organisms (e.g., strain 19 *Brucella abortus*).

Antimicrobial products are of two general types—inactivated or killed and attenuated or modified live agents. Killing the agent with chemicals or destroying its capacity to reproduce by irreversible damaging nucleic acid are the most straightforward approaches to eliminating pathogenicity. Inactivated viral vaccines are preferred primarily because they provide the best margin of medical safety. Although there are a few exceptions, the chief limitation to the widespread use of inactivated products for viruses is the general inability to confer the proper level or type of immunity as determined by field trial studies. This is most likely the result of the inability to provide sufficient antigenic mass for immunization.

The second method for development of a candidate vaccine is to artificially select for attenuated, non-disease-producing viral variants. This process is achieved by repeated passages through abnormal hosts (different species or embryonated eggs) or *in vitro*, by tissue culture methodology. These modified live virus (MLV) products are in widespread use today and provide the clinician with the ability to incite protective levels of immunity to the pathogens in question. T cell-mediated immunity is more readily induced by MLV because viral antigen is presented in context of class I MHC.

An ideal vaccine must stimulate effective and long-lasting immunity, must be safe, and must be cheap, stable, and easily transported and administered. Today, MLV products most closely realize this goal. However, MLVs are not ideal. The essential problem is that an attenuated virus is a living one, and therefore changeable and, under certain conditions, it can mutate back to a virulent form or can recombine with avirulent agents to produce a new virulent counterpart. Also, special handling is required to preserve the replicative ability of the virus. In vaccine formulations, this limitation may be overcome by increasing the number of viral infectious units per dose or by specialized processing (refrigeration, lyophilization, etc.). Further, application of MLV to pregnant animals, debilitated patients, the very young or very old, or those suffering from intercurrent endocrine, metabolic, or infectious disease, may result in MLV-induced disease in recipients. In addition, development of MLV products may be limited by the nature of the agent itself. Viruses (or bacteria) that are not easily grown, purified, or propagated in vitro limit the success of the attenuation process. Finally, unwanted and unforeseen interactions between MLV agents in multiagent vaccine preparations may result in clinical disease. For these reasons, attention has been redirected toward exploration of useful alternatives to MLVs. To be safe and efficacious, a number of variables in vaccine formulations must be considered. Advantages of modified-live versus killed products include decreased chances of developing hypersensitivity reactions.

Dosage is a second vaccine variable. The antigenic dose must be enough to stimulate immunity yet not massive enough to induce tolerance. For infectious canine hepatitis (ICH), a viral disease caused by canine adenovirus type, 1 (CAV-1), the viral dose is critical. Early vaccine formulations consisted of very small numbers of fully-CAV-1 virulent virions. Animals develop manifestations of ICH if too much virus is given. Today, this possibility is remote because use of avirulent canine adenovirus type 2, an upper respiratory virus, will provide complete protection from CAV-1-induced disease.

The route of vaccination is also important. Contagious ecthyma, a viral disease of sheep, produces multiple painful herpetic-type skin lesions around the face, lips, and coronary bands. The vaccine consists of fully virulent virus but is administered in the flank. A similar skin lesion develops at the vaccination site but not around the muzzle. Because this vaccine consists of virulent virus, it should never be administered to a flock before an outbreak, because once introduced this way, the virus persists in the flock or on the premises, requiring annual vaccination of lambs and new additions.

Age at the time of vaccination is another factor to consider. For diseases widespread in the animal population, such as canine distemper, the likelihood that the dam possesses protective antibodies transferable through colostrum to the neonate is high. Thus attempts to immunize animals possessing passively acquired antibody fail. It is axiomatic that for a vaccine to take, the animal must be susceptible to the disease in question.

Another example of the age factor is the use of strain 19 *B. abortus* in the bovine population. With brucellosis there is an age-related susceptibility to infection whereby younger animals are more susceptible than adults. Strain 19 is used prophylactically only in calves. Although immunization stimulates immunity in both calves and adults, agglutinin titers persist in the adults, making their sera similar to virulent *Brucella* spp. carriers. The age influences the response to immunization and consequently interferes with states and federal test and slaughter regulations instituted for control of the disease.

To be effective, a vaccine must induce the right type of immune response to the appropriate immunogen in the right location. For generalized infections, this requirement is not absolute; however, for local infections such as mastitis, this feature is critical. In Chapter 16, the immunobiology of the immune response to TGE of piglets was discussed. In that disease, an effective immunogen induces an IgA response. Virus-specific circulating IgG was not protective. In that same chapter, it was emphasized that the tetanus is caused not be infection with *Clostridium tetani* but rather by the toxin it elaborates in the tissue. Thus vaccination with tetanus toxoid and not vaccination against the microbe results in disease prevention.

Several types of vaccine formulations are currently available for use in veterinary medicine. Monovalent vaccines, such as the one used against canine distemper, are effective because field strains of distemper virus are all of one immunogenic type. Other viral diseases, such as foot-and-mouth disease, are caused by a number of different viral serotypes. Because immunization with one serotype does not protect against infection by other serotypes, polyvalent vaccines containing several different serotypes are used. Polyvalent vaccines must be distinguished from mixed vaccines. A mixed vaccine refers to a product containing immunogens obtained from different pathogens. Examples of this type are the DHL combination (distemper, hepatitis, leptospirosis) administered to dogs and the bovine combination vaccine for clostridial diseases (e.g., blackleg, malignant edema, black disease, enterotoxemia, and *Clostridium sordellii* infection). A homotypic vaccine product is one that contains the attenuated or killed agent identical to its disease-causing counterpart. Most products are of this type. A heterotypic vaccine is one that uses as immunogen a related but not identical agent to stimulate protective immunity. Examples of this type are the use of measles virus vaccines to protect dogs from virulent canine distemper and the use of turkey herpesvirus that successfully stimulates protective immunity against Marek's disease herpesvirus infection of chickens.

Because of convenience and economic considerations, there is a strong tendency to develop and market multiple agent vaccine formulations. Some products may contain as many as seven distant MLV agents. As their number increases, so does the possibility of untoward adverse interactions between individual MLVs and the host. Adverse consequences are likely to be infrequent and sporadic. The veterinary clinician must be constantly aware of the risk/benefit ratio for vaccination and should promptly report any suspected failures to the manufacturer. A complete list of products and product information can be found in an annual reference book, *Veterinary Pharmaceuticals and Biologicals*, published by F.A. Davis in Philadelphia, or may be obtained from sales representatives of the various biologic supply houses.

ACTIVE IMMUNITY: FUTURE DEVELOPMENTS IN VACCINE FORMULATION

In Figure 17-1, the general outline for design of current and future vaccine products (in this case viral) is outlined. The underlying principle is identical when vaccines for bacteria or various parasites are contemplated. The level of complexity of these higher life forms makes the process of selection and efficacy testing very arduous.

Vaccine products at levels 1 and 2 are in current use and have been delineated in the previous section.

Level 3: the noninfectious subunit vaccine

In order to understand the principle behind this type of vaccine and those of level 4, it is necessary to describe certain biochemical features of the viral proteins that induce the protective immune response in that host. Proteins on the exterior surface of the virus are responsible for specific attachment

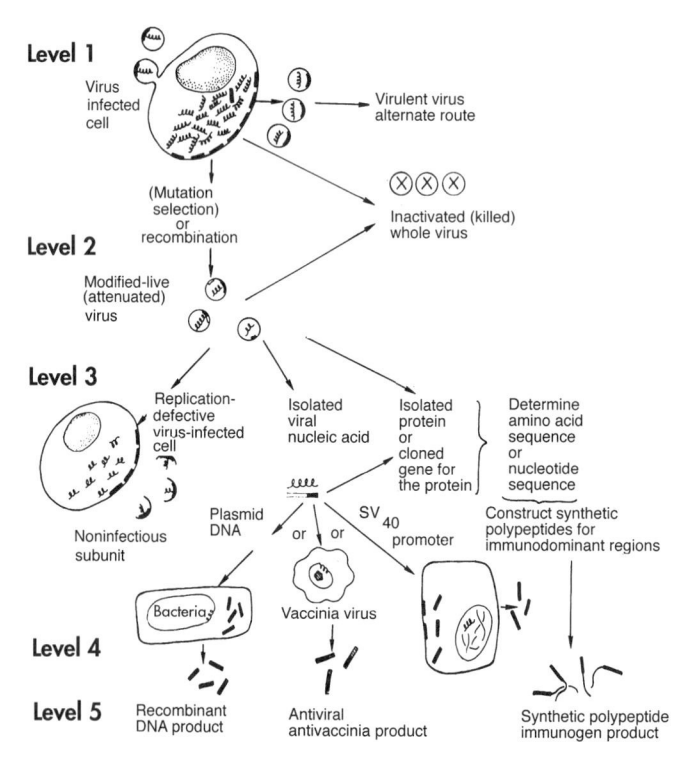

Figure 17-1 A schematic diagram that outlines the construction and evolution of viral vaccine products.

of the virus to the surface of susceptible cells and subsequent penetration of the cell by viral nucleic acid. These surface proteins are also necessary for assembly and release of virions from infected cells and thus are inserted into the host cell membrane *before* virion assembly. Specific antibody reacts with these proteins and either prevents attachment or retards assembly and release of newly synthesized virions. Cytotoxic-T lymphocytes also react with these proteins on cell surfaces and cause cell death, thereby eliminating the source of new virus within host tissues. These viral proteins are also glycosylated; that is, they contain carbohydrate residues on their surfaces, and these sugars provide conformational properties and cell membrane–binding properties to the protein. Envelope proteins are globular, in 3 dimensions, and may be several thousand amino acids in length. However, only certain portions of this folded molecule are hydrophilic and located on the exterior of the protein. At a topographic level, these critical regions or epitopes are the most important components for recognition by the immune system. Thus a successful noninfectious vaccine product must not only be devoid of viral nucleic acid but also must contain these exterior viral proteins (or at the very least, their specific epitopes).

Norden's Leukocell vaccine (and its second generation, Leukocell 2 manufactured by Smith Kline Beecham) for prevention of feline leukemia was the first commercially available, non-replicating, veterinary biologic to incorporate the above outlined principle of viral assembly. The concept behind the product is deceptively simple. It has been known for many years that antibody production to the feline oncornavirus cell-membrane antigen (FOCMA) is associated with resistance to feline leukemia virus (FeLV)-induced disease. This virus infection-induced envelope glycoprotein is synthesized and inserted into the cell membrane of virus-infected cells. Through several manipulations, a virus replication-defective cell line has been developed that releases formed precursor FOCMA proteins as extracellular soluble products. It is this material, harvested and concentrated, that is used for vaccination. The material is immunogenic, nonreplicative, and derived from a persistently infected cell line. It is called a *subunit product* and is distinguished from other subunit materials (see level 4) chiefly because the material is harvested from an infected cell line without genetic manipulation.

Level 4: genetically engineered vaccine products

In the last 10 years the techniques and promise of genetic engineering technology have virtually revolutionized our thinking in medicine and biology.

The technology is based on the fact that genetic information for life is encoded in the pattern sequence and arrangements of nucleotides within the DNA molecule. Regarding viruses, linear segments of DNA (RNA in the case of RNA viruses) or genes encode for each of the virion proteins. Viruses are the simplest of life forms. For DNA viruses, gene segments encoding for the protein of choice are isolated by the use of specialized sets of enzymes, called *endonucleases*, which cleave double-stranded DNA at specific nucleotide sequence sites on the molecule. Fragments are then separated on the basis of size and are ready for vector manipulations. The technology for RNA viruses is more complicated. Two approaches are used. In the first, viral genomic RNA is isolated, and then a complementary RNA strand is synthesized through an enzyme reaction with reverse transcriptase. From this mirror-image synthetic RNA, a DNA (cDNA) strand is synthesized. The resultant product is identical in sequence to the original, viral, genomic RNA. In the second approach, viral messenger RNAs (mRNAs) are complementary to genomic viral RNA. Complementary DNA to these mRNAs, once synthesized, now contains the correct sequence of information for coding of the viral protein. For either virus, the DNA segment specific for the viral protein of interest is then readied for expression by attachment to a vector (Figure 17-1).

For bacteria, the vector may be a plasmid (an extrachromosomal, circular, DNA segment first identified as the structure that transmits antibiotic resistance to bacteria) or a bacterial virus (phage). The wanted DNA segment is added to the plasmid/phage DNA by first enzymic cleavage of the circular DNA, and then the foreign DNA is inserted into the broken circle. Vectored DNA (frequently attached adjacent to a gene coding for antibiotic resistance) is then used to infect susceptible bacteria. These bacteria are then propagated in the presence of an antibiotic; resistance organisms containing both foreign viral DNA and the gene for antibiotic resistance are selected for further growth by subculture. As outlined in Figure 17-1, the modified bacterial then will produce the desired viral gene protein product (along with irrelevant bacterial protein) in copious amounts. Of course, the technology and concurrent difficulties are numerous. Nonetheless, this manipulation is now standard for all molecular genetics laboratories.

From this, it follows that the bacteria-free product (or even the live bacteria) could simply be harvested for use as the immunogen. Unfortunately, in spite of its great initial promise, the recombinant bacterial vaccine products are not particularly effective as immunogens. There are two reasons for this. Mention was made previously of the critical contributions of glycosylation to protein behavior and immunogenicity. Prokaryotes (bacteria) do not possess mammalian glycosylation enzyme systems, thus the protein products are not appropriately glycosylated. The second problem relates to the epitope concept. Selecting the correct segment of DNA coding for the important epitope is frequently not physically possible because the epitope has a spatial configuration and is not a linear DNA sequence.

To circumvent these conceptual problems, at least two variants of the bacterial cloning procedure have been developed and show great promise for future use. Instead of inserting foreign DNA into bacteria, investigators have recently focused their efforts toward insertion of the foreign DNA into mammalian-compatible delivery systems. Vaccinia (rox) virus is a large, complex, DNA virus with limited pathogenic capability. Vaccinia DNA, by ordinary virus standards, is large and can easily accommodate insertion of foreign genetic material (using the same endonuclease/ligase procedure developed for bacteria). Altered vaccinia virus is still an obligate intracellular parasite of mammalian (or avian) cells. Thus vaccinia-infected cells will produce the foreign protein that will be subsequently glycosylated by host-cell enzyme systems. The resultant isolated product is appropriately immunogenic. More importantly, a vaccinia virus containing foreign DNA from many different viral or bacterial pathogens can be constructed, and the altered vaccinia vaccine product can be used to direct immunize animals. Except for the vaccinia virus itself, there is no possibility that the resultant multiple vaccine construct will contain living viral materials. This has, in fact, been recently accomplished.

A vaccinia vector offers a number of important advantages. It carries a large genome for insertion of 12 or more foreign genes. It is attenuated, and stable, and is not integrated into host cellular DNA. Its construction as a modified-live agent provides a mechanism for amplification of the gene product through vaccinia-virus replication cycles. Possible shortcomings of this engineered product include the possibility that booster injections may not be applicable once initial exposure to the vaccinia agent has occurred and that the virus may be transmitted to unvaccinated animals. However, recent work indicates that these criticisms are not valid. A successful Rinderpest vaccine has been developed, using vaccinia as a vector by Dr. T. Yilma and colleagues.

Vaccinia recombinants still do not perform as well as their MLV counterparts in terms of quality of immune response. To improve immunogenicity, two approaches are contemplated. Insertion of multiple copies of the same gene should, in theory, provide more antigenic mass for purposes of immunization. Alternatively, an adjuvant gene such as those coding for interferon or interleukin 2 may be inserted into the vaccinia along with the desired gene. Again, in theory, the gene product(s) of the adjuvant would serve to stimulate the immune response to the recombinant gene.

A variant of the vaccinia story is the recent development of a feasible gene-transfer system for mammalian cells. For this, advantage is taken of the fact that certain DNA tumor viruses (e.g., simian virus 40 [SV40] adenovirus) contain gene sequences that will insert into normal, host cell DNA. By coupling the desired viral gene to the SV40 gene, it is possible to produce immortalized cells containing the wanted viral DNA, which, in theory, will be transcribed and produced by the altered cells. From this, the product can be harvested like FOCMA for immunization. The major difficulty in this system is that the level and complexity inherent in the regulation of genomic expression in eukaryotic (mammalian) cell systems are poorly understood and, hence, not easily manipulated.

Recently the insect virus baculovirus (*Autographa californica* nuclear polyhedrosis virus) has been used as a vector for mammalian and viral gene expression. Insertion of the desired gene into baculovirus followed by infection of insert cells (*Spodoptera frugiperda*) results in expression of the cloned gene. Several genes form viruses of veterinary importance, such as the fusion protein from bovine, respiratory, syncytial virus, have been expressed in this way. Infection of the larval insect with recombinant baculovirus can yield large amounts of expressed protein.

Level 5: synthetic immunogens

In addition to numerous technical obstacles and their limiting factors, genetic manipulation as a viable approach to vaccine production poses moral, ethical, and legal difficulties. These difficulties are concerned with what is, in essence, the creation of new life forms. Although remote, the possibility of creating aberrant and potentially dangerous altered pathogens exists. One way to avoid this regulatory and ethical morass is to bypass the need for recombinant technology entirely. This can be done by taking advantage of the recently developed capability to sequence both proteins and nucleic acids; from this, using automatic peptide synthesizers, completely synthetic vaccine products can be constructed.

After isolating the pivotal viral protein, the primary amino acid sequence is determined by sequential enzymatic digests. With the aid of a computer that takes into account binding angles and structural restraints of the amino acids involved, sites or patches on the surfaces of the molecule (e.g., epitope candidates) can be identified and their sequence deduced. In cases where protein isolation is not feasible, the gene coding for that protein can be isolated as described earlier and then sequenced through sequential, endonuclease digestion. Because the triplet code of three sequential nucleotide residues is (with a few exceptions) specific for one of the 20 amino acids, the primary amino acid sequence may be deduced. Using either approach, short peptides can be synthesized that are identical to epitope regions of the native molecule. This approach is not without the shortcomings noted earlier (inadequate glycosylation and linear versus spatial or discontinuous determinants). Nonetheless, these synthetic polypeptides, when coupled to carrier protein molecules to enhance immunogenicity, represent perhaps the ultimate in specifically engineered vaccines.

ANTI-IDIOTYPES AND THEIR POTENTIAL AS VACCINE IMMUNOGENS

The idiotype-anti-idiotype network, described by Jerne, is a result of the diversity and specificity of antibodies. The conceptual framework for delineation of this network is credited to the work of Henry Kunkel and Jacques Oudin. Oudin coined the word idiotype (individual) to describe an antibody molecule with binding specificity for the antigen combining site (variable [v]-region, hypervariable domains) of the inducing Ig-immunogen. Development of monoclonal antibody technology has greatly facilitated study and exploitation of this unique system of immunoregulation. Recently, delineation of idiotype interactions has resulted in the development of a novel approach to vaccine formulations. The essentials of the process are outlined in Figure 17-2.

The basic steps in the approach follow. Antibody is raised to the candidate immunogenic material. This substance may be protein, lipid, or carbohydrate. The latter feature is of great importance because immunogens prepared by recombinant or polypeptide synthesis methods are restricted to proteins only. Antibody 1 is then purified by affinity chromatography and used to immunize animals of the same species/strain. The result is an antibody that recognizes only V-region determinants or idiotypes and is referred to as the anti-idiotype. The V-region of the anti-idiotype antibody molecule is structurally identical to the original inciting immunogen. Thus this molecule, particularly if produced as a monoclonal, can be substituted as immunogen for the generation of protective antibody, the anti-idiotype. In this fashion, immunogens can be custom designed for many different materials of a proteinaceous or nonproteinaceous nature. This approach has been used experimentally but has not yet yielded any commercial products.

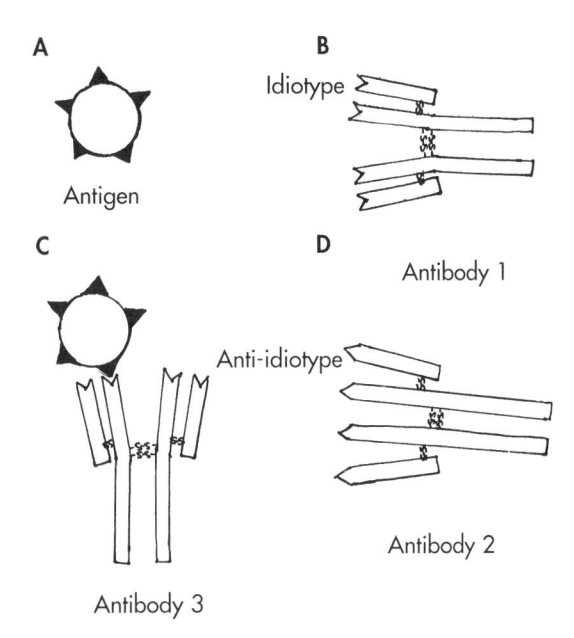

Figure 17-2 A scheme for design of a vaccine product using the idiotype-antidiotype regulatory network. In this scheme, antigen, **A** is used to evoke the production of antibody 1, **B**; this antibody is then used as the immunogen to evoke antibody 2, **C**. Antibody 2 is the "vaccine;" when injected into the host its variable region resembles the antigenic epitope on the original antigen. It will induce antibody 3, **D**, which is capable in binding to and neutralizing the antigen.

TYPES OF VACCINES AVAILABLE IN VETERINARY MEDICINE

Various types of vaccines are available for use in veterinary medicine. Monovalent vaccines, such as the one used against canine distemper, are effective because field strains of distemper virus are of one immunogenic type. Other viral diseases, such as foot-and-mouth disease, are caused by a number of different viral serotypes. Since immunization with one serotype does not protect against infection by other serotypes, polyvalent vaccines containing several different serotypes are used. Polyvalent vaccines must be distinguished from mixed vaccines. A mixed vaccine refers to a product containing immunogens obtained from different pathogens. Examples of this type are the DHL combination (distemper, hepatitis, leptospirosis) administered to dogs and the bovine combination vaccine for clostridial diseases (e.g., blackleg, malignant edema, black disease, enterotoxemia, and *clostridium sordellii* infection).

A homotypic vaccine product is one that contains the attenuated or killed agent immunologically identical to its disease-causing counterpart. Most products are of this type. A heterotypic vaccine is one that uses a related but not identical agent as immunogen to stimulate protective immunity. Examples of this type are the use of measles virus vaccines to protect dogs from virulent canine distemper and the use of turkey herpesvirus that successfully stimulates protective immunity against Marek's disease herpesvirus infection of chickens.

Tables 17-1 and 17-2 list the types of vaccines available for use by veterinarians in the United States. A complete list of products and product information can be found in an annual reference book, *Veterinary Pharmaceuticals and Biologicals*, published by Veterinary Medicine Publishing, Edwardsville, Kansas.

Table 17-1 Types of viral vaccines available for use in veterinary medicine

Domestic animal species	Disease and/or agent	Type of vaccine recommended
Canine	Canine distemper virus	MLV-DCV or MLV-MV CDV
	Infectious canine hepatitis	MLV
	Parainfluenza virus	MLV
	Rabies virus	MLV or killed
	Parvovirus	MLV or killed
Feline	Panleukopenia virus	MLV or killed
	Rhinotraceitis virus	MLV or killed
	Calicivirus	MLV or killed
	Rabies virus	MLV or killed
	Feline leukemia virus	Subunit
Bovine	Bovine virus diarrhea	MLV
	Bovine reovirus	MLV
	Infectious bovine rhinotracheitis virus	MLV
	Parainfluenza-3 virus	MLV
	Rabies virus	MLV
	Warts (papilloma virus)	Killed
	Blue tongue virus	MLV
	Bovine rotavirus	MLV
	Bovine coronavirus	MLV
Equine	Equine encephalomyelitis (Western, Eastern, Venezuelan)	MLV or killed
	Equine (influenza (A/1, A/2)	MLV or killed
	Equine rhinopneumonitis	MLV or killed
Porcine	Parvovirus	Killed
	Transmissible gastroenteritis	MLV
	Pseudorabies virus	MLV or killed
Ovine	Contagious ecythema	Live

Table 17-2 Types of bacterial or bacterial product vaccines available for use in veterinary medicine

Domestic animal species	Disease and/or agent	Type of vaccine recommended
Canine	Leptospirosis *(L. Canicola, L. icterohaemorrhagica)*	Killed
	Bordetella bronchiseptica	Attenuated
Feline	Chlamydia	Attenuated
Bovine	*Bordetella bronchiseptica*	Killed
	Pasteurella multocida, P. haemolytica	Killed, avirulent live
	Haemophilus somnus	Killed
	Clostridium chauvoei and C. septicum	Killed
	Campylobacter (Vibrio) fetus	Killed
	Staphylococcus aureus	Killed
	Leptospirosis (see Porcine)	Attenuated
	Bacillus anthracis (Anthrax)	Attenuated
	Brucella abortus (strain 19)	Attenuated
	Escherichia coli	Killed
	Anaplasma marginale (Anaplasmosis)	Killed
	Salmonella typhimurium	Killed
	Clostridium (spp.)	
	C. haemolyticum	Killed
	C. novyi	Killed, Toxoid
	C. chauvoei, C. septicum	Killed
	C. sordellii	Killed, Toxoid
	C. perfringens, C, D	Attenuated, Toxoid
	C. tetani	Toxoid
Equine	*Clostridium tetani*	Toxoid
	Streptococcus equii	Killed
	Streptococcus equi-M	Extract
Porcine	Leptospirosis *(L. canicola, L. grippotyphosa, L. hardjo, L. icterohaemmoragiae, L. pomona)*	Killed
	Haemophilus pleuropneumoniae	Killed
	Escherichia coli	Killed
	Pasteurella multocida A	Killed
	Salmonella choleraesuis	Killed
	Erysipelothrix rhusiopathiae	Attenuated, Killed

SUGGESTED READINGS

Arnon R, Shapira M, Jacob CO: Synthetic vaccines, *J Immunol Methods* 61:261-273, 1983.

Boyle DB: Poxviruses as vectors for veterinary vaccines, *Aust Vet J* 66:419-420, 1989.

Collins FM: Vaccines and cell-mediated immunity, *Bacteriol Rev* 38:371-409, 1974.

Esposito JJ, Murphy FA: Infectious recombinant vectored virus vaccines, *Adv Vet Sci Comp Med* 33:195-247, 1989.

Engleberg NC, Eisenstein BI: The impact of new cloning techniques on the diagnosis and treatment of infectious disease, *N Engl J Med* 311:892-901, 1984.

Kennedy RC, Melnick JL, Ressman GR: Anti-idiotypes and immunity, *Sci Am* 32:48-56, 1986.

Kohler H: Idiotypic network interactions, *Immunol Today* 1:18-21, 1980.

Krakowka S: Vaccines and vaccine products: progress and prospects. In *Immunology for the veterinary practitioner*, Amarillo Cell Culture Co., 6-9, 1986.

Loar AS: Feline leukemia virus immunization and prevention, *Vet clin of North Am Small Anim Prac* 23(1):193-211, 1993.

Mims CA: *The pathogenesis of infectious disease*, London, 1976, Academic Press.

Morein B, Hoglund S: Subunit vaccines against infection by enveloped viruses, *Adv Biotechnol Processes* 14:69-90.

Norcross NL: Immune response of the mammary gland and role of immunization in mastitis control, *J Am Vet Med Assoc* 170:1228-1233, 1977.

Norrby E: Viral vaccines: the use of currently available products and future developments, *Arch Virol* 76:163-177, 1983.

Perkus ME, Piccini A, Lipinskas BR, and others: Recombinant vaccinia virus: immunization against multiple pathogens, *Science* 299:981-984, 1985.

Poskitt IDC, Jean-Francis MF, Turnbull and others: Internal image (AB2 beta) antidiotype vaccines, theoretical and practical aspects, *Vaccine* 9:792-796, 1991.

Sissons JGP, Oldstone MBG: Host response to viral infections. In Fields BN, editor: Virology, New York, 1985, Raven Press.

Steward MW, Howard CR: Synthetic peptides: a next generation of vaccines?, *Immunol Today* 8:51-53, 1987.

Tickhonenko TI: Virion proteins and the perspectives of gene manipulation in vaccine preparation, *Acta Virol* 29:254-265, 1985.

Walker PD: Bacterial vaccines: Old and new, veterinary and medical, *Vaccine* 10:977-990 1992.

Yancy RJ: Recent advances in bovine vaccine technology, *Dairy Sci* 76:2418-2434, 1993.

Index

A

A45 lethal trait in cattle, 114-115
Abscess after *C. pseudotuberculosis* infection in sheep, MHC and, 59
Absorption, solid phase, to separate bound and unbound reactants, 92
Acquired immunity and innate immunity, interactions of, 5
Acquired immunodeficiency syndrome, 160
Activated B lymphocytes, products of, 30-39
Activation, complement; *see* Complement activation
Active immunity, 170-175
Addison's disease, 154
Adherence techniques to isolate antigen-specific leukocytes, 102
Adhesin deficiency, leukocyte
   bovine, 115
   canine, 117
Adhesions, 72-73
Adrenal gland, autoimmune diseases of, 154
Adrenal insufficiency, 154
Affinity in antigen-antibody interactions, 36
Affinity constant, 76
Agammaglobulinemia
   bovine, 115
   primary, equine, 114
Agglutination, 77-78
Agglutination test(s), 77-78
   advantages of, 77
   Coombs', 79-80
   2-mercaptoethanol, 80
   milk-ring, 78-79
   plate or card, 78, 79
   qualitative, 78-80
   quantitative, 80
   tube, 80
Agglutinins, 77
Agretope, epitope vs, 12
Aldehyde-fixed tissues, immunofluorescence assays in, 94
Alleles of MHC, 55
Allergenic pneumonitis, canine, 135
Allergen-specific IgE, direct skin test for, 130
Allergic alveolitis, bovine, 147
Allergic bronchitis, canine, 135
Allergic dermatitis, canine, 134-135
Allergic enteritis, canine and feline, 135
Allergic gastritis, canine and feline, 135
Allergic inhalant dermatitis in dogs, 134
Allergic reactions in type I hypersensitivity, late-phase, 133
Allergic response, haptens causing, 7
Allergic rhinitis
   bovine, 136
   canine, 135
Allergic wheals, equine, 136
Allergy, 129
   gastrointestinal, canine and feline, 135
   milk, bovine, 135
   respiratory, canine, 135
Alloantigens, lymphocyte glycoprotein (Lyt), 22, 23
Allograft, 10
Allograft rejection, T-lymphocyte-mediated, 103-104
Allotypic variation in immunoglobulin structure, 31
Alpha interferon, 5, 43
Alpha-beta T-cell receptor for antigen, 63-64
Alpha-fetoprotein, 11
Alveolar cells, macrophages becoming, 20
Alveolar macrophages as defense mechanism, 4
Alveolitis, allergic, bovine, 147
Ammonium sulfate fractionation, 92
ANA test to diagnose systemic lupus erythematosus, 155
Anaphylactic shock, 133-134
Anaphylactic type reactions, mediators of, 132-133
Anaphylaxis
   effector cells of, 26-28
   slow-reacting substance of, 133
   systemic, 132, 133-135
      species differences in, 135
Anaphylaxis test, passive cutaneous, 130
Anaplasma marginale, vaccine against, 177
Anaplasmosis, vaccine against, 177
"Ancestral antibody," 34
Anemia
   hemolytic
      autoimmune, 151
      Coombs positive, 151-152
      cryopathic immune mediated, 151
   infectious, equine, 145, 161, 166-167
      Coggins' test for, 83
      infection with, IgG(T) levels in, 36
Angioneurotic edema, 50, 53
Aniline dyes to label proteins, 90, 91
Animals, domestic; *see* Domestic animals
Anterior uveitis, 147-148
Anthrax, 159-160
   vaccine against, 177
Antibodies, 30; *see also* Immunoglobulins
   "ancestral," 34
   antigen and, union of, 76
   antigen reaction with; *see* Antigen-antibody reactions
   cellular origin of, 30
   diversity of, molecular basis of, 37
   formation of, 31
   IgE
      other antigens producing, 10
      production of, by parasitic antigens, 10
   last dilution of, yielding positive reaction, reciprocal of, 76-77
   monoclonal, 37-38
      production of, 37-38
   natural, autoimmune reactions and, 151
   reaginic; *see* Immunoglobulin E
   structural-functional relationships of, 32
   tetanus-resistant, 10
   valency of, antigen-antibody union and, 76
Antibody reactions, cytotoxic, 136
Antibody response to protein epitopes, 8
Antibody-antigen interactions, 36-37

Antibody-dependent cytotoxicity, 136, 137
Antibody-directed cellular cytotoxicity, 109
Antigen mixtures, antigenic analysis of, 82, 83
Antigen-antibody interactions, 36-37
Antigen-antibody reactions, 78
Antigen-binding site of immunoglobulin, 33
Antigen-induced selection, 37
Antigen-presenting cells, 62-63
  interaction of T cells and, 63
  macrophages as, 20, 21-22
Antigen-presenting function of phagocytic cells, 21-22
Antigen-specific leukocytes, isolation of, 102
Antigen-specific reactions of lymphocytes in vitro, 107
Antigenic analysis of antigen mixtures, 82, 83
Antigenic determinants, 7
Antigenic shift, 10
Antigenic variation, 10
Antigens; *see also* Immunogens
  alpha-beta T-cell receptor for, 63-64
  antibody and, union of, 76
  carcinoembryonic, 11
  cell membrane, oncornavirus-associated, feline, 122
  clusters of differentiation (CD), 11-12
  complete, 7
  definition of, 6
  endocytosis of, 63
  in environment, 8-10
    cross-reaction with, autoimmune reactions and, 150
  erythrocyte, 11
  F, 9
  FOCMA, 167
  Forssman, 11
  H, 9, 11
  histocompatibility, 55
    and blood group antigens, 55-61
  IgM response to, 12
  immunogens and, 6-12
  incomplete, 7
  leukocyte, dog, 57
  lymphocyte; *see* Lymphocyte antigen
  lymphocyte function-associated, 29
  major histocompatibility, allografts and, 10
  on mammalian cells, 10-12
  MHC, functions of, 58-59
  O, 9, 11
  oncofetal, 10, 11
  producing IgE antibodies, 10
  recognition and presentation of, 62-65
  sequestered, autoimmune reactions and, 150
  T-cell receptor for, 23
  T-cell-independent, 64
  T-dependent, 12
  Thy-1 or theta, 22
  tissue grafting and, 10
  tumor-associated, 10-11
  very late, 29
Antiglobulin for immunoassays and immunocytochemistry, 96
Antiglobulin test, Coombs, direct, 151
Anti-idiotypes as vaccine immunogens, 175
Arabian horses, combined immunodeficiency disease of, 113-114
Arthritis
  idiopathic nondeforming, 152
  immune-mediated, 152-153
  rheumatoid, 152
Arthus, Maurice, 139
Arthus reaction, 139, 140
Ascaris suum, late-phase allergic reaction in sheep caused by, 133

Assay(s)
  bactericidal, 73, 74
  C1q-binding, 146
  CH50, 75
  cytotoxic T-cell, 108-109
  enzyme-linked immunosorbent, 94-96, 130, 132
  for humoral immunity, 76-98
  immunofluorescence, 92-94
  immunologic, secondary, 77
  for innate immune defenses, 71-75
  interleukin 2, for lymphocyte function, 107
  for lymphocyte functions in mixed or purified cellular populations, 103-109
  monocyte function, 108
  natural killer cell, 109
  radioimmune, 94-96
  serologic
    choice of, 96-97
    primary, 90-97
  solid phase plate, 94-96
  for T lymphocyte function, 99-110
  target cell cytotoxicity, 108
  terminal deoxynucleotidyl transferase (TdT), 23
Asthma, feline, 135
Atopy, 132
Attenuated viral variants for vaccines, 170-171
Autoantibodies
  to glomerular basement membrane, glomerulonephritis mediated by, 144
  natural, 150
Autoimmune diseases
  adrenal gland, 154
  dermatologic, 154-155
  endocrine system, 153
  hematopoietic system, 151-153
  MHC class II association with, 155-156
  neuromuscular system, 153
  organ-specific, 151-156
  pancreatic, 153-154
  systemic, 155-156
  thyroid gland, 153
Autoimmune hemolytic anemia, 151
  Coombs positive, 151-152
Autoimmune thrombocytopenia, 152
Autoimmune thyroiditis, 153
Autoimmune type II disease, 136
Autoimmunity, 150-156
  causes of, theories on, 150-151
  definition of, 150
Avian species, lymphoid tissues in, 18-19
Avidity in antigen-antibody interactions, 37

B

B1H inhibitors, 22
B cell(s), 12
  antigens expressed by, 25
  structure and function of, 24-25
B-cell differentiation, 66
B-cell epitope, 12
B-cell stimulatory factor, 42
B lymphocyte(s)
  activated, products of, 30-39
  activation of, 66
  antigen presentation and, 63
  antigen recognition and presentation and, 64-65
  assays for, 103
  pokeweed mitogen-induced, 25
  structure and functions of, 24-25
B-lymphocyte differentiation, terminal, neoplasms of, 118-119

Index

Bacillus anthracis, vaccine against, 177
Bacteria, defenses against, complement and, 52
Bacterial antigens in environment, 8-10
Bacterial cloning procedures in genetically engineered vaccines, 174
Bactericidal assay, 73, 74
Baculovirus and genetically engineered vaccines, 174
BALT; *see* Bronchus-associated lymphoid tissue
Basement membrane, glomerular
   autoantibodies to, glomerulonephritis mediated by, 144
   immune complex deposition in, 143
Basic proteases, effects of, 133
Basophils
   cutaneous, hypersensitivity to, 137
   inflammatory mechanisms caused by, 140
   structure and functions of, 26-28
Basset-beagle crossbreeds, severe combined immunodeficiency syndrome in, 116
Beagle-basset crossbreeds, severe combined immunodeficiency syndrome in, 116
Beagles
   IgA deficiency in, 35
   primary IgA deficiency in, 116
Beta globulin fraction of serum, antibody activity in, 30
Beta inferferon, 5, 43
Binding immunoassays, primary, general amplification schemes used in, 96
Binding phases of antigen-antibody reaction, 77
Binding specificities of plant lectins, 106
Biochemical innate defenses, 3-4
Biologic activities of complement components, 50-52
Biotin for immunoassays and immunocytochemistry, 96
Birds
   disease resistance and MHC in, 59
   herpesvirus in, 125-126
   lymphosarcoma in, 125
   major histocompatibility complex in, 58
   serum immunoglobulin levels in, 36
Black Pied Danish cattle, A45 lethal trait in, 114-115
Blood
   peripheral
      isolation of lymphocytes from, using Ficoll-Hypaque, 100
      purification of mononuclear cells from, 99-100
   transfusions of; *see* Transfusions
Blood group antigens, histocompatibility antigens and, 55-61
Blood group systems, human, 59-60
Blood groups
   bovine, 60
   canine, 60
   caprine, 61
   equine, 60-61
   feline, 61
   ovine, 61
   porcine, 60
   and transfusion, 59-61
Blood typing in dogs, 60
"Blue eye," 147, 148
Blue tongue virus in cattle, vaccine for, 176
BoLA, 57
Bone marrow and lymphocyte development, 13-14
Bone marrow cells; *see* B cells
Bordetella bronchiseptica, vaccine against, 177
Bound and unbound reactants, separation of, 92
Bovine; *see also* Cattle
Bovine and human respiratory syncytial virus, cross-reactivity of, 8
Bovine leukocyte adhesion deficiency, 72-73
Bovine lymphocyte antigen complex, 57
Bovine shipping fever pneumonia, vaccination against, 9

Brittany spaniels, C3 deficiency in, 53
Bronchitis, allergic, canine, 135
Bronchus-associated lymphoid tissue (BALT), 18
Brucella abortus, vaccine against, 177
Brucella abortus infections in cattle
   IgM to identify, 35
   2-mercaptoethanol test to diagnose, 80
   milk-ring test to diagnose, 78-79
   plate or card test to diagnose, 78, 79
Brucella spp., 160
Brucellosis
   in cattle*see* *Brucella abortus* infections in cattle
   canine, glomerulonephritis associated with, 145
   complement fixation test to diagnose, 88
   vaccination against, 171
Bullous pemphigoid, 154
Burnet, McFarland, 62
Bursa of Fabricius as lymphoid organ, 16
Bursal-derived cells; *see* B cells
Bursopoietin, 16

C

C-reactive protein, 52
C-terminal end of immunoglobulin molecule, 30, 31
C1, 45-46, 49
   biologic activities of, 51
C1q, 45-46
C1q-binding assay, 146
C1q protein, 22
C1r, 45, 46
C1s, 45, 46
C2, 46, 49
   deficiency of, 53
C2 protein, 22
C2a, 46
C2b, 46
C3, 46, 49
   deficiency of, 53
      in dogs, 115-116
C3 activator, 49
C3 convertase, 48, 49
C3 protein, 22
C3 shunt system, 49
C3a, 46
   biologic activities of, 51
C3b, 46, 49
C3b inhibitors, 22
C3bBb, 49
C3c, 46
C3d, 46
C4, 46, 49
C4 protein, 22
C4-binding protein, 50
C4a, 46
C4b, 46
C5, 46
   deficiency of, 53
C5 protein, 22
C567, biologic activities of, 51
C5a, 46
   biologic activities of, 51
C5b, 46-47
C5b67 complex, 47
C6, 47
   deficiency of, 53
C7, 47
   deficiency of, 53
C8, 47
   deficiency of, 53

C9, 47
Cachectin, 43
Calicivirus, feline, vaccine for, 176
Campylobacter fetus, vaccine against, 177
Capillary tube precipitation test, 81, 82
Capsid proteins as immunogens, 10
Carcinoembryonic antigen, 11
Card agglutination test, 78, 79
Carriers, 6
Cats
  allergic enteritis in, 135
  allergic gastritis in, 135
  asthma in, 135
  blood groups in, 61
  bullous pemphigoid in, 154
  calicivirus in, vaccine for, 176
  Chédiak-Higashi syndrome in, 75, 117
  complement levels in, 53
  gastrointestinal allergy in, 135
  glomerulonephritis in, 145
  hyperthyroidism in, 153
  immunodeficiency diseases of, 117
  infectious peritonitis virus of, and transmissible
      gastroenteritis virus of swine, cross-reactivity of, 8
  leukemia in
    indirect complement fixation inhibition to diagnose, 89
    indirect fluorescent antibody test for, 95
    lymphocyte blast transformation test to diagnose, 106-107
    vaccine against, 173
  leukemia virus in, 160, 167
    lymphomas induced by, 122-123
    vaccine for, 176
  lymphocyte antigen of, 58
  major histocompatibility complex in, 58
  myasthenia gravis in, 153
  neutrophil dysfunction of, 72
  oncornavirus-associated cell membrane antigen, 122, 167
  panleukopenia in, 160
  panleukopenia virus in, vaccine for, 176
  picornavirus in, complement fixation test to diagnose, 88
  plasma cell of, 25
  plasma cell myelomas in, 120
  rhinotracheitis virus in, vaccine for, 176
  systemic anaphylaxis in, clinical signs of, 135
  vaccines available for, 176, 177
  viremia in, immunofluorescence assays to diagnose, 94
Cattle
  A45 lethal trait in, 114-115
  agammaglobulinemia in, 115
  allergic rhinitis in, 136
  atopy in, 132
  blood groups in, 60
  blue tongue virus in, vaccine for, 176
  Brucella abortus infections in
    IgM to identify, 35
    2-mercaptoethanol test to diagnose, 80
    milk-ring test to diagnose, 78-79
    plate or card test to diagnose, 78, 79
    vaccination against, 171
  coronavirus in, vaccine for, 176
  disease resistance and MHC in, 59
  extrinsic allergic alveolitis in, 147
  glomerulonephritis in, 145
  IgE-mediated disease in, 135-136
  immunodeficiency diseases of, 114-115
  immunoglobulin G deficiency in, 115
  infectious rhinotracheitis in, vaccine for, 176
  leukemia in, MHC and, 59
  leukemia virus in, 123-124

Cattle—cont'd
  leukemia virus in—cont'd
    lymphocyte blast transformation test to diagnose, 106-107
  leukocyte adhesin deficiency in, 72-73, 115
  lymphocyte antigen complex, 57
  lymphocytes of
    FACS analysis of, 24
    infection of, by *Theileria parva*, 121
  lymphomas in, 123-124
  major histocompatibility complex in, 57
  neutrophil dysfunction of, 72
  papilloma virus in, vaccine for, 176
  parainfluenza-3 virus in, vaccine for, 176
  potential applications of cytokines in, 45-46
  rabies in, vaccine for, 176
  reovirus in, vaccine for, 176
  respiratory syncytial virus in, 135
    and human respiratory syncytial virus, cross-reactivity of, 8
  rhinotracheitis, lymphocyte blast transformation test to diagnose, 106-107
  rotavirus in, vaccine for, 176
  serum immunoglobulin levels in, 36
  shipping fever pneumonia in, vaccination against, 9
  systemic anaphylaxis in, clinical signs of, 135
  vaccines available for, 176, 177
  virus diarrhea in, vaccine for, 176
  warts in, vaccine for, 176
CD antigens, 11-12
CD2, 23-24
  natural killer cells expressing, 26
CD3, 23
CD3 complex, antigen recognition and, 63-64
CD4, 23, 24
CD4 molecule, antigen recognition and, 64
CD4+ lymphocytes, histocompatibility restriction and, 58
CD4+ T lymphocyte, antigen recognition and, 62, 63
CD5, 23
CD8, 23, 24
CD8+ lymphocytes, histocompatibility restriction and, 58
CD21, 25
CD23, 36
CD25, 23
CD40, 25
Cell membrane antigen, oncornavirus-associated, feline, 122
Cell monolayer/tissue section absorption to separate bound and unbound reactants, 92
Cells; *see also* specific cells
  antigen-presenting, 62-63
    interaction of T cells and, 63
  B, 12
  immune system, 19-28
  involved in innate immunity, 4-5
  Kupffer's, 5
  lymphoid, interaction of microbes with, 160-161
  M, 18
  mammalian, antigens on, 10-12
  mast, inflammatory mechanisms caused by, 140
  mononuclear
    isolation of, 100-101
    from peripheral blood, purification of, 99-100
    separation of
      by immunologic method, 102-103
      by physical methods, 101-102
    structure and functions of, 20-21
  nurse, 16
  phagocytic, 19-22

Cells—cont'd
  T, 12
    helper, 12
    interaction of antigen-presenting cells and, 63
    suppressor, loss of, autoimmune reactions and, 151
Cellular adhesions, 72-73
Cellular cytotoxicity, lymphocyte-mediated, mechanisms of, 109
Cellular origin of antibody, 30
Cellular populations, mixed or purified, assays for lymphocyte functions in, 103-109
Central lymphoid organs, development of, 13-16
CH_1 domain, 33
CH_2 domain, 33
CH_3 domain, 33
CH_{50} method of complement titration, 53
CH_{100} method of complement titration, 53
CH50 assay, 75
Charge of immunogens, 6
Chemical defenses in gastrointestinal tract, 4
Chemiluminescence, neutrophil, 73, 74
Chemotactic factor(s)
  of complement, biologic activities of, 51
  for eosinophils, effects of, 133
  for neutrophils, effects of, 133
  produced by lymphocytes, 45
Chemotaxis, 73
Cheviot lambs, immune complex disease in, 146
Chickens; see also Birds
  lymphoid tissues in, 18-19
  lymphosarcoma in, 125
  Marek's disease in; see Marek's disease
  primary immunodeficiency disorder in, 117
Chlamydia, vaccine against, 177
Chondroitin sulfate, effects of, on basophils, 133
Chronic granulomatous disease, 73
Chronic obstructive pulmonary disease, equine, 136, 137-138
Chédiak-Higashi syndrome, 117
  in cats, 75
  neutrophil dysfunction in, 72
Circulating immune complexes, detection of, 146
Circulation, lymphocyte, 28-29
Clonal deletion, 6
Clonal expansion, 62
Clonal selection hypothesis, 37, 62
Clostridium chauvoei, vaccine against, 177
Clostridium novyi, vaccine against, 177
Clostridium perfringens, vaccine against, 177
Clostridium septicum, vaccine against, 177
Clostridium sordellii, vaccine against, 177
Clostridium tetani, 162
  vaccine against, 177
Cluster of differentiation terminology, 23
Clusters of differentiation antigens, 11-12
Coccidioidomycosis, 160
Coggin's test, 36
  for equine infectious anemia, 83
Colony-stimulating factors, 44
Colostrum, maternal immunoglobulins via, 169
Combined immunodeficiency disease of Arabian horses, 113-114
Combined immunodeficiency syndrome, severe, in dogs, 116
Complement, 71-75, 86
  components of, biologic activities of, 50-52
  defense against bacteria and, 52
  defense against viruses and, 52-53
  deficiency of, inherited, 53
  evaluation of, 75

Complement—cont'd
  immune responses and, 52-53
  inflammatory mechanisms caused by, 140
  as innate defense mechanism, 5
  levels of, in domestic animals, 53
  nomenclature for, 45
  third component of, deficiency of, in dogs, 115-116
  titration of, 86, 87
    general methods of, 53
  type II hypersensitivity and, 129
Complement activation
  alternate pathway of, 49-50
  other control mechanisms in, 50
  regulators of, 50
  soluble and membrane-bound inhibitors of, 50
Complement activation sequence, classical, 45-49
Complement fixation inhibition test, indirect, 89
Complement fixation tests, 77, 86-89
Complement fragments with biologic activities, 50-52
Complement reaction, 45-49
Complement receptor type 1, 50
  biologic activities of, 51
Complement receptor type 2, 50
  biologic activities of, 52
Complement receptor type 3, biologic activities of, 52
Complement receptor type 4, biologic activities of, 52
Complement receptors, 51-52
Complement system, 47-54
Complete antigens, 7
Complexity of immunogens, 6
Concanavalin A, binding specificity of, 106
Conformational epitopes, 7-8
Connective tissue, mast cells in, 27
Contagious ecythma; see Ecythma
Continuous epitopes, 7-8
Coombs' agglutination test, 79-80
Coombs antiglobulin test, direct, 151
Coombs positive autoimmune hemolytic anemia, 151-152
Coombs' reagent, 79, 80
Coronavirus
  bovine, vaccine for, 176
  cross-reactivity of, 8
Corpuscles, Hassall's, 14
Corynebacterium tuberculosis infection in sheep, abscess after, MHC and, 59
Cough reflex to remove foreign material, 4
CR1, 25
CR2, 25
Cross-reaction with environmental antigens, autoimmune reactions and, 150
Cross-reactivity, 8, 9
Cryopathic immune mediated hemolytic anemia, 151
Culicoides gnat, hypersensitivity to, 136
Culture test, mixed leukocyte, 107
Cutaneous anaphylaxis test, passive, 130
Cutaneous basophil hypersensitivity, 137
Cutaneous histiocytoma, canine, 126
Cyclic neutropenia, 72, 74-75
  canine, 117
Cystitis, treatment of, 4
Cytokine synthesis inhibitory factor, 43
Cytokines, 40-46
  biologic properties of, 40
  major, 41
  nomenclature for, 45
  potential applications of, in veterinary medicine, 45-46
  T-cell-derived, T-cell differentiation and, 64-65
  therapy with, 45
Cytotoxic antibody reactions, 136

Cytotoxic T-cell assay, 108-109
Cytotoxic T-cell responses to tumors, 10-11
Cytotoxicity
  antibody-dependent, 136, 137
  antibody-directed cellular, 109
  cellular, lymphocyte-mediated, mechanisms of, 109
  lymphocyte-mediated, analogous mechanisms between membrane attack and, 49
  NK-cell-mediated, 26
  T-cell, immune response and, 66
Cytotoxicity assays, target cell, 108
Cytotysin, 49

D

Dalmatian dogs, atopy in, 132
Deficiency
  adhesin, leukocyte
    bovine, 115
    canine, 117
  immune, 52
  immunoglobulin A, selective, in dogs, 116
  immunoglobulin G
    bovine, 115
    in sheep, 115
  immunoglobulin M, selective, of horses, 114
  of third component of complement in dogs, 115-116
Degradability of immunogens, 6
Delayed-type hypersensitivity reactions, features of, 45
Deletion, clonal, 6
Demodectic mange, lymphocyte blast transformation test to diagnose, 106-107
Dendritic macrophages, 20-21
Deoxyribonucleic acid
  genetically engineered vaccine products using, 173-174
  recombination of, during B-cell differentiation, 37
Dermatitis
  allergic, canine, 134-135
  allergic inhalant, in dogs, 134
  flea allergy, canine, 137
  immunologically mediated, 148
Dermatologic immune-mediated disorders, 154-155
Diabetes mellitus, 146-147, 153-154
Diagnostic reagents, haptens as, 7
Diarrhea
  bovine virus, vaccine for, 176
  as means to eliminate toxins and pathogens, 4
DiGeorge syndrome in humans, thymosin for, 16
Dilution
  of antibody yielding positive reaction, last, reciprocal of, 76-77
  optimal, 76
Dinitrophenol for immunoassays and immunocyto chemistry, 96
Direct Coombs' agglutination test, 79
Direct Coombs antiglobulin test, 151
Direct immunofluorescence assays, 92-94
Direct skin test for allergen-specific IgE, 130
Dirofilaria immitis, antigens of, 10
Dirofilaria immitis infection
  in dogs, 136
  glomerulonephritis associated with, 145
Discoid lupus, 155
Discontinuous epitopes, 7-8
Disease(s)
  Addison's, 154
  autoimmune, organ-specific, 151-156
  autoimmune type II, 136
  granulomatous, chronic, 73
  Graves', 153

Disease(s)—cont'd
  hemolytic, of newborn pigs, 61
  IgE-mediated
    bovine, 135-136
    equine, 136
  immune complex, 139-149; *see also* Immune complex diseases
  immune-mediated, immunologic mechanisms in, 129-138
  immunodeficiency; *see* Immunodeficiency diseases
  infectious; *see* Infectious diseases
  Johne's, complement fixation test to diagnose, 88
  Marek's, 121, 125
    MHC and, 59
  neoplastic, of lymphoreticular system, 117-118
  Newcastle, 160
  parasitic, IgE-mediated reactions in, 136
  pemphigus, 154
  pulmonary, chronic obstructive, equine, 136, 137-138
  resistance to, MHC and, 59
Distemper, canine
  complement fixation test to diagnose, 88
  IgG and IgM to test for, 35
  lymphocyte blast transformation test to diagnose, 106-107
  vaccination against, 171, 175, 176
Distemper virus, canine, 160
Distemper virus infection, canine, 163-166
Disulfide bonds of immunoglobulin molecule, 32-33
DLA, 57
DNA; *see* Deoxyribonucleic acid
Dogs
  allergenic pneumonitis in, 135
  allergic bronchitis in, 135
  allergic dermatitis in, 134-135
  allergic enteritis in, 135
  allergic gastritis in, 135
  allergic inhalant dermatitis in, 134
  allergic rhinitis in, 135
  atopy in, 132
  blood groups in, 60
  blood typing in, 60
  brucellosis in, glomerulonephritis associated with, 145
  bullous pemphigoid in, 154
  C3 deficiency in, 53, 115-116
  cutaneous mast cell tumor, 28
  complement levels in, 53
  cutaneous basophil hypersensitivity in, 137
  cutaneous histiocytoma in, 126
  cyclic neutropenia in, 72, 74-75, 117
  distemper in; *see* Distemper, canine
  distemper virus in, 160
  distemper virus infection in, 163-166
  flea allergy dermatitis in, 137
  gastrointestinal allergy in, 135
  glomerulonephritis in, 144-145
  granulocytopathy syndrome in, 117
  heartworm infection in, 136
  hepatitis in, complement fixation test to diagnose, 88
  hyperthyroidism in, 153
  IgA deficiency in, 35
  immunodeficiency diseases of, 115-117
  immunodeficient dwarfism in, 116
  infectious hepatitis in
    anterior uveitis associated with, 147-148
    vaccination against, 171, 176
  leukocyte adhesin deficiency in, 117
  leukocyte antigen system of, 57
  lymphoma in, 124-125
  major histocompatibility complex in, 57
  malignant histiocytosis in, 126

Dogs—cont'd
    myasthenia gravis in, 153
    nematode parasites in, 166
    neutrophil dysfunction of, 72
    neutrophil function defect in, 117
    NK cells of, 27
    parainfluenza virus in, vaccine for, 176
    parvovirus in, vaccine for, 176
    phytohemagglutinin-P-stimulated lymphocyte culture in, 105
    plasma cell myelomas in, 119-120
    polymyositis in, 153
    rabies in, vaccine for, 176
    respiratory allergy in, 135
    selective IgA deficiency in, 116
    serum immunoglobulin levels in, 36
    severe combined immunodeficiency syndrome in, 116
    systemic anaphylaxis in, clinical signs of, 135
    T-cell leukemia in, 124
    thyroiditis in, 153
    transmissible venereal sarcoma in, 126
    undefined immunodeficiency syndromes iln, 117
    vaccines available for, 176, 177
Domains, 32-33
    biologic activities of, 33
    in immunoglobulin superfamily, 37
Domestic animals
    complement levels in, 53
    immune complex glomerulonephritis in, 144-146
    lymphomas in, 122-123
Drugs, autoimmune reactions and, 151
Dwarfism, immunodeficient, canine, 116
Dyes, aniline, to label proteins, 90, 91

E
Eastern equine encephalomyelitis, vaccine for, 176
Ecisonoids, 133
Ecthyma, contagious, in sheep, vaccine for, 171, 176
Edema, angioneurotic, 50, 53
Effector cells of anaphylaxis, 26-28
Effector phase of immune response, 66-67
ELA, 58
Encephalomyelitis, equine, vaccine for, 176
Encephalopathy, mink, 161
Endocrine system, autoimmune diseases of, 153
Endocytosis of antigen, 63
Endonucleases, vaccine products utilizing, 173
Enteritis, allergic, canine and feline, 135
Environment, antigens in, 8-10
Environmental antigens, cross-reaction with, autoimmune reactions and, 150
Enzyme-linked immunosorbent assay, 94-96, 97, 130, 132
Enzymes
    to label proteins, 91-92
    proteolytic, as chemical defense, 4
Eosinophilia, 28
Eosinophils
    chemotactic factor for, effects of, 133
    horse, 29
    proteins in, 28
    structure and functions of, 28
Epitope mapping, 12
Epitopes, 7
    accessibility of, 7
    agretope vs, 12
    B-cell, 12
    and immunogenicity in synthesizing vaccines, 12
    protein, 7-8
        antibody response to, 8

Epitopes—cont'd
    shared, 8, 9
    T-cell, 12
Epstein-Barr herpesvirus infection, 121
Erysipelothrix rhusiopathiae, vaccine against, 177
Erythrocyte antigens, 11
Erythrocytes
    in bone marrow, 13
    sensitized, in complement titration, 53
Erythropoietin, 40, 44
Escherichia coli
    indigenous, 4
    vaccine against, 177
Extrinsic allergic alveolitis, bovine, 147

F
F antigen, 9
Fab, 32
F(ab)$_2$, 32
Fabricius, bursa of, as lymphoid organ, 16
FACS analysis of bovine lymphocytes, 24
FACSCAN, 24
Factor B, 22
    in complement activation, 49
Factor D, 22
    in complement activation, 49
Factor H in complement activation, 49, 50
Failure of passive transfer of maternal immunoglobulin, 169
Farmer's lung disease, 147
Fc, 32
Fc', 32
Ferritin to label proteins, 91
Ficoll-Hypaque
    to isolate lymphocytes from peripheral blood using, 100
    to isolate mononuclear cells, 100-101
50% method of complement titration, 53
Fixation, complement, tests for, 86-89
Fixed macrophages, 5
FLA, 58
Flea allergy dermatitis, canine, 137
Flora
    of gastrointestinal tract, normal, 4
    of skin, normal, 3-4
Fluorescence-activated cell sorter, 102
FOCMA antigen, 167
"Fog fever," 147
Formalin-fixed tissues, immunofluorescence assays in, 94
Forssman antigen, 11

G
GALT; *see* Gut-associated lymphoid tissue
Gamma globulin fraction of serum, antibody activity in, 30
Gamma interferon, 41, 43-44
    macrophage activation and, 66-67
Gastritis, allergic, canine and feline, 135
Gastroenteritis, transmissible, in swine, 163
    vaccine for, 176
Gastrointestinal allergy, canine and feline, 135
Gastrointestinal nematode parasites and mucosal immunity, 166
Gastrointestinal tract
    barrier function of, 4
    normal flora of, 4
    role of, in innate immunity, 4
Gel precipitation test, 81-82
Gene, immune response, 59
Genetically engineered vaccine products, 173-174
German measles, 160
German shepherds, IgA deficiency in, 35, 116

GLA, 57
Gland, thyroid, autoimmune diseases of, 153
Glomerular basement membrane
  autoantibodies to, glomerulonephritis mediated by, 144
  immune complex deposition in, 143
Glomerular filtration apparatus, renal, 142, 143
Glomeruli, renal, immune complexes in, detection of, 146-147
Glomerulonephritis
  bovine, 145
  canine, 144-145
  equine, 145
  feline, 145
  immune complex
    diagnosis of, 146
    in domestic animals, 144-146
  mediated by autoantibodies to glomerular basement membrane, 144
  mediated by immune mechanisms, 142-144
  ovine, 146
  porcine, 146
Gluteraldehyde-fixed tissues, immunofluorescence assays in, 94
Gnat, Culicoides, hypersensitivity to, 136
Goats
  blood groups in, 61
  complement levels in, 53
  lymphocyte antigen in, 57
  major histocompatibility complex in, 57
Graft-versus-host reaction, 104
Grafting, tissue, antigens and, 10
Granulocyte macrophage-colony stimulating factor, 40, 44
Granulocyte-colony stimulating factor, 40, 44
Granulocytes in bone marrow, 13
Granulocytopathy syndrome, canine, 117
Granulomatous disease, chronic, 73
Graves' disease, 153
Growth factor, pre-B-cell, 42
Guinea pig
  alternate pathway of complement activation in, 49-50
  complement deficiencies in, 53
  complement levels in, 53
Gut-associated lymphoid tissue, 16

H

H antigen, 9, 11
H-2 complex in mice, 55
Habronemiasis, 29
Haemophilus pleumopneumoniae, vaccine against, 177
Haemophilus somnus, vaccine against, 177
Haplotypes, definition of, 55
Hapten, 6, 7
Hardy test, 94
Hashimoto's thyroiditis, 153
Hassall's corpuscles, 14
Heartworm infection in dogs, 136
  glomerulonephritis associated with, 145
Heaves, equine, 136, 137-138, 147
Heavy chains, 30, 31, 32
Helix pomatia, binding specificity of, 106
Helminth infections, 166
Helper T cells, 12, 22-23
  types of, 42
Hemagglutinin of Influenzavirus, immune response caused by, 10
Hemal lymph nodes in ruminants, 19
Hematopoietic system, autoimmune diseases of, 151-153
Hemolytic anemia
  autoimmune, 151
    Coombs positive, 151-152

Hemolytic anemia—cont'd
  cryopathic immune mediated, 151
Hemolytic disease of newbown pigs, 61
Heparin, effects of, on mast cells, 133
Hepatitis, canine
  complement fixation test to diagnose, 88
  infectious
    anterior uveitis associated with, 147-148
    vaccination against, 171, 176
Herpesvirus(es), 121
  equine, 160
  in turkeys, 125-126
Herpesvirus-induced lymphomas, 125-126
Heterotypic vaccines, 176
Histamine, effects of, 133
Histiocytes, macrophages becoming, 20
Histiocytoma, cutaneous, canine, 126
Histiocytosis
  malignant, 126
  systemic, 126
Histocompatibility antigens, 55
  and blood group antigens, 55-61
  major, allografts and, 10
Histocompatibility complex, major; *see* Major histocompatibility complex
Histocompatibility restriction, 58
Histopaque to isolate mononuclear cells, 100-101
Histoplasmosis, 160
Hives in horses, 136
Holstein cows, atopy in, 132
Homotypic vaccines, 176
Horses
  blood groups in, 60-61
  bullous pemphigoid in, 154
  complement levels in, 53
  disease resistance and MHC in, 59
  encephalomyelitis in, vaccine for, 176
  eosinophil collection in, 29
  glomerulonephritis in, 145
  heaves in, 136, 137-138, 147
  herpesvirus infection in, 160
  IgE-mediated disease in, 136
  immunodeficiency diseases of, 113-114
  infectious anemia in, 145, 161, 166-167
    Coggins' test for, 83
  infectious anemia virus infection in, IgG(T) levels in, 36
  influenza in, vaccine for, 176
  lymphocyte antigen in, 58
  major histocompatibility complex in, 58
  neonatal isoerythrolysis in, 136
  plasma cell myelomas in, 120
  primary agammaglobulinemia in, 114
  queens itch in, 136
  rhinopneumonitis in, vaccine for, 176
  selective immunoglobulin M deficiency of, 114
  serum immunoglobulin levels in, 36
  strangles in, cross-reactivity in, 8
  systemic anaphylaxis in, clinical signs of, 135
  transient hypogammaglobulinemia in, 114
  vaccines available for, 176, 177
H-thymidine incorporation to assess T-lymphocyte function, 105
Human immunodeficiency virus, 160-161
Humans
  blood group systems of, 59-60
  complement levels in, 53
  IgA deficiency in, 35
  leukocyte antigen complex in, 55

Humans—cont'd
  respiratory syncytial virus in, and bovine respiratory syncytial virus, cross-reactivity of, 8
  serum immunoglobulin levels in, 36
  systemic anaphylaxis in, clinical signs of, 135
Humoral immunity, assays for, 76-98
Humoral response, immune response and, 67
Hybridoma, 37, 38
Hypersensitivity, 129
  to Culicoides gnat, 136
  cutaneous basophil, 137
  type I, 129, 131
    clinical syndrome of, 133-136
    late-phase allergic reactions in, 133
  type II, 129, 131, 136
  type III, 129-130, 131, 139
  type IV, 130, 131
Hypersensitivity pneumonitis, 147
Hypersensitivity reactions
  delayed-type, features of, 45
  mechanisms of, 129-130
  type II, from incompatible blood transfusions, 59
Hyperthyroidism, 153
Hypoadrenalcortism, 154
Hypogammaglobulinemia, transient, equine, 114
Hyposensitization therapy for dogs, 135

I

ICAM-1, 29
Identification methods for T lymphocyte function, in vivo, 99
Identity, partial, precipitin lines of, 83
Idiopathic nondeforming arthritis, 152
Idiotype, 175
Idiotypic variation in immunoglobulin structure, 31
IgA; *see* Immunoglobulin A
IgD; *see* Immunoglobulin D
IgE; *see* Immunoglobulin E
IgG(T) in horses, 36
IgG; *see* Immunoglobulin G
IgM; *see* Immunoglobulin M
IL; *see* Interleukin
Immune complex diseases, 139-149
  detection or diagnosis of, 146
  inflammatory mechanisms identified for, 140
  other clinical forms of, 147-148
  pathologic mechanism of tissue damage induced by, 139-141
  systemic, 141-142
Immune complex glomerulonephritis in domestic animals, 144-146
  diagnosis of, 146
Immune complexes
  circulating, detection of, 146
  deposition of, in glomerular basement membrane, 143
  in renal glomeruli, detection of, 146-147
  type III hypersensitivity and, 129-130
Immune defenses, innate, assays for, 71-75
Immune deficiency, 52
Immune function, methods to evaluate, 69-110
Immune mechanisms, glomerulonephritis mediated by, 142-144
Immune-mediated arthritides, 152-153
Immune-mediated disease, immunologic mechanisms in, 129-138
Immune-mediated hemolytic anemia, cryopathic, 151
Immune response, 62-67
  caused by hemagglutinin of influenzavirus, 10
  complement and, 52-53
  effector phase of, 66-67

Immune response—cont'd
  and infectious disease, 159-168
    general characteristics of, 161-162
  primary, 62
  secondary, 62
  soluble factors of, 40-46
Immune response gene, 59
Immune system
  cells of, 19-28
  interaction of microbes with, 160-162
Immunity
  acquired, and innate immunity, interactions of, 5
  active, 170-175
  examples of, 162-167
  humoral, assays for, 76-98
  innate; *see* Innate immunity
  mucosal, gastrointestinal nematode parasites and, 166
  passive, 169-170
Immunoassay
  binding, primary, general amplification schemes used in, 96
  reagents for, 96
Immunocytochemistry, reagents for, 96
Immunodeficiencies, inherited, 113-128
Immunodeficiency diseases
  bovine, 114-115
  canine, 115-117
  equine, 113-114
  feline, 117
  ovine, 115
  primary, in veterinary medicine, 113-118
    miscellaneous, 117
Immunodeficiency states, thymosin for, 16
Immunodeficiency syndrome
  acquired, 160
  canine, undefined, 117
  severe combined, in dogs, 116
  simian, 160
Immunodeficiency virus, human, 160-161
Immunodeficient dwarfism, canine, 116
Immunodiffusion
  Ouchterlony two-dimension, in gel test, 82
  radial, 85
Immunoelectrophoresis, 84-85
  rocket, 85-86
Immunofluorescence assays, 92-94
Immunogenicity
  characteristics determining, 6
  definition of, 6
  in synthesizing vaccines, epitopes and, 12
Immunogens; *see also* Antigens
  antigens and, 6-12
  capsid proteins as, 10
  effective, characteristics of, 6
  synthetic, 174-175
  vaccine, anti-idiotypes as, 175
Immunoglobulin A, 18, 30; *see also* Immunoglobulins
  biologic properties of, 34
  characteristics of, 35
  in colostrum and milk, 36
  deficiency of
    in dogs, 35, 116
    in humans, 35
  physicochemical properties of, 34
  structural features of, 33
Immunoglobulin D, 30; *see also* Immunoglobulins
  characteristics of, 35
Immunoglobulin E, 30; *see also* Immunoglobulins
  allergen-specific, direct skin test for, 130

Immunoglobulin E—cont'd
  biologic properties of, 34
  characteristics of, 34-35
  physicochemical properties of, 34
  production of, regulation of, 132
  structural features of, 33
  type I hypersensitivity and, 129, 130-132
Immunoglobulin E antibodies
  other antigens producing, 10
  production of, by parasitic antigens, 10
Immunoglobulin E-mediated disease
  bovine, 135-136
  equine, 136
Immunoglobulin E-mediated reaction, 132
  in parasitic disease, 136
Immunoglobulin G, 30; *see also* Immunoglobulins
  biologic properties of, 34
  characteristics of, 34
  in colostrum and milk, 36
  deficiency of
    bovine, 115
    in sheep, 115
  physicochemical properties of, 34
  structural features of, 33
  structure of, 31, 32
  to test for canine distemper, 35
  type II hypersensitivity and, 129
Immunoglobulin G1 in bovine colostrum, 36
Immunoglobulin M, 30; *see also* Immunoglobulins
  biologic properties of, 34
  characteristics of, 34-35
  in colostrum and milk, 36
  deficiency of, in horses, selective, 114
  identification of cattle infected with *Brucella abortus* using, 35
  physicochemical properties of, 34
  structural features of, 33
  to test for canine distemper, 35
  type II hypersensitivity and, 129
Immunoglobulin M response to antigens, 12
Immunoglobulins, 30-39; *see also* Antibody(ies)
  biologic properties of, 34
  classes of, 30
    characteristics of, 33-36
  in colostrum and milk, 36
  domestic animal, 36
    subclasses and nomenclature in, 34
  levels of, in piglets, 36
  maternal, passive transfer of, failure of, 169
  maternal transport to newborn, 169
  physicochemical properties of, 34
  secretory; *see* Immunoglobulin A
  structural features of, 30-33
  structure of, 30, 31
    in domains, 33
    variations in, 30-31
  subclasses of, 30
  superfamily of, 37
  thyroid stimulating, 153
Immunologic assays, secondary, 77
Immunologic defenses, methods of avoiding, 161
Immunologic mechanisms
  in immune-mediated disease, 129-138
  mixed, in hypersensitivity disorders, 136-138
Immunologic method to separate mononuclear cells, 102-103
Immunologically mediated dermatitis, 148
Immunology, principles of, 1-67
Immunomodulators, vaccines, and vaccination, 169-177
Immunopathology, 111-156

Immunoprophylaxis, principles of, 157-177
Immunosuppression, viral-induced, 160
In vitro assessment of T-lymphocyte function, 104-107
In vivo evaluation of T-lymphocyte function, 103-104
In vivo identification methods for T lymphocyte function, 99
Inactivated viral vaccines, 170
Incompatibility with blood transfusions, 59
Incomplete antigens, 7
Indirect complement fixation inhibition test, 89
Indirect Coombs' agglutination test, 80
Indirect immunofluorescence antibody tests, for feline leukemia, 95
Indirect immunofluorescence assays, 92-94
Infection
  of bovine lymphocytes by *Theileria parva*, 121
  Brucella abortus; see *Brucella abortus* infections
  canine distemper; *see* Distemper, canine
  heartworm, in dogs, 136
    glomerulonephritis associated with, 145
  herpesvirus, equine, 160
  leukemia virus, in mice, 125
  local, 159
  measles virus, lymphocyte blast transformation test to diagnose, 106-107
  Ostertagia, in sheep, 136
  respiratory syncytial virus, bovine, 135
  systemic, 159
Infectious anemia, equine, 145, 161, 166-167
  Coggins' test for, 83
Infectious bovine rhinotracheitis virus, vaccine for, 176
Infectious canine hepatitis
  anterior uveitis associated with, 147-148
  vaccination against, 171, 176
Infectious diseases
  general characteristics of, 159-162
  immune response and, 159-168
    general characteristics of, 161-162
Influenza, equine, vaccine for, 176
Influenzavirus, hemagglutinin of, immune response caused by, 10
Inhalant dermatitis, allergic, in dogs, 134
Inherited complement deficiencies, 53
Inherited immunodeficiencies, myelomas, and lymphomas, 113-128
Innate immune defenses, assays for, 71-75
Innate immunity, 3-5
  and acquired immunity, interactions of, 5
  cells involved in, 4-5
  complement and, 5
  macrophages and, 5
  molecules mediating, 5
  neutrophils and, 4-5
  system related, 3-4
Integrins, 29
Interferon
  alpha, 43
  beta, 43
  gamma, 41, 43-44
    macrophage activation and, 66-67
Interferons, 5, 43-44
Interleukin, 40-43
Interleukin 1, 21, 40, 41
  to assess monocyte function, 108
  biologic properties of, 41
Interleukin 2, 41-42
Interleukin 2 assay for lymphocyte function, 107
Interleukin 3, 41, 42, 44
Interleukin 4, 41, 42
Interleukin 5, 40, 41, 42

Interleukin 6, 40, 41, 42
Interleukin 7, 41, 42, 44
Interleukin 8, 41, 42
Interleukin 9, 41, 42-43
Interleukin 10, 41, 43
Intracellular adhesin molecule-1, 29
Intradermal skin test, 103
Irish setter
 granulocytopathy syndrome in, 117
 leukocyte adhesin deficiency in, 117
Isoerythrolysis, neonatal
 in cattle, 60
 in horses, 60-61, 136
Isotypic variation in immunoglobulin structure, 30-31
Itch, queens, 136

J

J chain
 in immunoglobulin A, 35
 in immunoglobulin M, 34
J substance in cattle, 60
Jenner, Edward, 3
Jersey cows, milk allergy in, 135
Johne's disease, complement fixation test to diagnose, 88

K

Kappa chains, 30
Kauffman-White classification system of Salmonella, 9
Kidney involvement in systemic lupus erythematosus, 141
Killing defects, 73-75
Kunkel, Henry, 175
Kupffer's cells, 5
Kuru, 161

L

Labeling reagents for primary serologic assays, 90-92
Lactobacilli, vaginal, as defense mechanism, 4
Lactoferrin as chemical defense, 4
Lactoperoxidase as chemical defense, 4
Lambda chains, 30
Langhan's cells, macrophages becoming, 20
Large granular lymphocytes, 22
Late-phase allergic reactions in type I hypersensitivity, 133
Lazy leukocyte syndrome, 73
Lectins
 for immunoassays and immunocytochemistry, 96
 plant, binding specificities of, 106
Leishmaniasis, 160
Lentil lectin, binding specificity of, 106
Leptospira canicola, vaccine against, 177
Leptospira grippotyphosa, vaccine against, 177
Leptospira hardjo, vaccine against, 177
Leptospira icterohaemmoragiae, vaccine against, 177
Leptospira pomona, vaccine against, 177
Leptospirosis
 complement fixation test to diagnose, 88
 vaccine against, 177
Leukemia
 bovine, MHC and, 59
 feline
  indirect complement fixation inhibition to diagnose, 89
  indirect fluorescent antibody test for, 95
  lymphocyte blast transformation test to diagnose, 106-107
  vaccine against, 173
 T-cell, in dogs, 124
Leukemia virus
 bovine, 123-124
  lymphocyte blast transformation test to diagnose, 106-107

Leukemia virus—cont'd
 feline, 160, 167
  lymphomas induced by, 122-123
  vaccine for, 176
Leukemia virus infection, murine, 125
Leukocell, 123, 173
Leukocell 2, 173
Leukocyte adhesin deficiency
 bovine, 115
 canine, 117
Leukocyte adhesion deficiency, 72-73
Leukocyte antigen complex, human, 55
Leukocyte antigen system, dog, 57
Leukocyte culture test, mixed, 107
Leukocytes
 antigen-specific, isolation of, 102
 as antigens, 11-12
 chemotactic ability of, 73
 phagocytosis and, 73
 polymorphonuclear; *see* Neutrophils
Leukosis, lymphatic, in chickens, 125
Leukotriene C4, 133
Leukotriene D4, 133
Leukotriene E4, 133
LFA-1, 29
Light chains, 30, 31, 32
Limulus polyphemus, binding specificity of, 106
Linear epitopes, 7-8
Lines of nonidentity, 82, 83
Local infections, 159
Long-acting thyroid stimulator, 153
L-selectin, 29
Lupus, discoid, 155
"Lupus band," 155
Lupus erythematosus, systemic, 141, 148, 155
Lymph nodes
 hemal, in ruminants, 19
 structure of
  and function of, 16-17
  of pig, 19
Lymphatic leukosis in chickens, 125
Lymphocyte antigen
 equine, 58
 feline, 58
 goat, 57
 ovine, 57
Lymphocyte antigen complex, bovine, 57
Lymphocyte blast transformation test, 106
Lymphocyte function-associated antigen, 29
Lymphocyte functions, assays for, in mixed or purified cellular populations, 103-109
Lymphocyte glycoprotein alloantigens (Lyt), 22, 23
Lymphocyte reactions, mixed, 107
Lymphocyte-mediated cellular toxicity, mechanisms of, 109
Lymphocyte-mediated cytotoxicity, analogous mechanisms between membrane attack complex and, 49
Lymphocytes
 activation of, 65-66
 antigen-specific reactions of, in vitro, 107
 B
  activated, products of, 30-39
  antigen presentation and, 63
  antigen recognition and presentation and, 64-65
  assays for, 103
  pokeweed mitogen-induced, 25
 in bone marrow, 13
 bovine, FACS analysis of, 24
 chemotactic factors produced by, 45
 circulation of, 28-29

Lymphocytes—cont'd
  culture of, phytohemagglutinin-P-stimulated canine, 105
  development of, 13-19
  functions of, 13
  interleukin 2 assay for, 107
  isolation of, from peripheral blood using Ficoll-Hypaque, 100
  large granular, 22
  in lymph nodes, 16
  in spleen, 17
  structure and functions of, 22-26
  T; *see* T lymphocytes
  thymic, 14-15
Lymphoid cells, interaction of microbes with, 160-161
Lymphoid nodules, 18
Lymphoid organs
  central, development of, 13-16
  peripheral, 16-18
Lymphoid system, 13-29
  development of, 13-19
Lymphoid tissue(s)
  bronchus-associated, 18
  gut-associated, 16
  species variation in structure of, 18-19
Lymphokines, 40
  assessment of T-lymphocyte function using, 107
  functions of, 41
  and intradermal skin tests, 103
Lymphoma(s), 120-126
  canine, 124-125
  in domestic animals, 122-123
  herpesvirus-induced, 125-126
  induced by feline leukemia virus, 122-123
  inherited, 113-128
  retrovirus viral, simian, 125
Lymphomatosis, visceral, in chickens, 125
Lymphopore, 49
Lymphoprep to isolate mononuclear cells, 100-101
Lymphoreticular neoplasms, 117-118
Lymphoreticular system, neoplastic diseases of, 117-118
Lymphosarcomas, 120-126
  associated with feline leukemia virus, 122-123
  avian, 125
  canine, 124-125
  porcine, 124
  thymic, 123
Lymphotoxin, 45
Lysozyme as chemical defense, 4

M

M cells, 18
Macrophage inhibition factor, 21, 41, 44
Macrophage-activating factor, 21
Macrophage-colony stimulating factor, 40, 44
Macrophages
  activation of, in immune response, 66-67
  alveolar, as defense mechanism, 4
  antigen presentation and, 63
  as antigen-presenting cell, 20, 21-22
  functions of, 5, 13
  innate immunity and, 5
  monocyte
    natural history of, 71
    phagocyte function of, 71
  structure and functions of, 20-21
  subsets of, 13
  types of, 20
Major histocompatibility antigens
  allografts and, 10
  class I, 10

Major histocompatibility antigens—cont'd
  class II, 10
  function of, 58-59
Major histocompatibility complex, 55-59
  alleles of, 55
  antigen recognition and, 62
  avian, 58
  bovine, 57
  canine, 57
  Class I molecules of, 55, 56
    characteristics of antigens produced by, 58
  class II, association with autoimmune disease and, 155-156
  Class II molecules of, 55, 56
    characteristics of antigens produced by, 58
  disease resistance and, 59
  in domestic animal species, 57-58
  equine, 58
  feline, 58
  goat, 57
  ovine, 57
  polymorphism of, detection of, 56-57
  porcine, 58
  protein products of, 55
Malaria, 160
Malignant histiocytosis, 126
Malignant lymphomas; *see* Lymphomas
Mammalian cells, antigens on, 10-12
Mammary gland, defense mechanisms of, 4
Mange, demodectic, lymphocyte blast transformation test to diagnose, 106-107
Marek's disease in chickens, 121, 125
  MHC and, 59
Marrow, bone, and lymphocyte development, 13-14
Mast cells
  inflammatory mechanisms caused by, 140
  structure and functions of, 26-28
  tumor of, canine, 28
Mastitis in cattle, MHC and, 59
Maternal immunoglobulin, passive transfer of, failure of, 169
Measles, German, 160
Measles virus infection, lymphocyte blast transformation test to diagnose, 106-107
Medullary macrophages, 20
Membrane, basement, glomerular
  autoantibodies to, glomerulonephritis mediated by, 144
  immune complex deposition in, 143
Membrane attack complex, 46-47
  analogous mechanisms between lymphocyte-mediated cytotoxicity and, 49
Membrane attack protein, 49
Membrane-bound inhibitors of complement activation, 50
Membrane cofactor protein, 50
2-Mercaptoethanol test, 80
Mice
  complement deficiencies in, 53
  complement levels in, 53
  H-2 complex in, 55
  leukemia virus infection in, 125
  plasma cell tumors in, 119
Microbes, interaction of, with immune system, 160-162
Milk allergy, bovine, 135
Milk-ring agglutination test, 78-79
Mink
  encephalopathy in, 161
  neutrophil dysfunction of, 72
Mitogen, pokeweed, binding specificity of, 106
Mixed cellular populations, assays for lymphocyte functions in, 103-109

Mixed immunologic mechanism in hypersensitivity disorders, 136-138
Mixed leukocyte culture test, 107
Mixed lymphocyte reaction test for Class II MHC molecules, 56
Mixed lymphocyte reactions, 107
Mixed vaccines, 171-172, 175-176
Modified live virus vaccines, 170-171
Molecular basis of antibody diversity, 37
Molecules mediating innate immunity, 5
Monkeys
  herpesvirus-induced lymphomas in, 125
  immunodeficiency syndrome in, 160
  retrovirus viral lymphoma in, 125
  T-lymphotropic virus-III in, 125
Monoclonal antibodies, 37-38
Monocyte/macrophages
  natural history of, 71
  phagocyte function of, 71
Monocytes
  in bone marrow, 13
  function of, assays for, 108
Monocytic origin, neoplasms of, 126
Monokines, 40
Mononuclear cells
  isolation of, 100-101
  from peripheral blood, purification of, 99-100
  separation of
    by immunologic method, 102-103
    by physical methods, 101-102
  structure and functions of, 20-21
Mononuclear phagocytes, interaction of microbes with, 160
Monovalent vaccines, 171, 175-176
Mucociliary blanket to remove foreign material, 4
Mucosal immunity, gastrointestinal nematode parasites and, 166
Mucosal surfaces, mast cells lining, 27
Mushroom worker's disease, 147
Myasthenia gravis, 153
Mycobacterium avis, 163
Mycobacterium bovis, 163
  skin testing for, 7
Mycobacterium spp., 160
Mycobacterium tuberculosis, 163
Myeloma protein, 118-119
Myelomas
  inherited, 113-128
  plasma cell, 118-120
    canine, 119-120

N
Natural antibodies, autoimmune reactions and, 151
Natural autoantibodies, 150
Natural killer cell assay, 109
Natural killer cell-mediated cytotoxicity, 26
Natural killer cells, 22
  canine, 27
  structure and function of, 26
Nematode parasites, gastrointestinal, and mucosal immunity, 166
Neonatal isoerythrolysis
  in cattle, 60
  equine, 60-61, 136
Neoplasms
  lymphoreticular, 117-118
  of monocytic origin, 126
  of terminal B-lymphocyte differentiation, 118-119
Neoplastic diseases of lymphoreticular system, 117-118
Neuromuscular system, autoimmune diseases of, 153
Neutralization test, 89, 90

Neutropenia, 72
  cyclic, canine, 117
Neutrophil activation protein-1, 42
Neutrophil chemiluminescence, 73, 74
Neutrophil function defect, canine, 117
Neutrophil phagocytes, interaction of microbes with, 160
Neutrophils, 71-75
  chemotactic factor for, effects of, 133
  functions of, 4-5
    evaluation of, 72
  inflammatory mechanisms caused by, 140
  innate immunity and, 4-5
  isolation of, 71-72
  natural history of, 71
  phagocyte function of, 71
  quantitation of, 72
  structure and functions of, 19-20
  type III hypersensitivity and, 130
Newcastle disease virus, 160
Nitroblue tetrazolium reduction test, 73, 74
NK cells; *see* Natural killer cells
Nodes, lymph; *see* Lymph nodes
Nodules, lymphoid, 18
Nondeforming arthritis, idiopathic, 152
Nonidentity, lines of, 82, 83
Noninfectious subunit vaccine, 172-173
N-terminal end of immunoglobulin molecule, 30, 31
Nurse cells, 16

O
O antigen, 9, 11
OLA, 57
Oncofetal antigens, 10, 11
Oncornavirus-associated cell membrane antigen, feline, 122
Oncornavirus-induced lymphoma in cattle, 123-124
Opaque substances to label proteins, 91
Opsonins, biologic activities of, 51
Opsonization, effect of, on phagocytosis, 5
Optimal dilution, 76
Organ-specific autoimmune diseases, 151-156
Organs, lymphoid; *see* Lymphoid organs
Ostertagia infection in sheep, 136
Ouchterlony precipitation test, 81-82
Oudin, Jacques, 175
Ovine lymphocyte antigen, 57

P
Pan T-cell marker, 22
Pancreas, autoimmune diseases of, 153-154
Panleukopenia, feline, 160
Panleukopenia virus, feline, vaccine for, 176
Papain, proteolytic digestion of IgG by, 32
Papilloma virus in cattle, vaccine for, 176
Parainfluenza virus, canine, vaccine for, 176
Parainfluenza-3 virus in cattle, vaccine for, 176
Parasites, nematode, gastrointestinal, and mucosal immunity, 166
Parasitic antigens in environment, 10
Parasitic disease, IgE-mediated reactions in, 136
Parasitic index, 73
Partial identity, precipitin lines of, 83
Parvovirus
  in dogs, vaccine for, 176
  porcine, vaccine for, 176
Passive cutaneous anaphylaxis test, 130
Passive immune protection, 169-170
Passive transfer of maternal immunoglobulin, failure of, 169
Pasteurella haemolytica, vaccine against, 177
Pasteurella multocida, vaccine against, 177

Pasteurellosis, pneumonic, 160
Patches, Peyer's, 18
Pathogens, phagocytes, macrophages, and neutrophils against, 71
Pemphigoid, bullous, 154
Pemphigus, 148
Pemphigus complex, 154
Pemphigus diseases, 154
Pemphigus erythematosus, 154
Pemphigus foliaceous, 154
Pemphigus vegetans, 154
Pemphigus vulgaris, 154
Pepsin, proteolytic digestion of IgG by, 32
Peptide, viral, 66
Perforin, 49
Peripheral lymphoid organs, 16-18
Peristaltic reflexes as means to eliminate toxins and pathogens, 4
Peroxidase-antiperoxidase for immunoassays and immunocytochemistry, 96
Peyer's patches, 18
pH
　of stomach as chemical defense, 4
　of urinary tract as defense mechanism, 4
Phagocytes
　function of, evaluation of, 71-75
　mononuclear, interaction of microbes with, 160
　neutrophil, interaction of microbes with, 160
Phagocytic cells, 19-22
　functions of, 21-22
Phagocytic index, 73
Phagocytosis, 21, 73
　effect of opsonization on, 5
Physical innate defenses, 3-4
Physical methods to separate mononuclear cells, 101-102
Phytohemagglutinin, binding specificity of, 106
Phytohemagglutinin-P-stimulated canine lymphocyte culture, 105
Picornavirus, feline, complement fixation test to diagnose, 88
Pigeon breeder's disease, 147
Piglets, transmissible gastroenteritis of, 163
Pigs; see Swine
Plant lectins, binding specificities of, 106
Plasma cells
　feline, 25
　myelomas of, 118-120
　　canine, 119-120
　structure and function of, 25-26
　tumors of, murine, 119
Plasmacytomas in mice, 119
Plate or card agglutination test, 78, 79
Platelet activating factor, 133
Platelets, inflammatory mechanisms caused by, 140
Pneumonia, bovine shipping fever, vaccination against, 9
Pneumonic pasteurellosis, 160
Pneumonitis
　allergenic, canine, 135
　hypersensitivity, 147
Pokeweed mitogen, binding specificity of, 106
Pokeweed mitogen-induced B lymphocytes, 25
Polyethylene glycol preparation to separate bound and unbound reactants, 92
Polymorphism, MHC, detection of, 56-57
Polymorphonuclear leukocytes; see Neutrophils
Polymyositis, 153
Polyvalent vaccines, 171-172, 175-176
Positive selection of thymocytes, 15
Prausnitz-Küstner test, 130
Pre-B-cell growth factor, 42
Precipitation, 80-81

Precipitation test(s), 77, 80-81
　capillary tube, 81, 82
　gel (Ouchterlony), 81-82
　quantitative, 85-86
Precipitin tests, qualitative, 81-85
Preperdin, 49
Primary agammaglobulinemia, equine, 114
Primary binding immunoassays, general amplification schemes used in, 96
Primary binding phase of antigen-antibody reaction, 77
Primary immune response, 62
Primary immunodeficiency diseases in veterinary medicine, 113-118
Primary immunoglobulin A deficiency in dogs, 116
Primary serologic assays, 90-97
Properdin, 22
Prostaglandin D2, 133
Proteases, basic, effects of, 133
Protein
　C-reactive, 52
　capsid, as immunogens, 10
　of complement system, macrophage production of, 22
　in eosinophils, 28
　membrane attack, 49
　membrane cofactor, 50
　myeloma, 118-119
Protein A for immunoassays and immunocytochemistry, 96
Protein epitopes, 7-8
　antibody response to, 8
Protein products of MHC, 55
Proteinuria in renal glomerular disease, 146
Proteoglycan, effects of, 133
Proteolytic enzymes as chemical defense, 4
Pseudomonas aeruginosa, 160
Pseudomonas haemolytica, 160
Pseudorabies, porcine, vaccine for, 176
Pulmonary disease, chronic obstructive, equine, 136, 137-138
Purification of mononuclear cells from peripheral blood, approach to, 99-100
Purified cellular populations, assays for lymphocyte functions in, 103-109

Q

Qualitative agglutination tests, 78-80
Qualitative precipitin tests, 81-85
Quantitative agglutination tests, 80
Quantitative precipitation tests, 85-86
Queens itch in horses, 136

R

Rabbits
　complement deficiencies in, 53
　complement levels in, 53
Rabies
　bovine, vaccine for, 176
　in dogs, vaccine for, 176
　immunofluorescence assays to diagnose, 94
Radial immunodiffusion, 85
Radioallergosorbent test, 130, 132
Radioimmune assay, 94-96
Radioisotopes to label proteins, 90, 91
Rats, complement levels in, 53
Reactants, bound and unbound, separation of, 92
Reaction(s)
　allergic, in type I hypersensitivity, late-phase, 133
　anaphylactic type, mediators of, 132-133
　antibody, cytotoxic, 136
　antigen-antibody, 78
　antigen-specific, of lymphocytes in vitro, 107
　complement, 45

Reaction(s)—cont'd
  graft-versus-host, 104
  IgE-mediated, 132
    in parasitic disease, 136
  lymphocyte, mixed, 107
  tetanus toxin-antitoxin, 162-163
Reagents
  Coombs', 79, 80
  diagnostic, haptens as, 7
  immunoassay and immunocytochemistry, 96
  labeling, for primary serologic assays, 90-92
Reaginic antibody; *see* Immunoglobulin E
Reciprocal of last dilution of antibody yielding positive reaction, 76-77
Reflex(es)
  cough, to remove foreign material, 4
  peristaltic, as means to eliminate toxins and pathogens, 4
Regulators of complement activation, 50
Rejection, allograft, T-lymphocyte-mediated, 103-104
Renal glomerular filtration apparatus, 142, 143
Renal glomeruli, immune complexes in, detection of, 146-147
Reovirus, bovine, vaccine for, 176
Respiratory allergy, canine, 135
Respiratory syncytial virus, human and bovine, cross-reactivity of, 8
Respiratory syncytial virus infection, bovine, 135
Respiratory tract, role of, in innate immunity, 4
Response
  humoral, immune response and, 67
  immune; *see* Immune response
Restriction, histocompatibility, 58
Restriction fragment length polymorphisms, 56-57
Retrovirus viral lymphoma, simian, 125
Rheumatoid arthritis, 152
Rheumatoid factor, 152
Rhinitis, allergic
  bovine, 136
  canine, 135
Rhinopneumonitis, equine, vaccine for, 176
Rhinotracheitis, bovine
  infectious, vaccine for, 176
  lymphocyte blast transformation test to diagnose, 106-107
Rhinotracheitis virus, feline, vaccine for, 176
Ribonucleic acid, genetically engineered vaccine products using, 173-174
Ricinus communis, binding specificity of, 106
Rinderpest vaccine, 174
RNA, genetically engineered vaccine products using, 173-174
Rocket immunoelectrophoresis, 85-86
Rosette formation
  to separate mononuclear cells, 102-103
  T cells involved in, 23-24
Rotavirus, bovine, vaccine for, 176
Rous sarcoma virus, in chickens, MHC and, 59
Ruminants, hemal lymph nodes in, 19
Russel bodies, 26

S
Salmonella
  Kauffman-White classification system of, 9
  O antigen in, 9
Salmonella cholerasuis, vaccine against, 177
Salmonella typhimurium, 160
  vaccine against, 177
Sarcoid in horses, MHC and, 59
Sarcoma, venereal, transmissible, in dogs, 126
Sarcoma virus, Rous, in chickens, MHC and, 59
Schistosoma mansoni, 136
Scrapie, 161
  in sheep, MHC and, 59

Secondary binding phase of antigen-antibody reaction, 77
Secondary immune response, 62
Secondary immunologic assays, 77
Secretory functions of phagocytic cells, 22
Secretory immunoglobulin; *see* Immunoglobulin A
Selectins, 29
Selection, positive, of thymocytes, 15
Selective IgA deficiency in dogs, 116
Selective immunoglobulin M deficiency of horses, 114
Sensitized erythrocytes in complement titration, 53
Separation strategies in primary serologic assays, 92
Sequential epitopes, 7-8
Sequestered antigens, autoimmune reactions and, 150
Serolog, 103
Serologic assays
  choice of, 96-97
  primary, 90-97
Serologic typing for Class I MHC molecules, 56
Serology, 76
Serum sickness, 141-142
Severe combined immunodeficiency syndrome in dogs, 116
Shar Pei dogs
  IgA deficiency in, 35
  primary IgA deficiency in, 116
Shared epitopes, 8, 9
Sheep
  blood groups in, 61
  bovine leukemia virus in, 124
  complement levels in, 53
  contagious ecythema in, vaccine for, 176
  disease resistance and MHC in, 59
  ecthyma in, vaccination against, 171
  glomerulonephritis in, 146
  immunodeficiency diseases of, 115
  late-phase allergic reaction in, from *Ascaris suum*, 133
  major histocompatibility complex in, 57
  nematode parasites in, 166
  Ostertagia infection in, 136
  serum immunoglobulin levels in, 36
  vaccines available for, 176
Shift, antigenic, 10
Shock, anaphylactic, 133-134
Siberian tiger, immunodeficiency disorder of, 117
Sickness, serum, 141-142
Simian immunodeficiency syndrome, 160
Sinusoidal macrophages, 20
Skin
  autoimmune diseases of, 154-155
  barrier function of, 3
  normal flora of, 3-4
  role of, in innate immunity, 3-4
Skin test
  direct, for allergen-specific IgE, 130
  intradermal, 103
  for *Mycobacterium bovis*, 7
Slow-reacting substance of anaphylaxis, 133
Solid phase absorption with protein A or carrier beads to separate bound and unbound reactants, 92
Solid phase plate absorption to separate bound and unbound reactants, 92
Solid phase plate assays, 94-96
Soluble factors of immune response, 40-46
Soluble inhibitors of complement activation, 50
Species differentiation in eosinophils, 28
Species variation in structure of lymphoid tissues, 18-19
Spleen, structure and function of, 17-18
Stable structure of immunogens, 6
Staphylococcus aureus, vaccine against, 177
Stomach, pH of, as chemical defense, 4
Streptococcus equii, vaccine against, 177

Streptococcus equi-M, vaccine against, 177
Streptococcus spp., 160
Stress syndrome, porcine, 61
Superantigens, 12
Superfamily, immunoglobulin, 37
Suppressor T cells, loss of, autoimmune reactions and, 151
Swine
  blood groups in, 60
  complement levels in, 53
  glomerulonephritis in, 146
  lymph node structure of, 19
  lymphosarcoma in, 124
  major histocompatibility complex in, 58
  parvovirus in, vaccine for, 176
  plasma cell myelomas in, 120
  pseudorabies in, vaccine for, 176
  serum immunoglobulin levels in, 36
  stress syndrome in, 61
  systemic anaphylaxis in, clinical signs of, 135
  transmissible gastroenteritis of, 163
    vaccine for, 176
  transmissible gastroenteritis virus of, and feline infectious peritonitis virus, cross-reactivity of, 8
  vaccines available for, 176, 177
Swiss Bernese mountain dogs, systemic histiocytosis in, 126
Syndrome
  Chédiak-Higashi, 117
  granulocytopathy, canine, 117
  immunodeficiency
    acquired, 160
    canine, undefined, 117
    severe combined, in dogs, 116
    simian, 160
Synthetic immunogens, 174-175
Synthetic vaccines, requirements for, 12
System-related innate defenses, 3-4
Systemic anaphylaxis, 132, 133-135
  species differences in, 135
Systemic autoimmune diseases, 155-156
Systemic histiocytosis, 126
Systemic immune complex disease, 141-142
Systemic infections, 159
Systemic lupus erythematosus, 141, 148, 155

T
T cells, 12
  categories of, 22-23
  helper, 12, 22-23
    types of, 42
    interaction of antigen-presenting cells and, 63
  suppressor, loss of, autoimmune reactions and, 151
T-cell-activating factor to assess monocyte function, 108
T-cell assay, cytotoxic, 108-109
T-cell cytotoxicity, immune response and, 66
T-cell–derived cytokines, T-cell differentiation and, 64-65
T-cell differentiation and T-cell–derived cytokines, 64-65
T-cell epitope, 12
T-cell-growth factor to assess lymphocyte function, 107
T-cell-independent antigens, 64
T-cell leukemia in dogs, 124
T-cell receptor (TCR) for antigen, 23
  alpha-beta, 63-64
T-dependent antigens, 12
T lymphocytes
  activation of, 65-66
  antigen recognition and presentation and, 62-64
  CD4+, antigen recognition and, 62, 63
  function of
    assays for, 99-110

T lymphocytes—cont'd
  function of—cont'd
    in vitro assessment of, 104-107
    in vivo evaluation of, 103-104
    in vivo identification methods for, 99
  in spleen, 17-18
  structure and functions of, 22-24
  subsets of, 40-41
  type IV hypersensitivity and, 130
T-lymphotropic virus-III, simian, 125
Target cell cytotoxicity assays, 108
Terminal B-lymphocyte differentiation, neoplasms of, 118-119
Terminal deoxynucleotidyl transferase (TdT) assay, 23
Test(s)
  agglutination; *see* Agglutination tests
  anaphylaxis, passive cutaneous, 130
  antiglobulin, Coombs, direct, 151
  Coggin's, 36
    for equine infectious anemia, 83
  complement fixation, 77, 86-89
  Hardy, 94
  indirect complement fixation inhibition, 89
  lymphocyte blast transformation, 106
  mixed leukocyte culture, 107
  neutralization, 89, 90
  nitroblue tetrazolium reduction, 73, 74
  Prausnitz-Küstner, 130
  precipitation; *see* Precipitation tests
  precipitin, qualitative, 81-85
  radioallergosorbent, 130, 132
  skin
    direct, for allergen-specific IgE, 130
    intradermal, 103
    for *Mycobacterium bovis*, 7
Tetanus, antibodies resistant to, 10
Tetanus toxin-antitoxin reaction, 162-163
TGE; *see* Transmissible gastroenteritis virus of swine
Theileria parva, infection of bovine lymphocytes by, 121
Theileriasis in cattle, MHC and, 59
Therapy, hyposensitization, for dogs, 135
Theta antigen, 22
Thrombocytopenia, autoimmune, 152
Thrush, 3
Thy-1 antigen, 22
Thymic lymphocytes, 14-15
Thymic lymphosarcoma, 123
Thymocytes, 14
  differentiation of, 16
  positive selection of, 15
Thymopoietin, 16
Thymosin, 16
Thymulin, 16
Thymus
  histologic anatomy of, 15
  location of, 15
  and lymphocyte development, 14-16
Thymus derived cells; *see* T cells
Thyroid gland, autoimmune diseases of, 153
Thyroid stimulating immunoglobulin, 153
Thyroid stimulator, long-acting, 153
Thyroiditis
  autoimmune, 153
  Hashimoto's, 153
Ticks, resistance to, MHC and, 59
Tissue
  connective, mast cells in, 27
  lymphoid
    bronchus-associated, 18
    gut-associated, 16
    species variation in structure of, 18-19

Tissue damage induced by immune complex diseases, pathologic mechanism of, 139-141
Tissue grafting, antigens and, 10
Titer, 76-77
Titration, complement, 86, 87
TNF; *see* Tumor necrosis factor
Tonsils, 18
Total hemolytic method of complement titration, 53
Toxins, autoimmune reactions and, 151
Transfer, passive, of maternal immunoglobulin, failure of, 169
Transfusion
   blood groups and, 59-61
   incompatibility with, 59
Transient hypogammaglobulinemia, equine, 114
Transmissible gastroenteritis of piglets, 163
Transmissible gastroenteritis virus of swine, 163
   and feline infectious peritonitis virus, cross-reactivity of, 8
   vaccine for, 176
Transmissible venereal sarcoma in dogs, 126
Trichinella spiralis in sheep, MHC and, 59
Trypanosoma cruzi, antigenic variation by, 10
Trypanosomiasis, 160
Tube agglutination test, 80
Tuberculosis, 163
   intradermal skin test to diagnose, 103
Tumor(s)
   mast cell, canine, 28
   plasma cell, murine, 119
Tumor-associated antigens, 10-11
Tumor necrosis factor, 5, 28, 43
Tumor necrosis factor alpha, 41, 43
Tumor necrosis factor beta, 41, 43
Turkeys, herpesvirus in, 125-126
Type I interferon, 5
Type II interferon, 5

U

Unbound and bound reactants, separation of, 92
Undefined canine immunodeficiency syndromes, 117
Urinary tract, pH of, as defense mechanism, 4
"Urner pneumoniae," 147
Urogenital tract, role of, in innate immunity, 4
Urticaria in horses, 136
Uveitis, anterior, 147-148

V

Vaccination
   against bovine shipping fever pneumonia, 9
   current principles of, 170-172
   vaccines, and immunomodulators, 169-177
Vaccine immunogens, anti-idiotypes as, 175
Vaccines
   attenuated viral variants for, 170-171
   epitopes and immunogenicity in synthesizing, 12
   future developments in formulation of, 172-175
   genetically engineered, 173-174
   heterotypic, 176
   homotypic, 176
   inactivated, 170
   mixed, 171-172, 175-176
   modified live virus, 170-171
   monovalent, 171, 175-176
   noninfectious subunit, 172-173
   polyvalent, 171-172, 175-176
   preparation of, 170
   Rinderpest, 174
   synthetic, requirements for, 12
   types of, in veterinary medicine, 175-177

Vaccines—cont'd
   vaccination, and immunomodulators, 169-177
   viral, construction and evolution of, 172
Vaccinia virus and genetically engineered vaccines, 174
Vagina, lactobacilli of, as defense mechanism, 4
Valency of antibody species, antibody-antigen union and, 76
Variable-heavy loops, 33
Variable-light loops, 33
Variation, antigenic, 10
Vasoactive factors of complement, biologic activities of, 51
Venereal sarcoma, transmissible, in dogs, 126
Venezuelan equine encephalomyelitis, vaccine for, 176
Very late antigen, 29
Veterinary medicine
   primary immunodeficiency diseases in, 113-118
   vaccines in, 175-177
Vibrio fetus, vaccine against, 177
Viral antigens in environment, 10
Viral-induced immunosuppression, 160
Viral lymphoma, retrovirus, simian, 125
Viral peptide, 66
Viral vaccine products, construction and evolution of, 172
Viremia, feline, immunofluorescence assays to diagnose, 94
Virus(es)
   avoiding immunologic defenses by, 161
   blue tongue, in cattle, vaccine for, 176
   bovine leukemia, lymphocyte blast transformation test to diagnose, 106-107
   defenses against, complement and, 52-53
   distemper, canine, 160
      infection with, 163-166
   feline infectious peritonitis, and transmissible gastroenteritis virus of swine, cross-reactivity of, 8
   immunodeficiency, human, 160-161
   leukemia
      bovine, 123-124
      feline, 160, 167
         lymphomas induced by, 122-123
         vaccine for, 176
      infection with, in mice, 125
   measles, infection with, lymphocyte blast transformation test to diagnose, 106-107
   Newcastle disease, 160
   panleukopenia, feline, vaccine for, 176
   parainfluenza, canine, vaccine for, 176
   respiratory syncytial, bovine, 135
      human and, cross-reactivity of, 8
   rhinotracheitis, feline, vaccine for, 176
   Rous sarcoma, in chickens, MHC and, 59
   transmissible gastroenteritis, of swine and feline infectious peritonitis virus, cross-reactivity of, 8
   vaccinia, and genetically engineered vaccines, 174
Virus neutralization test, 89, 90
Visceral lymphomatosis in chickens, 125
VLA-4, 29
Vomiting as means to eliminate toxins and pathogens, 4

W

Warts, bovine, vaccine for, 176
Weimaraner dogs, neutrophil function defect in, 117
West Highland white terriers, atopy in, 132
Western equine encephalomyelitis, vaccine for, 176
Wheals, allergic, equine, 136

X

Xenograft, 10

Z

Zeta potential, 77